"This is the breakthrough we've been waiting for regarding the primary care of those with mental health problems. This should be essential reading for anyone in this field, and certainly anyone going through medical school."
DR. ANDRÉ TYLEE, *Professor of Primary Care Mental Health, Institute of Psychiatry, King's College London*

"It is time that medical science and practice takes nutrition seriously as one of the key factors that determines the health of the brain."
PROFESSOR DAVID SMITH, *Deputy Head, Division of Medical Services, University of Oxford*

"This book will make a tremendous difference to the millions of people who suffer unnecessarily from mental health problems. Nutritional medicine is the future."
DR. HYLA CASS, *Assistant Clinical Professor of Psychiatry, UCLA School of Medicine*

"This excellent book gives us a most powerful weapon in our fight against mental disease."
DR. ABRAM HOFFER, *psychiatrist*

"This book is of groundbreaking significance. You've got to read it."
HAZEL COURTENEY, *Daily Mail*

"If you care about keeping your mind sharp and your mood good, the undeniable message of this book is that you can change how you think and feel by what you eat."
GLORIA HUNNIFORD, *TV and radio presenter*

"We need psychiatrists to take up nutrition as part of their weaponry against disease. If they follow the advice in this book, they will be a good step along the way of helping their patients to get a lot better than many who are now on drug treatment alone."
GWYNNETH HEMMINGS, *Schizophrenia Association of Great Britain*

"This book makes it clear that a nutritionally ignorant psychiatrist is about as useful as a claustrophobic plumber. Everyone else knows that food can make you happy or sad, why do psychiatrists keep ignoring the fact? They have ignored nutrition for far too long."
JEROME BURNE, *Medicine Today*

"If you care about your mind, your moods or even your mental alertness, this book will change your attitudes to the foods you eat—for the better! This comprehensive work will provide you with food for thought, as you learn about foods for the mind. An excellent book."
DR. CHRIS STEELE, *This Morning* (ITV)

About the Author

Patrick Holford began his academic career in experimental psychology. While at the University of York he became interested in the biochemistry of mental illness. His research led him to two pioneers in the field, the late Dr. Carl Pfeiffer from Princeton's Brain Bio Center, and Dr. Abram Hoffer, former director of psychiatric research for Saskatchewan, Canada. Both claimed that nutritional therapy gave outstanding results in treating mental health problems. He became their student and later, that of twice Nobel prize winner Dr. Linus Pauling.

In 1984 Patrick Holford founded the Institute for Optimum Nutrition (ION). A charitable and independent educational trust for furthering education and research in nutrition, ION is now one of the most respected training colleges offering degree accredited training for nutritional therapy.

At ION he researched the role of nutrition in intelligence, culminating in a landmark trial in 1987 proving that nutritional supplementation can raise IQ. He also researched nutritional approaches to depression, schizophrenia and eating disorders, and developed a method for assessing a person's optimal nutrition requirements that has been tested on more than 100,000 people.

Since 1997 he has written more than 20 popular books, now translated into 23 languages. The first, *The Optimum Nutrition Bible*, has sold over a million copies worldwide.

Backed by more than 20 years of research and clinical experience, Patrick Holford is committed to bringing this radical, new and proven approach to mental health to those who need it. With that aim in mind he is the Chief Executive of the Food for the Brain Foundation, an educational non-profit group, and director of the Brain Bio Centre, the Foundation's outpatient clinic in Richmond, Surrey, specializing in the nutritional treatment of children with ADHD and autistic spectrum disorders, and nutritional solutions for depression, schizophrenia, dementia, and Alzheimer's disease (see page 475).

Other books by Patrick Holford

The New Optimum Nutrition Bible
100% Health
Optimum Nutrition for Your Child's Mind (with Deborah Colson)
Smart Food for Smart Kids (with Fiona McDonald Joyce)
The Alzheimer's Prevention Plan
Food Is Better Medicine Than Drugs (with Jerome Burne)
Beat Stress and Fatigue
Say No to Cancer
Say No to Heart Disease
Say No to Arthritis
Improve Your Digestion
Balancing Hormones Naturally (with Kate Neil)
Boost Your Immune System (with Jennifer Meek)
Supplements for Superhealth
The Optimum Nutrition Cookbook (with Judy Ridgway)
The 30-Day Fatburner Diet
Six Weeks to Superhealth
Natural Highs (with Dr. Hyla Cass)
500 Health and Nutrition Questions Answered
The Holford Low-GL Diet
The Holford Low-GL Diet Cookbook (with Fiona McDonald Joyce)
The Holford Low-GL Diet Made Easy

The definition of insanity:

To keep doing the same things
and expect different results.

Patrick Holford's

NEW OPTIMUM NUTRITION NUTRITION FOR THE MIND

Basic
Health
PUBLICATIONS, INC.

Published by
Basic Health Publications, Inc.
28812 Top of the World Drive
Laguna Beach, CA 92651
949-415-4327 • www.basichealthpub.com

Published in the United Kingdom by Piatkus Books Ltd.,
an imprint of Little, Brown Book Group Ltd.

Published by arrangement with Little, Brown Book Group Ltd., London, England

Library of Congress Cataloging-in-Publication Data

Holford, Patrick.
   New optimum nutrition for the mind / Patrick Holford.
     p. cm.
   Rev. ed. of: Optimum nutrition for the mind. c2004.
   Includes bibliographical references and index.
   ISBN 978-1-59120-259-2
   1. Brain—Popular works. 2. Nutrition—Popular works. 3. Mental illness—Nutritional aspects—Popular works. 4. Nootropic agents—Popular works. 5. Dietary supplements—Popular works. I. Holford, Patrick. Optimum nutrition for the mind. II. Title.
   QP376.H68   2009
   612.8'2—dc22

2009037222

Edited by Barbara Kiser • Text design by Paul Saunders

Printed in the United States of America.

10   9   8

Contents

Foreword

No one can question the massive adaptive stress all human beings are facing as we enter the 21st century. As the pace of life accelerates, with mobile phones, email, and instant news, there are a number of big questions at hand. Can we cope? Do we have the brains to adapt? In many cases, the answer is no. Fatigue, anxiety, sleeping problems, mood swings, memory problems, and the blues are the hallmarks of our age. Those even less well adapted become mentally ill. ADHD, autism, schizophrenia, and suicide are all on the increase. How can we stay mentally sharp and happy in our hectic times?

When the needs are very great, the solution may be just around the corner. The needs of the majority, and especially the mentally ill, are enormous—and they are not being met. But the solution is, in fact, already visible and developing rapidly. Patrick Holford, a skillful and insightful writer and nutritionist, has provided the necessary information in this excellent and important book. If the methods he outlines were widely practiced, they would go a long way towards meeting the problems of our modern mental health crises. People suffering from mental illnesses, who today receive too little help, will find this book just what they need to take to their mental health providers to show them highly safe and successful treatments, backed by considerable research.

Recently King County, in the state of Washington, passed legislation making their state institutions accountable for the treatment of the mentally ill. Their new mission is to vastly improve the recovery rates of their patients. This book contains the very information needed to persuade their psychiatrists that only by following orthomolecular or nutritional psychiatry will they be able to reach recovery rates that are greater than 10 percent. Tranquilizer use alone helps well under 10 percent of schizophrenic patients to fully recover.

I have been practicing psychiatry for the past 50 years, and have seen it develop from our use of one vitamin, B3, to treat schizophrenia, to its present state, which is much more comprehensive and applicable to a large variety of psychiatric conditions. My clinical observations fully confirm what Patrick Holford describes so well in this book.

Patrick Holford's New Optimum Nutrition for the Mind fulfills a major modern need for information about the causes, prevention, and treatment of diseases, including psychiatric disorders, which today make up the massive wave of illness that is sweeping the globe. At the same time, affluent malnutrition is spreading across all the high-tech nations. Is it a coincidence, or is such malnutrition triggering the massive deterioration in our nations' health?

About half the population of Canada, the U.S. and the U.K. suffers from one or more degenerative disease such as schizophrenia, the bipolar psychoses, depression, anxiety, Alzheimer's, arthritis, diabetes, neurological disease, obesity, immune deficiency, addictions, cancer, cardiovascular disease, and so on. It is difficult to pick up a daily paper without some reference to the serious health crises facing nations. In some of the wealthiest countries, like the U.S. and Canada, governments are more and more concerned over the costs of heathcare and disease treatment and are making strenuous but mostly futile efforts to control costs—without any attempt to really reduce them by getting their people well.

We do know what should be done. We must provide information to the public and to the healing professions which will halt the continual spread of disease due to malnutrition. And this is another area where Patrick Holford's book will be a key element. As a student and follower of Dr. Carl Pfeiffer, one of the pioneers in nutritional medicine, Holford has followed the development of this new field assiduously, and it shows.

At the beginning of the orthomolecular era it was very difficult for physicians to enter the field. There were a small number of very good books which specialized in certain aspects of the entire program. Some went very heavily into the question of hypoglycemia and carbohydrate metabolism. Some dealt much more with the allergic reactions that can create any psychiatric syndrome whatever. Some emphasized the vitamins, some the minerals. But most of the publishers were small, with small advertising budgets, and these books were never promoted very well. Only within the past 10 years have we had books which covered the whole field.

This is one of the better ones because of its wide coverage of every aspect of orthomolecular practice, with descriptions of all the syndromes with which psychiatrists must deal. For interested physicians, this makes it much easier to enter the field, as they can find the information they need in one or two books.

We desperately need doctors to transform their practices as quickly as possible in order to slow the ever-increasing rate of disease development. The curve that relates prevalence of serious chronic illness against time is not linear. It is curvilinear upward, and if unchecked we will see over 75 percent of our populations suffer from one or more serious chronic illness in the next decade or two. *Patrick Holford's New Optimum Nutrition for the Mind* gives us a most powerful weapon in our fight against mental disease. It is also essential reading for anyone wanting to stay in top mental health throughout life, free from depression, memory decline, and, even worse, senility.

Dr. Abram Hoffer M.D., Ph.D.

Dr. Abram Hoffer, former Director of Psychiatric Research in Saskatchewan, Canada, ran the first ever double-blind controlled trial in the history of psychiatry in the 1950s, proving the power of vitamins in treating schizophrenia. Even though his ideas were attacked and ridiculed he has persevered, and now in his nineties, he continues to help hundreds of people with mental health problems get better through optimum nutrition.

Introduction to the new edition

The first edition of this book inspired many changes and gave birth to the Food for the Brain Foundation, for whom I now work. It all happened when I sent the book to André Tylee, Professor of Primary Care Mental Health at the Institute of Psychiatry, King's College, London. He was so excited by the growing evidence of nutrition's power to promote mental health and reverse mental health problems that we started a think tank. People from all the relevant fields—psychiatry, nutrition, brain chemistry, psychotherapy, psychology, and so on—were invited to our meetings. Finally, we founded the non-profit Food for the Brain Foundation, whose stated aim is:

> 66 To promote awareness of the link between learning, behavior, mental health, and nutrition. To educate and provide educational material to children, parents, teachers, schools, universities, the public, health professionals, caterers, and the government thereby promoting mental health through optimum nutrition. 99

I'd like to share our vision, because it's to this that this book is dedicated—to create a future where optimum nutrition as a way to mental health is understood by all, and implemented by many—a future where:

- Babies are optimally nourished for brain development during pregnancy and infancy

- Nurseries and schools, from infancy to university, actively encourage optimum nutrition for brain function

- Governments actively encourage optimum nutrition to promote learning and prevent behavioral and mental health problems from childhood to old age

- The treatment of mental health problems involves correcting nutritional imbalances as a first-line procedure

- The public has easy access to information about optimum nutrition for mental health.

The Foundation has an unparalleled scientific advisory board made up of nine professors in fields such as psychiatry, education, nutrition, brain chemistry, and so on. Their names appear on its website, www.foodfor thebrain.org, and are also scattered throughout this book in testament to their pioneering research in this field.

Over the past five years this collective wisdom, backed up by hundreds of new and important published research studies, has put more flesh on the bones of the original book, and also fleshed out the theories that define a radical new approach to mental health: optimum nutrition for the mind. One of these is the growing awareness that faulty methylation—a body process that happens a billion times a second and is intimately linked to nutrition—lies behind many mental health problems, from depression to schizophrenia.

Nutrition is the key to well-being of mind and mood, but not the only one. Insightful, effective psychotherapy and an understanding of the genetics are as vital. This idea—that most mental health problems can be made better by resolving psychological issues, correcting biochemical imbalances through nutritional therapy, and comprehending the genetic makeup that makes each of us different and some of us more prone to mental health disorders—has also been the vision of two great men of science.

They are the late Dr. Carl Pfeiffer, with whom I was honored to study; and Dr. Abram Hoffer, now in his nineties and going strong. Hoffer has successfully treated more people with schizophrenia than anyone else in the world, and his tireless dedication to science has given birth to a whole new approach—the optimum nutrition approach—in psychiatry. His autobiography, *Adventures in Psychiatry*, makes for fascinating reading.

These two men, between them, have made more than a dozen essential discoveries which even today continue to unfold. These include:

- The discovery of the importance of zinc in mental health

- The power of vitamin B3 (niacin) to reverse psychosis

- The importance of vitamins B6, B12, and folic acid in mental health, now known to be the lynchpins of methylation, one of the hottest new discoveries in this field

- The discovery of the mauve factor, an abnormal chemical in urine that indicates increased brain oxidation and a need for specific nutrients, often found in those with autism and schizophrenia

- The discovery that food allergies can cause mental illness.

Carl Pfeiffer's work took place at the Brain Bio Center in Princeton. To honor it, we have named our own outpatient clinic for the Foundation the Brain Bio Centre. Dr. Hoffer's work is carried on through the International Schizophrenia Foundation (www.orthomed.org).

This book is my way of showing these giants of medicine and psychiatry that their work goes on, and of showing you what has been learnt so far about how to protect and promote your mind, mood, memory, and sanity through optimum nutrition in what often seems an increasingly mad world. The definition of insanity is to keep doing the same things and expect different results, and I hope this book will help wake up patients and professionals alike to the insanity of relying on drugs for the treatment of our children, elders, and everyone suffering depression, anxiety or more severe forms of mental illness, when a better, safer, and cheaper way is already in place—optimum nutrition.

Wishing you the best of health and happiness,

Patrick Holford

Acknowledgments

This book would not have been possible without the help, support and research of many people. Firstly, I would like to thank Dr. Abram Hoffer and the late Dr. Carl Pfeiffer with all my heart. I consider these great men my mentors, the first pioneers of a badly needed mental health revolution, from whom I have learnt so much about mental health and nutrition. I am indebted to both for their contributions to various chapters of this book, posthumously in the case of Dr. Carl Pfeiffer.

I am also deeply indebted to Shane Heaton, both for his help with the research, editing, and moral support, and for his contributions to Chapters 27, 28, and 29. Many thanks also to Jane Nodder for her contribution to Chapter 33, Dr. Geoffrey and Lucille Leader for their contributions to Chapter 35 on Parkinson's, to Imogen Caterer for her help with Chapters 24, 30, and 34, to Natalie Savona for her help with Chapter 18, to Tuula Tuormaa for her help with the sections on allergies, to Dr. Alex Richardson and Madeleine Portwood for all their help and invaluable research on essential fats, to Jerome Burne for his help with Chapter 22, and to Dr. Hyla Cass for keeping me up to date with new and interesting research. I am also indebted to Sarah Carolides, Amanda Moore, and Carolyn Bird for generously sharing their research, and to the graduates of the Institute for Optimum Nutrition, the front-line troops, who are putting this essential knowledge into practice for the benefit of those who suffer from mental health problems. Finally, I would like to thank my staff—Bebe, Cath, and Murali, Charlotte, and particularly Sarah Hanson, for all the new research—and my publishers Piatkus, especially Gill, Jo, Helen, and Barbara on editorial, as well as Philip, Jana, and Judy for their support, encouragement, and enthusiasm.

Guide to abbreviations and measures

Most vitamins are measured in milligrams or micrograms. Vitamins A, D, and E are also measured in International Units (IUs), a measurement designed to standardize the various forms of these vitamins, which have different potencies.

1 gram (g) = 1,000 milligrams (mg) = 1,000,000 micrograms (mcg)

1 mcg or retinal (1 mcg RE) = 3.3 IUs of vitamin A
1 mcg RE of beta carotene = 6 mcg of beta carotene
100 IUs of vitamin D = 2.5 mcg
100 IUs of vitamin E = 67 mg

A note on notes, recommended reading, and resources

In each part of the book, you'll find numbered references. These refer to notes gathered in the References section that starts at the back of the book on page 436. The research papers listed here are for those readers who want to study this subject in depth. I also refer to books and websites that are more oriented to the layperson throughout the book. Details of these can be found in Recommended Reading (page 471) and Useful Addresses (page 474) at the back of the book. Many of these books and research papers are available at the Institute for Optimum Nutrition library in Richmond, Surrey.

PART 1

Food for Thought

How you think and feel is directly affected by what you eat. This idea may seem strange, yet the fact is that eating the right food has been proven to boost your IQ, improve your mood and emotional stability, sharpen your memory and keep your mind young. In this part of the book, you will discover the Five Brain Foods that will keep you in tip-top mental health.

CHAPTER 1

You think what you eat

How sharp is your mind, how balanced is your mood, how consistent is your energy, how happy are you—and what, if anything, do these qualities have to do with what you eat? These are some of the questions we set out to answer in Britain's biggest-ever health survey—known as ONUK for Optimum Nutrition UK—which involved 37,000 people and took place in 2004.[1] What we found was sobering stuff. Here, for instance, are the proportion of people who said they suffer frequently or 'always' from certain conditions:

- Become impatient quickly   82%
- Have low energy level   80%
- Energy is less than it used to be 76%
- Feel have too much to do   67%
- Become anxious or tense easily   64%
- Have PMS/PMT (women only)   63%
- Easily become angry   53%
- Suffer from depression   44%

- Have difficulty concentrating   43%
- Become nervous/hyperactive   38%
- Have poor memory/difficulty learning   32%

Does this sound like anyone you know? Welcome to the 21st century. Despite improvements in diet and better standards of living, the average person is, as one child said in an exam howler, a knackered ape, not a naked ape! So what's going wrong?

Our minds and bodies have been shaped over millions of years of evolution. Our species, *Homo sapiens*, learned to adapt to changing climates, to changing food supplies and to a changing world. But it takes time to adapt and change can be painful. Right now we have a problem. Humanity is struggling to adapt to life in a phase that makes the Industrial Revolution seem like child's play. Our physical environment is changing, for instance. We have invented some 10 million new chemicals, thousands of which are added to our food, are found in common household products, and are in the water we drink and the air we breathe.

Our psychological environment is changing even faster. This layer of our environment consists of concepts of who we are, who we're with, and what we do. Memories of times and places. Thoughts and feelings. All these make up the fabric of our psychological world. You can't see it or touch it, but it is no less real. We tell the story of our life across a matrix of time and space.

Yet in the last 50 years, our whole experience of time and space has changed fundamentally. What we could do in a week, we can do in a day. The distance we would have covered in a day we can cover in an hour. You want to speak to a friend while strolling through a park? Dig out your cellphone. You want to send a letter? Write an email and get a reply in a minute or less. You want to go somewhere? Jump on a plane. We no longer live in towns and cities, we live in the world. Global news reaches us in seconds. We can even fly almost anywhere in a day. Every culture is exposed to every other culture.

But this cross-culturalization is placing untold strains on all of us, from America to Africa, Asia, Australia, and Europe. Many of us are struggling to survive, let alone thrive, in the new millennium. Putting the squeeze on time and space isn't making us happy.

The high cost of living

So these are exceptionally challenging times. Some of us are rising to the challenge, but most of us are struggling to keep up and are living with fatigue, anxiety, stress, depression, and sleeping problems. Too many people are suffering from mental health problems ranging from autism and attention deficit disorder to Alzheimer's, depression, and schizophrenia. In fact, recent research shows that each year in the U.K., 350,000 elderly people are diagnosed with cognitive impairment, while 185,000 develop dementia. That is 500 people every day—the equivalent of four packed double-decker buses.[2]

The outlook on children's disorders is just as worrying. One in 6 children have special educational needs, while 1 in 3 live with behavior, attention, and learning problems.[3] The rise in cases of autism is positively alarming: current research indicates that 1 in 86 children in the U.K. now have the condition.[4] In the U.S., an estimated 1 in 10 women are on antidepressants.[5] In fact, the world over there's been a massive increase in the incidence of mental health problems, especially among young people. Suicide, violence and depression are on the rise, according to the World Health Organization (WHO). Mental health problems, says the WHO, are fast becoming the number one health issue this century, with 1 in 10 people suffering from them at any point in time, and 1 in 4 hit by them at some point in their life.[6]

Having worked with thousands of people struggling with these problems, and researched the underlying causes, I've come to the conclusion that most can be prevented, and in many cases reversed, by a fundamentally new approach to mental well-being.

This has nothing to do with today's therapeutic front-runners, drugs or psychotherapy. By drugs I include the staggering array we prescribe for ourselves—from caffeine to chocolate. We've all been down this route. Tired? Choose caffeine, sugar, or a cigarette. We drink 1.5 billion caffeinated drinks a week in Britain, including tea, coffee, and cola, and we eat 6 million kilos of sugar and 2 million kilos of chocolate every week. We also smoke 1.5 billion cigarettes in that time. Anxious or depressed? Have a drink. We drink 120 million alcoholic drinks a week—and smoke 10 million marijuana joints. And if things get really bad? Go to the doctor for a prescribed drug. In Britain we're popping 532 million tranquilizers, 463 million sleeping pills and 823 million antidepressants every year. All of these work to some extent, but at what cost, in terms of side effects and dependence?

A more hopeful development, potentially at least, is that psychotherapy is becoming increasingly popular. More people are now seeking professional help, and more and more frequently, with at least 10 million visits a year. Alternatively, you can do a life-changing course, read a self-help book, or change your state of mind through yoga or meditation. All of these can help.

But meanwhile, aren't we forgetting something? Any intelligent person can recognize that our diets have changed radically in the last 100 years, along with our environment. When you consider that the body and brain are made entirely from molecules derived from food, air, and water, and that simple molecules like alcohol can fundamentally affect the brain, isn't it unlikely that changes in diet and the environment have had no effect on our mental health?

I believe that most of us are not achieving our full potential for mental health, happiness, alertness, and clarity because we are not achieving optimum nutrition for the mind, and this book presents ample evidence for my case. I also believe that a significant proportion of mentally unwell people are suffering from a chemical imbalance brought on by years of poor nutrition and exposure to environmental pollutants. For them, drugs are not the answer—after all, they are hardly suffering from a lack of drugs—and their longstanding imbalance may actually hamper the success of any therapy they're receiving.

As Einstein said, "The problems we have created cannot be solved at the same level of thinking we were at when we created them." We need a new way of thinking about mental health that includes the role of nutrition and the chemical environment and how these affect the way we think and feel.

Mind and body are not separate

One of the most limiting concepts in the human sciences is the idea that the mind and the body are separate. Try asking an anatomist, a psychologist, and a biochemist where the mind begins and the body ends. It is a stupid question, and yet that is exactly what modern science has done by separating psychology from anatomy and physiology.

But it's not just the scientists who live by this false distinction. It's us. When you're having difficulty concentrating, when your mood is low, when you struggle to find a memory, do you consider that you may be poorly nourished? Why not? Every one of these states—your thinking, feeling, mental energy, and focus—happens across a network of interconnecting brain cells, each one of which depends on an optimal supply of nutrients to work efficiently. Consider these experiments:

- Dr. David Benton measured the IQ scores of 90 schoolchildren and then gave 30 of them a high-dose multivitamin, 30 a dummy pill and 30 nothing. After eight months we re-evaluated their IQ. Only those children on the vitamins had a staggering increase in their non-verbal IQ of over ten points![7] Since this study, published more than a decade ago, 10 other studies have confirmed that supplements boost children's IQ. The effect is real.

- Dr. Thomas Crook from the Memory Assessment Clinic in Maryland in the U.S. gave 149 people with age-related memory impairment a daily dose of 300 mg of a nutrient called phosphatidylserine. When they were tested after 12 weeks, their memory had improved to the level of those 12 years younger.[8]

- Dr. Bernard Rimland from California compared the results of 1,591 hyperactive children treated with drugs to those of 191 hyperactive children given nutritional supplements. The nutritional approach was 18 times more effective.[9] Yet, despite this, drug prescriptions for children are almost doubling every year.

- Dr. Carl Birmingham from the Eating Disorders Clinic in Vancouver, Canada, gave people with anorexia a zinc supplement or a placebo. Those taking zinc increased their body weight twice as rapidly as those given the dummy pills.[10]

- Dr. Abram Hoffer from Canada has treated 5,000 people diagnosed with schizophrenia with high-dose multinutrients, especially large doses of vitamin B3 and vitamin C. His published 40-year follow-up reports reveal a 90 percent cure rate—defined as free of symptoms, able to socialize with family and friends, and paying income tax.[11] Despite this lifetime of research and results, Hoffer's approach to schizophrenia has been largely sidelined.

- Dr. Walter Poldinger and colleagues from Basel University in Switzerland gave depressed patients either a state-of-the-art SSRI antidepressant or a nutrient called 5-HTP. 5-HTP outperformed the drug on every measure, resulting in greater improvements in their depression, anxiety, and insomnia, and no side effects.[12] This is in sharp contrast to the estimated one suicide every day caused directly by adverse reactions to this class of antidepressant drug (see Chapter 22).

- Bernard Gesch of the University of Oxford gave prison inmates supplements of vitamins, minerals, and essential fats, or placebos, and demonstrated a dramatic 35 percent decrease in aggressive acts only in those taking the supplements.[13]

- Dr. Jane Durga from Wageningen University in the Netherlands gave 818 people from ages 50 to 75 either a supplement containing 800 micrograms of folic acid a day, or a dummy pill, for three years. On memory tests, the supplement users had scores comparable to people 5.5 years younger.[14]

- A recent trial published in the *American Journal of Psychiatry* tested the effects of giving 20 people suffering from depression, who were already on antidepressants but still depressed, a highly concentrated form of the omega-3 fat EPA or a placebo. By the third week the patients taking EPA were showing major improvements in mood, while those on the placebo were not.[15]

The evidence is there if you look for it. You can change how you think and feel by changing what you put into your mouth. Whatever your state of mind now, you will notice gradual improvements in your mind and mood as you follow the guidelines in this book.

You don't have to be clinically depressed, anxious, unable to concentrate, hyperactive, or losing your memory or your mind to benefit from this book, but it helps! Even if you feel all right, optimum nutrition can significantly boost your psychological well-being—because feeling *just* all right isn't all right. You should, and can, feel alert, energetic, happy, and unstressed, with a clear mind and a sharp intelligence.

Optimum nutrition and psychotherapy work wonders

Of course, as I've mentioned, improving our mental health isn't only about nutrition. While most psychotherapists ignore the role of nutrition and the brain's chemistry in how we think and feel, let's not make the same mistake of omission. I believe the solution to the mental health problems that plague our society lies in a combination of optimum nutrition and good psychological support, which includes having a place you can call home, being treated with respect and dignity, and counseling. Certain kinds of counseling are highly effective for depression, for example, but far too infrequently prescribed or available. In fact, as the evidence for this grows, the U.K. National Health Service is actually cutting back on psychotherapists in an attempt to save money, yet spending more on less effective drugs.

The combination of optimum nutrition and psychotherapy works wonders for a wide variety of mental health problems, from depression to schizophrenia—and it works much better than drugs. Most of the psychiatrists I work with find that while drugs can be lifesaving in the short term, they become unnecessary when people are receiving the right combination of nutrients and psychological support.

We need a radical new approach based on science

With mental health problems rising at such a pace, we need a new way of thinking about the state of our minds. As Marcel Proust said, 'The real act of discovery consists, not in finding new lands, but in seeing with new eyes.' We need to wake up to the realization that poor nutrition and chemical imbalances probably underlie the majority of mental health problems. You can't just psychoanalyze away deficiencies in essential fats, vitamins, minerals and other key brain nutrients. We must think our way out of the box and come to grips with the fact that chemistry directly affects how we think and feel.

This means a new basis for both diagnosing and treating problems, and a new way of living and eating that supports our mental health, rather than eroding it. I believe we already have solutions to most forms of mental illness. We just have to look with new eyes. This book is dedicated to that vision.

SUMMARY

In summary, we can now say with confidence that:

- Most people are achieving well below their full potential for intelligence, memory, concentration, emotional balance, and happiness.

- The right combination of nutrients works better than drugs, and without the side effects.

- Psychotherapy works best if you're optimally nourished.

- Most mental health problems can be solved, or at least considerably relieved, with the right nutrition, together with the right psychological support and guidance.

CHAPTER 2

The five essential brain booster foods—check yourself out

Whether you're in good shape or are currently dealing with depression, mood swings, or another mental health problem, there are five essential foods you need to tune up your brain.

- **Balance your glucose**—it's fuel for the brain.

- **Essential fats**—these keep your brain well oiled.

- **Phospholipids**—these memory molecules give oomph to the brain.

- **Amino acids**—these are the brain's messengers.

- **Intelligent nutrients**—these include vitamins and minerals that fine tune your mind.

Knowing a few simple facts about your amazing brain shows you why these foods are so important for your mind. Every day we have around 6,000 thoughts—most of them repeats! Every single thought you have is represented by a ripple of activity across the network of nerves called your brain. Here's how it works.

What we call the brain is a network of neurons—special nerve cells that connect to other neurons. You've got 100 billion neurons, each connecting to thousands of others. To get an idea of just how complex that is,

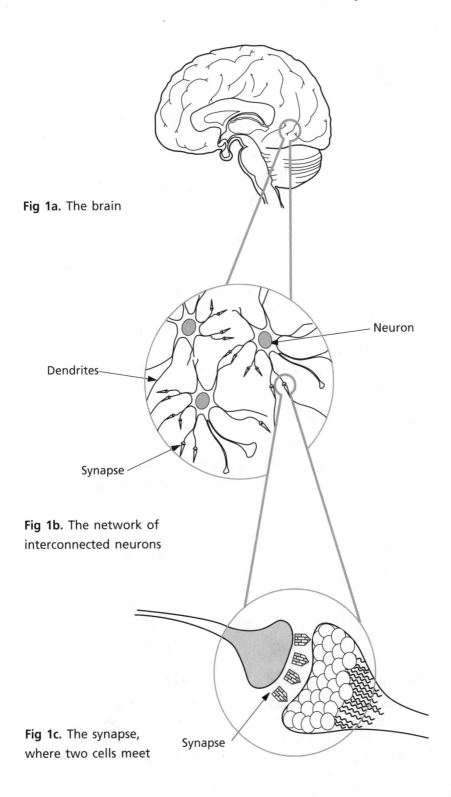

Fig 1a. The brain

Neuron

Dendrites

Synapse

Fig 1b. The network of
interconnected neurons

Fig 1c. The synapse,
where two cells meet

Synapse

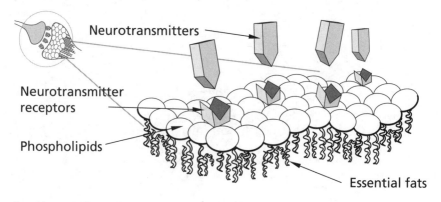

Fig 1d. How the brain receives a message

let's look at the Amazon rainforest. The Amazon stretches for 2.7 million square miles and contains about 100 billion trees. So there are as many cells in our brain as trees in the entire Amazon rainforest, and as many connections as leaves!

The connections between neurons are called dendrites. Where one dendrite meets another neuron, there's a gap, like the spark gap in a spark plug. This gap is called a synapse and it's across this gap that messages are sent from one neuron to another.

The message is sent from a sending station and received in a receiving station, called a receptor. These sending and receiving stations are built out of **essential fats,** found in fish and seeds; **phospholipids,** present in eggs and organ meats; and **amino acids,** the raw material of protein.

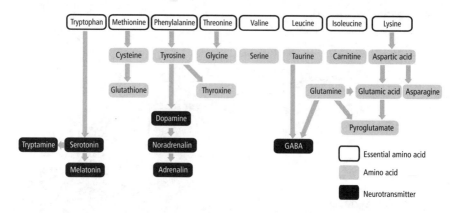

Fig 1e. Neurotransmitters are made from amino acids

The message itself, the neurotransmitter, is in most cases made out of amino acids. Different amino acids make different neurotransmitters. For example, the neurotransmitter serotonin, which keeps you happy, is made from the amino acid tryptophan. Adrenalin and dopamine, which keep you motivated, are made from phenylalanine (see Fig 1e on the previous page).

Turning an amino acid into a neurotransmitter is no simple job. Enzymes in the brain that depend on intelligent nutrients do it. These include vitamins, minerals, and special amino acids.

You are what you eat, but that goes beyond the physical body. How you think and feel also depends on what you eat. You can check out whether you are getting enough of these essential brain foods using the Brain Food Check below.

Brain food check

In each section there are ten questions. Check the box for *yes*. If you check five or more in the *yes* column, the chances are you're not getting enough of this essential brain food factor.

❓ GLUCOSE CHECK

☐ Do you usually eat white bread, rice, or pasta instead of brown/wholegrain?

☐ Do you crave certain foods such as carbohydrates?

☐ Do you have tea, coffee, and sugary foods or drinks, or cigarettes, at regular intervals during the day?

☐ Do you usually eat fruit, vegetables, or other carbohydrates without protein foods at the same time?

☐ Do you sometimes skip meals, especially breakfast?

☐ Do you wake unrefreshed or need something to get you going in the morning, like tea, coffee, or a cigarette?

☐ Do you often feel drowsy during the day?

☐ Do you sometimes lose concentration?

☐ Do you get dizzy or irritable if you don't eat often?

☐ Do you avoid exercise because you don't have the energy?

❓ FAT CHECK

☐ Do you eat oily fish (salmon, trout, sardines, herring, mackerel, or fresh tuna) less than once a week?

☐ Do you eat seeds or their cold-pressed oils less than three times a week?

☐ Do you eat meat or dairy products most days?

☐ Do you eat processed or fried foods (such as ready meals, chips, crisps) three or more times a week?

☐ Do you have dry or rough skin or a tendency to eczema?

☐ Do you have a poor memory or difficulty concentrating?

☐ Do you suffer from PMS or breast tenderness?

☐ Do you suffer from water retention?

☐ Do you suffer from dry, watery, or itchy eyes?

☐ Do you have inflammatory health problems such as arthritis?

❓ PHOSPHOLIPID CHECK

☐ Do you eat fish (especially sardines) less than once a week?

☐ Do you eat fewer than three eggs per week?

☐ Do you eat liver, soy/tofu, or nuts less than three times per week?

☐ Do you take less than 5g of lecithin each day?

☐ Is your memory declining?

☐ Do you sometimes go looking for something and forget what it was you were looking for?

☐ Do you find it hard to do calculations in your head?

☐ Do you sometimes have difficulty concentrating?

☐ Do you have a tendency towards depression?

☐ Are you a slow learner?

❓ AMINO ACID CHECK

☐ Do you eat less than one portion of protein-rich foods (meat, dairy, fish, eggs, tofu) each day?

☐ Do you eat fewer than two servings of vegetable sources of protein (beans, lentils, quinoa, seeds, nuts, wholegrains, and so on) each day?

☐ If you're vegetarian, do you rarely combine different protein foods such as those mentioned above?

☐ Are you very physically active or do you work out a lot?

☐ Do you suffer from anxiety, depression, or irritability?

☐ Are you frequently tired or do you lack motivation?

☐ Do you sometimes lose concentration or have poor memory?

☐ Do you have very low blood pressure?

☐ Do your hair and nails grow slowly?

☐ Are you constantly hungry and do you frequently get indigestion?

❓ INTELLIGENT NUTRIENT CHECK

☐ Do you eat fewer than five servings of fresh fruits and vegetables (excluding potato) every day?

☐ Do you eat fewer than one portion of dark green vegetables a day?

☐ Do you eat fewer than three portions of fresh or dried tropical fruit a week?

☐ Do you eat seeds (such as pumpkin, sunflower, tahini) or unroasted nuts less than three times a week?

☐ Are you currently not taking a multivitamin/mineral supplement every day?

☐ Do you usually eat white bread, rice, or pasta instead of brown/wholegrain?

☐ Do you consume more than one unit of alcohol most days?

☐ Do you suffer from anxiety, depression, or irritability?

☐ Do you suffer from muscle cramps?

☐ Do you have white marks on more than two fingernails?

The gut-brain connection

It used to be thought that all our thinking is done by neurons in the brain. We now know that the digestive system contains 100 million neurons, and produces as many neurotransmitters as the brain. The gut, for example, produces two-thirds of the body's serotonin, the happy neurotransmitter. So in essence, you're feeding two brains. Every time you eat something it sends signals to the brain because the gut and the brain are in permanent communication. This is why the right foods can make you happy and the wrong foods can make you feel anxious or depressed.

The following five chapters tell you how to feed your brain the right food to make it sing!

CHAPTER 3

Complex carbohydrates— the best brain food

The most important nutrient of all for the brain and nervous system is glucose, the fuel they run on. We humans are solar-powered. We use plants to collect the Sun's energy for us in the form of glucose. The plants absorb hydrogen and oxygen (H_2O—water) from the soil, and carbon and oxygen (CO_2—carbon dioxide) from the air, and combine these atoms together using the Sun's energy to make carbohydrate (COH).

We then digest the carbohydrate down into glucose and deliver this into both our brain and body cells. The glucose is then 'burned' within our cells, liberating the Sun's energy, which is what keeps us alive. Some of the excess is stored as a substance called glycogen, in our muscles and liver.

Your brain consumes more glucose than any other organ. In a sedentary day your brain can consume up to 40 percent of all the carbohydrate you eat. That's why you get hungry after exams! Any imbalance in the supply of glucose to the brain and you can experience fatigue, irritability, dizziness, insomnia, excessive sweating (especially at night), poor concentration and forgetfulness, excessive thirst, depression and crying spells, digestive disturbances and blurred vision.

Basically, the more carbohydrates you eat, and the more regularly you eat them, the healthier you are and the better your brain works. But it's not quite that simple. Some carbohydrates are better at fuelling the body properly than others.

Research at the Massachusetts Institute of Technology found a massive 25 percent difference between the IQ scores of children who were in the top fifth of the population for consumption of refined carbohydrates, compared with children who were in the bottom fifth.[16] So staying away from white bread, processed cereals, and sugar seems to be crucial to having a higher IQ.

But that's not all. To maximize mental performance, you need an *even* supply of glucose to the brain. This has been well proven by Professor David Benton at Swansea University in Wales, who has found that dips in blood sugar are directly associated with poor attention, poor memory, and aggressive behavior.[17] That's why children who fail to eat breakfast can't think straight at school.[18] So what kind of carbohydrates will fit the bill?

Food for fuel

Although we can make energy from protein, fat, and carbohydrate, carbohydrate-rich foods are the best kind of fuel. This is because when fat and protein are used to make energy there is a buildup of toxic substances in the body. Carbohydrates are the only 'smokeless' fuel.

But they need to be slow-releasing too. Complex carbohydrates like wholegrains, vegetables, beans, or lentils, or simpler carbohydrates such as fruit, take longer to digest than refined carbohydrates. So when you eat, say, brown rice, your body does exactly what it's designed to do. It digests it and releases its potential energy steadily and gradually.

Why refined is bad

What's so bad about refined carbohydrates, though—sugars, white bread, white rice, and the like?

When we refine sugars, we are in essence cheating nature by isolating the sweetness in a food (such as beets) and discarding the rest. All forms of concentrated sugar—white sugar, brown sugar, malt, glucose, honey, and syrup—are fast-releasing or, to put it another way, have a high glycemic load (GL), which triggers a rapid increase in blood-sugar levels. (See page 21 for the lowdown on GL.) The way the body responds to a sudden onslaught of sugar in the blood is to release the hormone insulin, which then escorts the sugar out into the cells. But there is only so much fuel they can take at any one time, so excess sugar is first put into storage in the liver and muscles as a substance called glycogen, and when that has reached its limits, as fat. So eating a lot of sugar regularly can leave you with a lot of stored fat.

Most concentrated forms of sugar are also devoid of vitamins and minerals, unlike natural sources such as fruit. White sugar has had around 90 percent of its vitamins and minerals removed. Without vitamins and minerals, our metabolism becomes inefficient, contributing to poor energy levels, concentration, and weight control.

Too much sugar also sends your adrenalin, the stress hormone, sky-high. Researchers at Yale University in the U.S. gave 25 healthy children a drink containing the amount of glucose found in a can of a popular soft drink. The rebound blood-sugar drop (which happens when too much sugar in the blood causes insulin to overcompensate by taking too much sugar out) boosted their adrenalin to over five times their normal level for up to five hours after ingesting the sugar. Most of these children had difficulty concentrating and were irritable and anxious, which are normal reactions to too much adrenalin in the bloodstream.[19] A similar study involving 404 Finnish children 10 to 11 years old showed that withdrawal, anxiousness, depression, delinquency, and aggression were twice as frequent in those consuming 30 percent more sucrose in the form of ice cream, sugary snacks, and soft drinks.[20]

Other refined carbohydrates such as white bread, white rice and processed cereals have an effect similar to that of refined sugar. The process of refining or even cooking starts to break down complex carbohydrates into simple carbohydrates, in effect predigesting them. When you eat them you get a rapid increase in blood-sugar level and a corresponding surge in energy. The surge, however, is followed by a drop as the body scrambles to balance your blood-sugar level.

Fruit sugars—a mixed bag

But it's not just about added or even refined sugar. The main sugar in most fruit is the simple sugar fructose. This enters the bloodstream fast, but is classified as slow-releasing because your body has to convert it to glucose before it can be used as fuel, and this process slows down its effect on the body.

Some fruits however, such as grapes and dates, contain almost pure glucose, putting the carbohydrates they contain in the fast-releasing category. Apples, on the other hand, contain mainly fructose and so are relatively

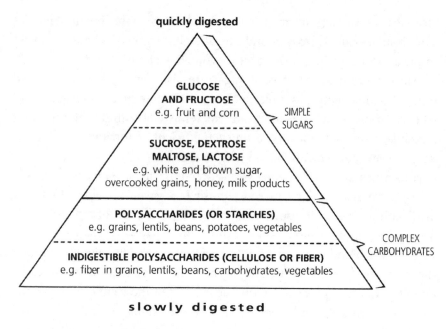

quickly digested

GLUCOSE
AND FRUCTOSE
e.g. fruit and corn

SIMPLE
SUGARS

SUCROSE, DEXTROSE
MALTOSE, LACTOSE
e.g. white and brown sugar,
overcooked grains, honey, milk products

POLYSACCHARIDES (OR STARCHES)
e.g. grains, lentils, beans, potatoes, vegetables

COMPLEX
CARBOHYDRATES

INDIGESTIBLE POLYSACCHARIDES (CELLULOSE OR FIBER)
e.g. fiber in grains, lentils, beans, carbohydrates, vegetables

slowly digested

Fig 2. The sugar family

slow-releasing. Bananas contain both, and raise blood-glucose levels quite speedily. But all fresh fruit does have two big advantages. One is fiber, which slows down the release of the sugars contained in the fruit. (This is why drinking juice, which is processed to remove most of the fiber, is a less desirable way of consuming fruit.) The other is vitamins, which as we'll see in Chapter 7 are essential for physical and mental health.

What about dried fruit? In a nutshell, it's problematic. This is because, weight for weight, it obviously has much less water than fresh fruit, and this both concentrates the sugar and makes it much smaller and less filling—so you can end up packing away quite a lot of it without realizing. More, the fiber in dried apples, say, is less effective at slowing down sugar release. So don't make dried fruit a substitute for fresh. And when you do eat dried fruit, soak it first—when it's plumped up and rehydrated it will be more filling, so you're likely to eat less of it.

Carbohydrates to concentrate on

By this time you'll have an idea of how important the release rate of carbohydrates is. But how can you tell which is fast-releasing and which slow?

As a general rule, you can assume that whole, unprocessed foods are the slowest to release their sugar. Beyond this, you can use a measure called glycemic load or GL.

GL describes both how much carbohydrate a food contains and how fast-releasing that carbohydrate is. So in essence, it measures a food's effect on blood-sugar levels. Foods with a GL of less than 10 are good and should be the staple foods of your diet. A GL of 11 to 14 is okay, and can be eaten in moderation. A GL higher than 15 should be avoided. Beware of combining two moderate-GL foods in one meal. When they're eaten together, their GL adds up to high. For example, a crumpet with unsweetened peanut butter (moderate with very low GL) remains moderate, but the GL score of a crumpet with a teaspoon of honey (moderate with moderate) shoots up.

The chart below gives GL scores for average servings of a range of common foods. You can start to use this now by checking out what you eat for breakfast.

If you start the day with cornflakes, which have a high GL score, you're getting rocket fuel first thing in the morning—and that means that a couple of hours later your blood glucose, and energy, will plummet. But have oat flakes, sweetened with a chopped apple—both of which are slow-releasing—and your energy and concentration will last right through to lunch.

Glycemic load of common foods

Food	Serving size (in g)	Serving size	GLs per serving
Bakery products & cakes			
Low-carb muffin	-	1 muffin	5
Apple and almond cake	-	1 medium slice	5
Carrot and walnut cake	-	1 medium slice	5
Muffin—apple, made without sugar	60	1 muffin	9
Muffin—apple muffin, made with sugar	60	1 muffin	13
Crumpet	50	1 crumpet	13
Muffin—apple, oat, sultana, made from packet mix	50	1 muffin	14
Muffin—bran	57	1 muffin	15
Banana cake, made without sugar	80	1 medium slice	16

Food	Serving size (in g)	Serving size	GLs per serving
Muffin—blueberry	57	1 muffin	17
Muffin—banana, oat, and honey	50	1 muffin	17
Croissant	57	1 croissant	17
Doughnut	47	1 plain doughnut	17
Sponge cake, plain	63	1 slice	17
Muffin—carrot	57	1 muffin	20
Breads & crackers			
Volkenbrot wholemeal rye bread	20	1 slice	5
Rice bread, high-amylose	20	1 small slice	5
Rice bread, low-amylose	20	1 small slice	5
Wholemeal rye bread	20	1 thin slice	5
Wheat tortilla (Mexican)	30	1 tortilla	5
Chapatti, white wheat flour, thin, with green gram	30	1 chapatti	5
Rye kernel (pumpernickel) bread	30	1 slice	6
Sourdough rye bread	30	1 slice	6
White, high-fiber bread	30	1 thick slice	9
Wholemeal (wholewheat) wheat flour bread	30	1 thick slice	9
Gluten-free fiber-enriched bread	30	1 thick slice	9
Gluten-free multigrain bread	30	1 slice	10
Light rye bread	30	1 slice	10
White wheat-flour bread	30	1 slice	10
Pita bread, white	30	1 pita	10
Wheat flour flatbread	30	1 slice	10
Gluten-free white bread	30	1 slice	11
Corn tortilla	50	1 tortilla	12
Middle Eastern flatbread	30	1 slice	15
Baguette, white, plain	30	⅓ loaf	15
Bagel, white, frozen	70	1 bagel	25
Rough Oat Cakes	10	1 oat cake	2
Fine Oat Cakes	9	1 oat cake	3
Cheesey Oat Cakes	8	1 oat cake	3
Cream cracker	25	2 cookies	11
Rye crispbread	25	2 cookies	11
Water cracker	25	3 cookies	17
Puffed rice cakes	25	3 cookies	17

Food	Serving size (in g)	Serving size	GLs per serving
Dairy products			
Cottage cheese	120	½ medium tub	2
Plain yogurt (no sugar)	200	1 small container	3
Non-fat yogurt (plain, no sugar)	200	1 small container	3
Soy yogurt	200	1 large bowl	7
Soy milk (no sugar)	(250ml)	1 glass	7
Low-fat yogurt, fruit, sugar	150	1 small container	7.5
Fruits			
Blackberries	120	1 medium bowl	1
Blueberries	120	1 medium bowl	1
Raspberries	120	1 medium bowl	1
Strawberries, fresh, raw	120	1 medium bowl	1
Cherries, raw	120	1 medium bowl	3
Grapefruit, raw	120	½ medium	3
Pear, raw	120	1 medium	4
Melon/cantaloupe, raw	120	½ small	4
Watermelon, raw	120	1 medium slice	4
Peaches, raw (or canned in natural juice)	120	1	5
Apricots, raw	120	4 apricots	5
Oranges, raw	120	1 large	5
Plum, raw	120	4	5
Apples, raw	120	1 small	6
Kiwi fruit, raw	120	1	6
Pineapple, raw	120	1 medium slice	7
Grapes, raw	120	16	8
Mango, raw	120	1 ½ slices	8
Apricots, dried	60	6 apricots	9
Fruit cocktail, canned (Del Monte)	120	Small can	9
Papaya, raw	120	Half a small papaya	10
Prunes, pitted	60	6 prunes	10
Apple, dried	60	6 rings	10
Banana, raw	120	1 small	12
Apricots, canned in light syrup	120	1 small can	12
Lychees, canned in syrup and drained	120	1 small can	16
Figs, dried, tenderized	60	3	16
Sultana grapes	60	30	25

Food	Serving size (in g)	Serving size	GLs per serving
Raisins	60	30	28
Dates, dried	60	8	42
Spreads & jams			
Pumpkin seed butter	16	1 tbsp	1
Peanut butter (no sugar)	16	1 tbsp	1
Blueberry spread (no sugar)	10	2 teaspoons	1
Apricot fruit spread, reduced sugar	10	2 teaspoons	2
Orange marmalade	10	2 teaspoons	3
Strawberry jam	10	2 teaspoons	3
Snack foods			
Hummus	200	1 small tub	6
Olives, in brine	50	7	1
Peanuts	50	2 medium handfuls	1
Cashew nuts, salted	50	2 medium handfuls	3
Potato chips, plain, salted	30	1 small packet	7
Popcorn, salted	25	1 small packet	10
Pretzels, oven-baked, traditional wheat flavor	30	15	16
Corn chips, plain, salted	50	18	17
ReBar fruit and veg bar	50	1	8
Apricot fruit bar (dried apricot filling in wholemeal pastry)	35	1	12
Muesli bar with dried fruit	30	1	13
Chocolate bar, milk, plain (Mars/Cadbury/Nestlé)	50	1	14
Twix® biscuit and caramel bar (Mars)	60	1 bar (2 fingers)	17
Snickers® bar (Mars)	60	1	19
Polos peppermint sweets (Nestlé)	30	16	21
Jelly beans, assorted colors	30	9	22
Kellogg's Pop-Tarts™, double choc	50	1	24
Mars Bar®	60	1	26

A comprehensive list of the GL of foods is available in the New Optimum Nutrition Bible *and* The Holford Low-GL Diet, *or online at www.holforddiet.com.*

How to stay in perfect balance

As you can see in the chart on the previous pages, the GL of some foods is through the roof. So it will be bound to play havoc with your blood-sugar balance and, in turn, your state of mind. You may have had a few shocks: baguettes and bagels have quite a high GL, for instance. But as you'll discover, it's amazingly easy to find delicious and thoroughly satisfying substitutes. Here are some examples of what you should and should not be eating to keep your blood glucose, and your brain, in balance.

Bad news and good news foods

Instead of...	eat
White toast and jam	Wholegrain toast and baked beans
Sweetened cornflakes	Hot cereal with raspberries
Croissants and baguettes	Wholegrain rye bread
White rice	Wholemeal spaghetti
Chocolate bars	Raw vegetable crudités with hummus or low GL fruit bars
Bananas	Berries, apples, or oranges
Crackers or rice cakes	Oatcakes

Picking the right carbs is vital, but you'll also need to follow a few other steps to achieve that perfect blood-sugar balance.

The long goodbye to sugar

It's best to decrease the sugar content of your diet slowly. Gradually get used to less sweetness. For example, sweeten cereal with fruit. Dilute fruit juices with water by at least half to halve their GL score. Avoid foods with added sugar. Limit dried fruit, and cut down on fast-releasing, high-GL fruits like bananas—or combine them with slow-releasing, low-GL carbohydrates such as oats.

The one exception to this rule is if you have just done some intense exercise, such as a one-hour run. You'll need to boost your blood-sugar levels fast, as your blood will be largely depleted of glucose and your glycogen levels will be low too. So at those moments there is no harm in snacking on a fast-releasing fruit such as a banana: any excess glucose in the blood will go to replenish your body's empty storage facilities rather than build up into high blood sugar.

Stay away from sugar substitutes

While they won't raise blood-sugar levels, sugar substitutes shouldn't be part of your plan to cut down on sugar in your diet. Aspartame, the most widely used, is particularly bad. Some studies have shown it to have adverse effects on health. One study into its effects showed that it caused nightmares, memory loss, bad temper, and nausea.[21] Besides the dangers of additives, there is another good reason not to use them. And that is that they don't help you adjust to less sweetness in our diet. For all of us, adults and children alike, staying away from sugar becomes easier and easier as our cravings for sugar subside. Artificial sweeteners simply keep the cravings alive.

One sugar substitute worth a mention is xylitol. It is derived from a natural source and is abundant in plums, which have a very low GL as a result. Xylitol has a fraction of the effect on blood sugar compared with regular sugar or even fructose. For example, 9 teaspoons of xylitol have the same effect on your blood sugar as 4 teaspoons of fructose—or 1 teaspoon of sugar! I still suggest you reduce your taste for sweet foods, but when some sweetness is really essential, for example if you're whipping up dessert for a special occasion meal, then xylitol is the best alternative to sugar. Xylitol can be found in most natural food stores..

Dynamic duo—protein and fiber

The more fiber and protein you include with any meal or snack, the slower the release of any carbohydrates you eat. Fiber does the job by actually getting in the way of the carbohydrate, impeding its interaction with digestive enzymes and effectively slowing its passage into the intestines, where it is absorbed into the bloodstream. Meanwhile, protein slows down the speed at which the stomach empties its contents of partially digested food into the intestines. Foods with high fiber and protein naturally have a lower GL.

As we've seen, anything that slows the passage of carbohydrate into the bloodstream is good for blood-glucose balance. So combining protein-rich foods with high-fiber, low-GL carbohydrates is an excellent rule of thumb in this context. Luckily, there are plenty of simple ways to do it.

- Have seeds or nuts when eating a fruit snack.

- Add seeds or nuts to carbohydrate-based breakfast cereals.

- Serve salmon, chicken, or tofu with brown basmati rice.

- Add kidney beans to sauces served with wholemeal pasta.

- Put cottage cheese on oatcakes, or hummus on rye bread.

Don't go without breakfast

Eating a decent breakfast really is essential for all of us—for children to be able to concentrate at school and adults at work. In one study, 29 school-children were given different breakfast cereals, a glucose drink, or no breakfast on different days. Their attention and memory were tested before breakfast, and again 30, 90, 150, and 210 minutes later. Children who had had the glucose drink or no breakfast showed poorer attention and memory compared to children eating the cereal.[22]

SUMMARY

In summary, here are some general guidelines to ensure you get enough low-GL carbohydrates, the best brain fuel:

- Choose wholefoods—wholegrains, lentils, beans, nuts, seeds, fresh fruit, and vegetables. Eat five or more servings of fruits and vegetables per day. Choose dark green, leafy, and root vegetables such as watercress, carrots, sweet potatoes, broccoli, Brussels sprouts, spinach, green beans or peppers, either raw or lightly cooked, and limit your consumption of starchier vegetables such as potatoes. Choose fresh fruit such as apples, pears, berries, melon, or citrus fruit. Have bananas in moderation. Dilute fruit juices and only eat dried fruits infrequently in small quantities, preferably soaked.

- Avoid sugar and foods containing sugar. This means anything with added glucose, sucrose, or dextrose, malt sugar, or honey.

▶

Keep fructose consumption within limits. Don't be tempted to go for sugar substitutes—most are detrimental to health and they all keep sugar cravings alive. If you need to sweeten something, use xylitol.

- Combine protein foods with carbohydrate foods by eating cereals and fruit with nuts or seeds, and having carbohydrate-rich foods (potatoes, bread, pasta, or rice) with protein-rich foods such as fish, chicken, lentils, beans, or tofu.

- Avoid overly processed foods.

- Choose wholegrains such as rice, buckwheat, millet, rye, oats, wholewheat, corn, or quinoa in cereal, breads, and pasta. Avoid refined white foods.

- If you want to drink juice, make it yourself with a juicer or choose real fruit juices (never fruit drinks) from the refrigerator and dilute 50/50. Steer clear of the highly processed kind with a long shelf life.

- Eat breakfast every day.

CHAPTER 4

Smart fats—the architects of higher intelligence

If you squeezed out all the water from your brain, a whopping 60 percent of the dry weight would be made up of fat. These fats are always being replenished, so it's crucial to know which kind will feed your brain the best.

Some fats are not only positively good for you, they are absolutely vital for mental health. Not only do you need them to stay free from disease—and depression, dyslexia, attention deficit disorder, fatigue, memory problems, Alzheimer's, and schizophrenia have all been linked to deficiency—you also need them in optimal amounts if you want to maximize your intelligence.

Our ability to perform in this world depends upon a balance of mental, emotional, and physical intelligence. Mental intelligence we are well aware of, with IQ tests that determine a person's ability to make intellectual connections and deal with complex concepts. But emotional intelligence is no less important. Your 'EQ' is a measure of your ability to respond emotionally to situations in an appropriate and sensitive way. If you lose your temper easily, and oscillate between depression and hyperactivity, lacking emotional balance and perspective, there's room for improvement—however bright you are.

Then there's physical intelligence. Your 'PQ' is all about your brain-body coordination. For example, a lot of children diagnosed with attention deficit disorder are clumsy by nature and have trouble with skills such as handwriting, reading, and taking notes in class, or keeping themselves organized. This is called *dyspraxia* or developmental coordination disorder.

Each type of intelligence is affected by our intake of essential fats, known as omega-3 and omega-6. Animals low in essential fats perform poorly on mental intelligence tasks, showing poor memory. Children deficient in essential fat levels have more learning difficulties, while children who are breastfed have higher IQs at age eight than bottle-fed babies, which is thought to be due to the higher levels of essential fats in breast milk.

The bottom line is that fat, at least the right kind, is good for you. As well as improving your mental health, the essential fats reduce the risk of cancer, heart disease, allergies, arthritis, eczema, and infections.

Good fats, bad fats

Conclusive research now clearly shows that the amount and type of fat consumed during fetal development, infancy, childhood, adolescence, adulthood, old age—and indeed every day of your life—has a profound

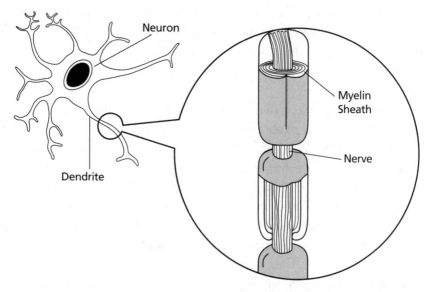

Fig 3. Close-up of a neuron

effect on how you think and feel. The brain and nervous system are totally dependent on a family of fats. These include:

- Saturated and monounsaturated fat

- Cholesterol

- Omega-3 (polyunsaturated) fat—especially EPA and DHA

- Omega-6 (polyunsaturated) fat—especially GLA and AA.

The first two types of fat can be made in the body. The omegas, however, have to be topped up through diet.

To understand why these fats are so important, let's take a closer look at a brain cell. If you remember from Chapter 2, the making of intelligence involves the careful connecting up of billions of nerve cells, each one of

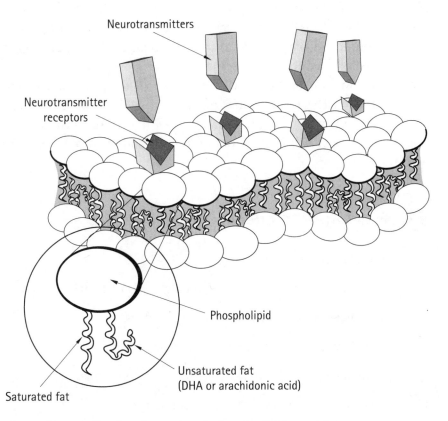

Fig 4. The myelin sheath, made of phospholipids and fats

which links to as many as 20,000 others. The messengers—neurotransmitters—deliver their messages across connection points called synapses into receptor sites. These receptor sites are contained within the myelin sheath, a membrane surrounding every neuron in the brain. It's a bit like a layer of insulation around an electrical wire and is roughly 75 percent fat. But what kind of fat?

The myelin sheath is made out of phospholipids (more on these in the next chapter), that each have a saturated and unsaturated fatty acid attached (see figure, page 31). The unsaturated fatty acid (the bent one) is usually an omega-3 or omega-6 fat. It is this balance that seems to be critical for the brain's structure and function. So for brain health, both omega-3 and omega-6 fat families must be present in your diet.

Are you fat deficient?

If you are fat-phobic you are depriving yourself of essential, health-giving nutrients. The same is true if you eat too much hard fat, either from saturated fat found in dairy products or meat, or damaged (trans) fats found in processed or fried foods and some margarines. In fact, unless you go out of your way to eat the right kind of fat-rich foods, or supplement essential fats, the chances are you're missing out. Most people in the West are eating too many saturated killer fats, and are undernourished in essential, healing fats. Check yourself out on this questionnaire, scoring 1 for each *yes* answer.

❓ ESSENTIAL FATS CHECK

☐ Do you have difficulty learning?

☐ Do you have a poor memory or difficulty concentrating?

☐ Do you have poor coordination or impaired vision?

☐ Do you have dry, unmanageable hair or dandruff?

☐ Do you have dry or rough skin or a tendency to eczema?

☐ Do you have brittle, easily frayed, or soft nails?

☐ Do you have excessive thirst and/or frequent urination?

☐ Do you suffer from PMS or breast tenderness?

☐ Do you suffer from dry, watery, or itchy eyes?

☐ Do you have inflammatory health problems such as arthritis?

☐ Do you have high blood pressure or high blood lipids?

☐ Do you have slow/poor wound healing?

☐ Do you have obsessive or compulsive behavior?

☐ Do you have phobias, extreme fears, or night terrors?

☐ Do you suffer from anxiety or depression?

☐ Do you suffer from travel or motion sickness?

☐ Do you experience fits or convulsions?

If you have answered *yes* to more than four questions, you are very likely deficient in essential fats. Check that your diet contains enough seeds, seed oils, and fish.

Ultimately, the most precise way to know your fat status is to have a blood test. This gives you a complete breakdown of all the essential fats and what you're lacking. These tests are available through nutritional therapists.

Fat figures

How much fat do you need to eat? It is best to consume no more than 20 percent of overall calories as fat. The current average in Britain is around 36 percent. In countries with a low incidence of fat-related diseases, like Japan, Thailand, and the Philippines, people consume only about 15 percent of their total calorie intake as fat. For example, Japanese people eat 40g of fat a day. British people eat over 100g of fat a day.

Most authorities now agree that, of our total fat intake, no more than a third should be saturated (hard) fat, and at least a third should be polyunsaturated oils providing the two essential fat families, omega-3 and omega-6. (More on these on page 34.) These two essential fat families also need to be roughly in balance—in other words, 1:1, which is the ratio our pre-Industrial Revolution ancestors achieved. Nowadays, an average balance is

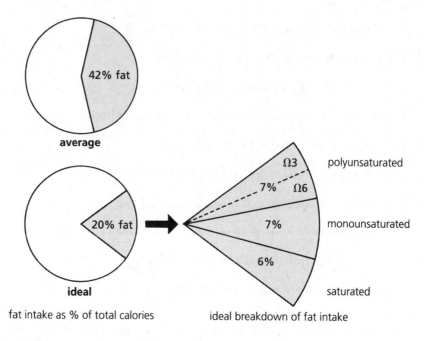

Fig 5. What we eat vs what we need

more like 1:20 in favor of omega-6. It may be not just gross deficiency in these fats, but also the gross imbalance between the two types, that is contributing to the mental and other health problems we see today.

Most people are deficient in both omega-6 and omega-3 fats. In addition, a high intake of saturated fats and damaged polyunsaturated fats, known as trans fats, stops the body from making good use of the little essential fat the average person does eat in a day.

Fantastic fats: the essential omegas

By now you'll have gathered how important the omega-fat families are to mental and emotional health. Let's delve deeper, first taking a closer look at the essential fats so many of us lack—the omega-3s.

The omega-3s

Why is the modern-day diet likely to be more deficient in omega-3 fats than in omega-6s? It's all because the grandmother of the omega-3 family, alpha-linolenic acid, and her metabolically active grandchildren EPA (eicosapentaenoic acid) and DHA (docosahexaenoic acid), are more unsaturated and so more prone to damage by cooking, heating, and food processing. In fact, the average person today eats a mere sixth of the omega-3 fats found in the diet of people living in 1850. This decline is partly due to food choices, but mainly to food processing.

Omega-3 fats are not only important because they are part of myelin. It's from these fats that our body and brain makes **prostaglandins,** extremely active hormonelike substances. More and more functions of prostaglandins are being found every year, but for now we know that they relax blood vessels and so lower blood pressure, help to maintain water balance in the body, boost immunity, decrease inflammation and pain, and help insulin to work—which is good for blood-sugar balance. In the brain they regulate the release and performance of neurotransmitters, and low levels are known to be involved in various conditions, including depression and schizophrenia. You'll see evidence throughout this book that shows how omega-3 fats improve learning, behavioral problems, attention deficit disorder, depression, and schizophrenia.

As these fats get converted in the body to more active substances, they become more unsaturated, and generally the word referring to them gets longer. Take oleic acid—that's one degree of unsaturation. Then there's linoleic—two degrees of unsaturation; linolenic—three degrees; eicos-apentaenoic—five degrees; and so on. You can see this increasing complexity as we move up the food chain.

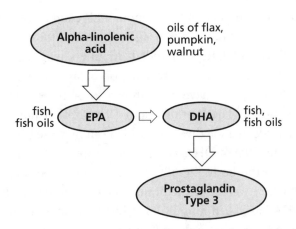

Fig 6. Omega-3 fats

For example, plankton, the staple food of small fish, is rich in alpha-linolenic acid. Carnivorous fish such as mackerel or herring eat the small fish that have converted some of their alpha-linolenic acid to more complex fats. The carnivorous fish continue the conversion. Seals eat them and have the highest EPA and DHA concentration, and then the Inuit people eat the seals and benefit from the ready-made meal of EPA and DHA. That's why the Inuit have the lowest risk of heart disease, despite eating a diet high in cholesterol.

The primary, most direct source of EPA and DHA is coldwater fish, especially fish that eat fish, namely herring, mackerel, salmon, and tuna (fresh, not canned). We normally need 300 to 400 mg of both DHA and EPA a day, and perhaps double or triple this to correct a problem, for example a learning difficulty or heart disease.

If you are vegetarian, the picture becomes a bit more complex. Our bodies struggle to convert alpha-linolenic acid into DHA and EPA—in fact, hardly any ALA is converted to DHA, while only about 5 percent of it is converted to EPA. For this reason, vegetarians rarely have sufficient EPA and DHA levels unless they eat significant quantities of flaxseeds (also known as linseeds), which are the richest source of ALA. The small amount of EPA that your body will make from flax has some positive effect, but you do have to eat a lot of the seeds. For example, 10g of ALA lowers blood pressure as effectively as 1.5g of EPA plus DHA, but to get this amount of ALA you'd have to eat three tablespoons of ground seeds or one tablespoon of flax oil. So while flaxseeds are good for you, they are no substitute for fish oils.

In any case, it is important to get enough EPA and DHA, whether from a direct source like coldwater fish or fish oils, or an indirect source such as flaxseeds or flaxseed oil. Regular added amount s are particularly recommended for women who are pregnant or breastfeeding, as these vital brain-friendly omega-3s have been shown to be important in fetal and infant development. The World Health Organization now recommends that formula feeds include these oils, which can increase babies' blood levels of DHA and EPA.[23] DHA is especially important in pregnancy and infancy because the body literally uses it to build the brain—in fact, a quarter of the dry weight of the brain is DHA. Mothers with the highest intake of DHA have been found to give birth to children with the highest intelligence and speed of thinking.[24] In fact, the level of DHA at birth correlates with the speed of thinking at age eight![25] That's how strong the link is. A high DHA intake later in life has also been found to cut the risk of developing dementia by over 40 percent.[26]

The best diet from the point of view of omega-3 fats is a *fishitarian* diet, where you eat fish three times a week, or at least a seed-eating vegan diet. Eggs of chickens fed a high omega-3 diet (usually flaxseeds) can also provide significant quantities of omega-3, but nothing like as high as fish or fish oil supplements. And as we'll see later, not only is it important to get enough omega-3s; it's equally vital to eat less saturated and processed fat.

It's not all bad news for vegans. An ongoing research program at Hammersmith Hospital in London has identified that the babies of vegan breastfeeding mothers are brainier, probably because their breast milk, compared to infant formula or the breast milk of dairy-eating vegetarians or omnivores, provides more of the essential fatty acids needed for the development of neural membranes. According to Louise Thomas, a member of the Hammersmith team, the balance of saturated vs polyunsaturated fat in fat tissue could act as a marker for intelligence.[27] However, in my opinion, the best way to get omega-3s is to eat a diet that contains both fish and seeds.

The omega-6s

The other essential fat family is omega-6. Of all the tissues of the body, the brain has the highest proportion of omega-6 fats.

The grandmother of the omega-6 fat family is linoleic acid. Linoleic acid is converted by the body into gamma-linolenic acid (GLA). Evening primrose oil and borage oil (also known as borage oil) are the richest known sources of GLA.

Supplementing GLA, usually from evening primrose oil, has proven effective in a wide variety of mental health problems. Numerous studies have shown that schizophrenics have low levels of omega-6 fats.[28–31] A large-scale placebo-controlled trial using evening primrose oil showed significant improvement in this debilitating condition.[32] However, results became even more spectacular when vitamins B6, zinc, niacin, and vitamin C were added, all of which are needed by the body to turn essential fats, both omega-3 *and* 6, into prostaglandins.[33] This produced marked improvements in memory, the symptoms of schizophrenia and also tardive dyskinesia, a side effect of some medication for psychiatric disorders.

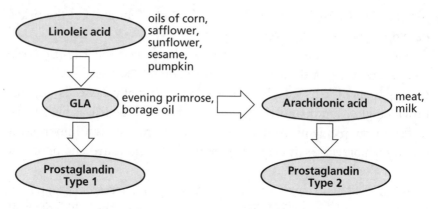

Fig 7. Omega-6 fats

Adding evening primrose oil to the diet of alcoholics going through withdrawal dramatically reduces symptoms, and in the long term improves memory.[34-38] Due to its reported effects on memory, evening primrose oil was given to Alzheimer's patients in a controlled trial and once again, highly significant improvements in memory and mental function were found.[39] Evening primrose oil has also been well proven to reduce pre-menstrual symptoms.

One omega-6 fat has something of a Jekyll and Hyde nature: arachidonic acid. While there is no question that it is essential for brain function, too much is bad news and associated with promoting inflammation. It can be derived either directly from meat or animal produce, or indirectly from linoleic acid or GLA. The latter may be preferable because, as well as producing arachidonic acid, they produce anti-inflammatory substances that balance its inflammatory effects.

In other words, let your body make its own arachidonic acid by eating seeds and their oils, rather than lots of meat and dairy produce.

Where to find omega-3 and omega-6 fats

As we've seen, the seeds with the highest levels of omega-3 fats are flaxseeds. Hemp and pumpkin seeds are rich sources too. Remember, though, that these have to be converted into EPA and DHA by the body and that fish, especially coldwater fish, are the best *direct* source of these brain boosters. This is why fish-eaters like the Japanese have three times the omega-3 fats in their body fat as the average American. Vegans, who eat more seeds and nuts, have twice the omega-3 fat level in their body fat as the average American. More on all this in a moment.

Some nuts and seeds are crossovers that contain both omegas. So along with sunflower, safflower, sesame, and corn, the best seeds for omega-6 fats are hemp and pumpkin.

Best foods for brain fats

Omega-3	Omega-6
Flax (linseed)	Safflower
Hemp	Sunflower
Pumpkin	Sesame
Walnut	Hemp
	Pumpkin
EPA & DHA	**GLA**
Salmon	Evening primrose
Mackerel	Borage oil
Herring	Blackcurrant seed
Sardines	
Anchovies	**Arachidonic Acid**
Tuna (fresh)	Meat
Marine algae	Dairy produce
Eggs	Eggs
	Squid

So what should you eat to get an optimal intake of these essential fats? There are three possibilities: eat seeds and fish; eat seed oils, which are more concentrated in essential fats but don't provide other nutrients such as minerals which are abundant in the whole seeds, and are less efficient at delivering omega-3s; or supplement concentrated fish oils along with seed oils such as evening primrose or starflower (borage) oil, high in GLA.

Getting the balance right

Before we look at how you can put your omega eating plan into action, a word about balance. There is significant evidence that the appropriate balance between omega-3 and omega-6 fats is 1 to 1, which reflects the diet of our ancestors before the Industrial Revolution. But the average balance these days is more like 1 to 20, or even as much as 1 to 30.

Although people these days tend to be deficient in both families of fats, they are relatively more deficient in omega-3s. It may be the imbalance between these two families of fats, in addition to overall deficiency, that affects brain function.

Seeds and fish

If you want to eat seeds to help boost your omegas, put one measure each of sesame, sunflower, and pumpkin seeds, and three measures of flaxseeds, in a sealed jar. Keep it in the fridge, away from light, heat, and oxygen. Simply adding one heaping tablespoon of these seeds, ground in a coffee grinder, to your breakfast each morning sets the scene for a good daily intake of essential fatty acids, particularly omega-6s. Along with this I'd recommend also eating 100g of oily fish twice a week (and please see the box below if you're a vegetarian or vegan).

A note to vegetarians

As explained earlier, relying solely on nuts and seeds to make complex brain fats such as DHA is close to useless. If you're a vegetarian this is vital to know. Vegetarians rarely have sufficient DHA levels, which can lead to health problems. India, for example, has one of the largest vegetarian populations and also has one of the highest rates of blindness, which is associated with deficiency in omega-3s, since both the eye and the brain are built out of DHA. Getting a direct source of EPA and DHA—whether from fish or algae—is incredibly important. There are now some specialist supplements that derived both DHA and EPA from marine algae. At this point in time the concentration of EPA or DHA is low and expensive but, as the technology develops, marine algae-derived EPA and DHA will become a viable source for strict vegans.

I'm not knocking seeds and nuts. They are a good source of fiber, minerals, and protein, and I eat them most days. However, I wouldn't recommend neglecting oily fish or fish oils. A direct source of DHA is essential, especially for pregnant or breastfeeding women. We are currently the third or fourth generation with inadequate DHA intakes, and experts now think this could have a lot to do with the increasing rates of neurological and mental health problems.

Seed oils

Keeping in mind what I've said about the body's difficulty in converting ALA into DHA and EPA, seed oil can be an option in helping boost your omegas. The best place to start is an oil blend that offers a 1:1 ratio of omega-3 and omega-6 fats. You want a blend that is cold-pressed, preferably organic, and kept refrigerated before you buy it. These are now widely available in health food stores. You need about a 2 teaspoons a day of such an oil and can add it to salads and other foods (without heating) or just take it neat. Hemp-seed oil is the next best thing. It provides 19 percent alpha-linolenic acid (omega-3), 57 percent linoleic acid and 2 percent GLA (both omega-6).

Essential fat supplements

As far as supplements are concerned, for omega-6 your best bet is starflower (borage) oil or evening primrose oil. Borage oil provides more GLA and you need at least 100 mg of GLA a day. Fish oils are best for omega-3 and you need at least 200 mg of EPA and 200 mg of DHA—or 400 mg of these two combined. So, either supplement one GLA capsule and one fish oil capsule rich in EPA and DHA, or find a supplement that combines EPA, DHA, and GLA and take one or two a day.

These levels of essential fats promote brain function and health. Quantities should be doubled if you scored high on the Essential Fats Check (see page 32), until your symptoms go away. (If you have a mental health problem that responds well to essential fats you may even need more, but this is explained in later chapters.)

Beware the fat anti-nutrients

A number of factors affect our ability to convert and use essential dietary fats. A diet high in fried food, meat, sugar, and alcohol, as well as stress, smoking, obesity, and a deficiency in antioxidant nutrients, is a recipe for neurological problems.

Perhaps the biggest culprit is trans fats, found in deep-fried foods and foods containing hydrogenated vegetable oil. Once eaten, trans fats are delivered directly to the brain and appear in the same position as DHA in nerve cell membranes. Twice as many trans fats appear in the brains of people deficient in omega-3 fats. So a combined deficiency in omega-3 fats and an excess of trans fats—the hallmark of the French fry genera-tion—is a bad scenario.

Another negative factor is alcohol. It not only blocks the conversion of fats into DHA, but dissolves fatty acids within the brain's membranes and replaces DHA with a poor substitute—docosapentaenoic acid (DPA). This may be one of the main reasons why alcohol consumption is associ-ated with mental impairment.

SUMMARY

In summary, here are some general guidelines to ensure you get enough brain fats:

- Eat seeds and nuts—the best seeds are flax, hemp, pumpkin, sunflower and sesame. You get more goodness out of them by grinding them first and sprinkling on cereal, soups, and salads.

- In addition, eat coldwater carnivorous fish—a serving of her-ring, mackerel, or organic or wild salmon two or three times a week provides a good source of omega-3 fats. Fresh tuna is another one to go for, but limit it to once a month because of mercury contamination.

- Use cold-pressed seed oils—choose either an oil blend or hemp oil for salad dressings, and drizzle on vegetables instead of butter.

- Minimize your intake of fried food, processed food, and satu-rated fat from meat and dairy.

- Supplement fish oil for omega-3 fats and borage or evening primrose oil for omega-6 fats.

In practical terms, you may want to pursue a combined strategy to ensure an optimal intake of brain fats. Here's what I recommend:

A tablespoon of ground seeds	– most days (five out of seven)
Cold-pressed seed oil blend	– on salad dressings and on vegetables
Coldwater carnivorous fish	– twice a week
EPA/DHA/GLA supplement	– once a day

CHAPTER 5

Phospholipids—your memory's best friends

Phospholipids are the intelligent fats in your brain. They are the insulation experts, helping make up a substance called myelin that sheathes all nerves and so promotes a smooth run for all the signals in the brain. Phospholipids also help make acetylcholine, the brain's memory neurotransmitter, as well as supplying nutrients that are involved in a key body process called methylation, which is how body and brain keeps thousands of critical biochemicals, including neurotransmitters, in balance (see Chapter 8). Not only do phospholipids enhance your mood, mind, and mental performance, they also protect against age-related memory decline and Alzheimer's disease.

There are three main kinds of phospholipids—phosphatidylcholine, phosphatidylserine, and phosphatidyl dimethylethanolamine, abbreviated to DMAE. Let's take a look at each in turn.

Superbrain builder—phosphatidylcholine

Supplementing phosphatidylcholine has some very positive benefits for your brain. Research on rats at Duke University Medical Center in the U.S. demonstrated that giving choline during pregnancy creates the equivalent of superbrains in the offspring.

The researchers fed pregnant rats choline halfway through their pregnancy. The infant rats whose mothers were given choline had vastly superior brains with more neuronal connections, and consequently, improved learning ability and better memory recall, all of which persisted into old age. This research showed that giving choline helps restructure the brain for improved performance in the long term.[40]

No such study has been carried out so far on pregnant women and their babies, so we can't automatically assume that the same applies in humans. But having said that, I'd certainly recommend that pregnant women have a spoonful of lecithin granules or a lecithin capsule (one of the best sources of phosphatidylcholine) a day.

According to Dr. Richard Wurtman of the Massachusetts Institute of Technology, if your choline levels are depleted, your body will grab the choline you need to build your nerve cells to make more acetylcholine.[41] So, Wurtman believes, providing the brain with enough of this smart nutrient is essential for preventing damage. This might also explain why the brains of poorly nourished women can shrink in size during pregnancy—because the fetus literally robs the mother's brain of essential fats and phospholipids to build its own. It's a case of "Mummy I shrank your brain," and could be the reason behind the forgetfulness some women report during pregnancy.

Phospholipids are something you need every day, and if you achieve the optimal intake your memory improves. In one study, 80 college students given a single 25g dose of phosphatidylcholine (3.75g of choline) found a significant improvement in explicit memory 90 minutes later. Slow learners responded particularly well.[42] Because the memory transmitter acetylcholine is made directly from choline, a deficiency in it is probably the single most common cause for declining memory.

The homocysteine connection

As well as being the critical building blocks for your neurons, and the raw material from which the brain makes acetylcholine, phosphatidylcholine is an important nutrient for keeping your level of the problematic amino acid homocysteine in check. A high blood level of homocysteine is an indicator for a number of degenerative diseases, including Alzheimer's.[43-44] Choline manages the job by converting into trimethylglycine (also called betaine), which then donates a methyl group to homocysteine, at which

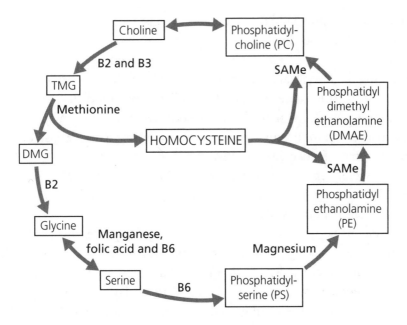

Fig 8. The phospholipid cycle

point homocysteine becomes the vital brain nutrient SAMe which, in turn, can help make more phosphatidylcholine and DMAE (see figure above). (More on methylation in Chapter 8.) The lower your homocysteine, the better you are at making phospholipids.

PS: don't forget the phosphatidylserine

The positive effects of supplementing phosphatidylserine (PS) are just as amazing as those from phosphatidylcholine. In one study, supplementing PS improved the subjects' memories to the level of people 12 years younger. Dr. Thomas Crook from the Memory Assessment Clinic in Bethesda, Maryland, in the U.S. gave 149 people with age-associated memory impairment a daily dose of 300 mg of PS or a placebo. When tested after 12 weeks, the ability of those taking PS to match names to faces (a recognized measure of memory and mental function) had vastly improved.[45]

The brain-boosting benefits of PS have been shown in more than 35 human studies spanning three decades, together with numerous animal studies. PS has proven highly beneficial, for instance, in animals with age-related memory decline.[46] Sixteen clinical trials indicate that PS can help counter measurable cognitive functions which tend to decline with age, including memory, learning, vocabulary skills, and concentration, as well as mood, alertness, and sociability. Studies have found that PS supplementation can also benefit those with only mild memory impairment,[47] and in addition to improving memory can alleviate depressive symptoms and seasonal affective disorder (SAD).[48–49]

The secret behind the memory-enhancing properties of PS is probably its ability to help brain cells communicate, as it is a vital element in the receptor sites of brain cells.

While the body can make its own PS, we need to get some directly from what we eat, making PS a semi-essential nutrient. The trouble is that modern diets are deficient in PS unless you happen to eat a lot of organ meats, in which case you may take in 50 mg a day. A vegetarian diet is unlikely to achieve even 10mg a day. So supplementing 100–300 mg of PS a day can make a real difference.

DMAE—a natural brain stimulant

DMAE, the final phospholipid in our trio, is abundant in sardines—indicating once again that eating fish really does feed the brain. It synthesizes phosphatidylcholine in the brain and accelerates the production of acetylcholine and, as it is much easier for DMAE to travel from bloodstream to brain than it is for phosphatydilcholine to make the trip, it has been the focus of a number of recent studies. Slight chemical variations of DMAE, marketed under various names, have proven highly effective in numerous double-blind trials in helping people with learning problems, attention deficit disorder, and memory and behavior problems. DMAE has been shown to reduce anxiety, stop the mind racing, improve concentration, and promote learning.

The ability of DMAE to tune up your brain was well demonstrated in a German study from 1996 that looked at a group of adults with cognitive problems.[50] The EEG brain waves of the participants were measured, and they were then given either placebos or DMAE. There were no changes in EEG for those on the placebos, but those taking DMAE showed improvements in brain wave patterns in those parts of the brain that play an important role in memory, attention, and flexibility of thinking. This research was recently followed by a study in which 80 volunteers watched emotional films.[51] Some were given DMAE and others, placebos. Both their brain-wave patterns and their subjective feelings were monitored. The researchers noted that the volunteers taking DMAE experienced more feelings of well-being despite suffering "borderline emotional disturbance."

People supplementing DMAE have reported a number of remarkable improvements in mind and mood, from a boost in concentration to differences in alertness and energy level and a need for less sleep. As shown in cases reported in *Smart Drugs II: The Next Generation* by Ward Dean, John Morgenthaler, and Steven Fowkes (Smart Publication), the effects can be dramatic:

> *"I've been taking DMAE for several weeks and I've noticed*
> *an amazing difference in mood and concentration level."*
> AFB, Austin, Texas

> *"I am currently taking 100 mg of DMAE per day and notice a real*
> *difference in my alertness, energy level, and decreased need for sleep."*
> RS, Seattle, Washington

> *"I've been using DMAE with pantothenic acid and a good*
> *multivitamin for two months now. One of the first things I noticed*
> *was that I fall asleep faster and wake up with a clearer mind.*
> *I experience a much sounder, more restful sleep. I constantly*
> *feel more attuned to my creative potential and I'm always*
> *in a good mood. I truly feel alive and awake."* PW [52]

But does DMAE deliver a result for those with worsening memory, perhaps with dementia? While animal studies have shown positive results,[53] to date there have been no impressive reversals in memory decline in people with Alzheimer's, although one study found improvement in mood, and a lessening in anxiety and irritability.[54] And if you take too much DMAE, above 1,500 mg a day, it may even have a worsening effect. One possible reason for this is that it can block the receptors for acetylcholine. I take 400 mg of DMAE a day and find it helps keep my mind and mood sharp and stable. Although the evidence in relation to Alzheimer's prevention is not there yet, there's good reason to add 100–500 mg to your daily supplement regime. There is certainly no evidence of any downside at these kinds of daily doses. DMAE is found in a number of brain-food formulas available in health food shops.

The lowdown on phospholipids

Although your body can make phospholipids, getting some extra from your diet is even better. The richest sources of phospholipids in the average diet are choline, abundant in egg yolks and organ meats, and DMAE, which as we've seen you can get from sardines as well as other fish. These sources also provide small amounts of phosphatidylserine. Nowadays we eat much less of these foods than we did a few decades ago, though. Since egg phobia set in, amid the unfounded fears that dietary cholesterol was the major cause of heart disease, our intake of phospholipids has gone down dramatically. At the same time, the number of people suffering from memory and concentration problems has gone up.

Now you can understand why lions and other animals at the top of the food chain eat the organs and brain first. And why the favorite meal of foxes—one of the most adaptive of all animals in Britain—is the heads of chickens. They're not stupid.

Why eggs are good for you

But we are, or at least are in danger of becoming so, unless we include phospholipids in our diet. One way to do this is to eat more eggs. But aren't they high in fat and cholesterol? As we learned in the last chapter, essential fats are good for you. The kind of fat in an egg depends on what you feed the chickens. If you feed them a diet rich in omega-3 fats, for example flaxseeds or fishmeal, you get eggs high in omega-3. An egg is as healthy as the chicken that laid it. As long as you don't fry them, eggs are a great brain food, and the richest dietary source of choline.

As for cholesterol, we forget that it is essential for good health. Your brain contains vast amounts of it and it is used to make the sex hormones estrogen, progesterone, and testosterone. It is simply a myth that eating eggs high in cholesterol gives you heart disease.

Here's one of many studies that prove it. Dr. Roslyn Alfin-Slater from the University of California gave 25 healthy people with normal blood-cholesterol levels two eggs per day (in addition to the other cholesterol-rich foods they were already eating as part of their normal diet) for eight weeks. A further 25 healthy people were given one extra egg per day for four weeks, then two extra eggs per day for the next four weeks. The results showed no change in blood cholesterol.[55] Other studies show the same thing. Eating eggs neither significantly raises blood cholesterol, nor is proven to increase the risk of heart disease.[56] A free-range, organic, omega-3 rich egg is a superfood.

Lecithin—a direct source of phospholipids

Lecithin is the best source of phospholipids, and widely available in health food shops, sold either as lecithin granules or capsules. 'Lecithin is practically a wonder drug as far as cognitive impairment is concerned,' says Dr. Dharma Singh Khalsa, author of *Brain Longevity* and an expert in nutrition and its role in enhancing memory. The ideal daily intake to keep your brain in top shape is 5g of lecithin, or half this if you take high PC (phosphatidylcholine) lecithin. The easiest and cheapest way to take this is to add a tablespoon of lecithin, or a heaping teaspoon of high-PC lecithin, to your cereal in the morning. Or you can take lecithin supplements. Most capsules provide 1200 mg, so you would need four a day. In case you were wondering, lecithin doesn't make you fat. In fact, quite the opposite: it helps the body digest fat.

While an optimal intake of phospholipids helps your brain sing by improving the insulation around nerves, choline and serine are also brain nutrients in their own right.

Other ways to increase your intelligent fats

We've seen how eggs are a great source of choline. Fish, especially sardines, followed by liver, soybeans, peanuts, and other nuts are also useful dietary sources. Or you might decide to supplement this valuable phospholipid. Aside from all the vital tasks it does, such as making acetylcholine,[57] choline also boasts a side benefit—it improves liver function.[58] An excellent way of getting your choline, as well as measuring your PS and DMAE, is to take a good brain-food formula that contains all of them.

SUMMARY

In summary, here are some general guidelines to help ensure you have an optimal intake of phospholipids, the memory molecules:

- Add a tablespoon of lecithin granules, or a heaping teaspoon of high-PC lecithin, to your cereal every day.

- Or eat an egg—preferably free-range, organic, and high in omega-3s.

- Supplement a brain-food formula providing phosphatidyl-choline, phosphatidylserine, and DMAE.

CHAPTER 6

Amino acids—the alphabet of mind and mood

Phospholipids improve the brain's hearing, so to speak, by keeping neurons' receptor sites in good condition. Amino acids, which are the building blocks of protein, improve the brain's talking. The words the brain uses to send messages from one cell to another are called neurotransmitters and the letters they use are built from are amino acids.

Deficiency in amino acids isn't at all uncommon and can give rise to depression, apathy, and lack of motivation, an inability to relax, and poor memory and concentration. Supplementing amino acids has been proven to correct all these problems. For example, a form of the amino acid tryptophan has proven more effective in double-blind trials than the best antidepressant drugs.[59] The amino acid tyrosine improves mental and physical performance under stress better than coffee.[60] The amino acid GABA is highly effective against anxiety.[61]

But to understand why amino acids are your brain's best friends, we need to explore what neurotransmitters actually do.

There are hundreds of different kinds of neurotransmitters in the brain and body, but here are the main players:

- **Adrenalin, noradrenalin, and dopamine** make you feel good, stimulating you, motivating you, and helping you deal with stress.

- **GABA** counteracts these stimulating neurotransmitters, relaxing you and calming you down after stress.

- **Serotonin** keeps you happy, improving your mood and banishing the blues.

- **Acetylcholine** keeps your brain sharp, improving memory and mental alertness.

- **Tryptamines** keep you connected. For example, melatonin keeps you in sync with day and night and the seasons.

There are many other substances in the brain that act much like neurotransmitters, such as endorphins, which give you a sense of euphoria. But these are the big five—the key players in the orchestra of your brain. Your mood, your memory, and your mental alertness are all affected by the activity of different kinds of neurotransmitters. If serotonin is up, for example, you are likely to be happy; if dopamine and adrenalin are down you are likely to feel unmotivated and tired. Having the right balance of these key neurotransmitters is a must if you want to be in tip-top mental health.

How neurotransmitters work

Neurotransmitters are released from one neuron and sent across the gap, the synapse, to deliver their message to the next neuron. Each neurotransmitter

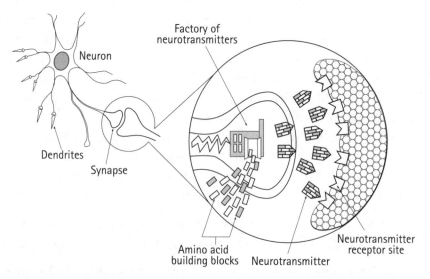

Fig 9. How neurotransmitters work

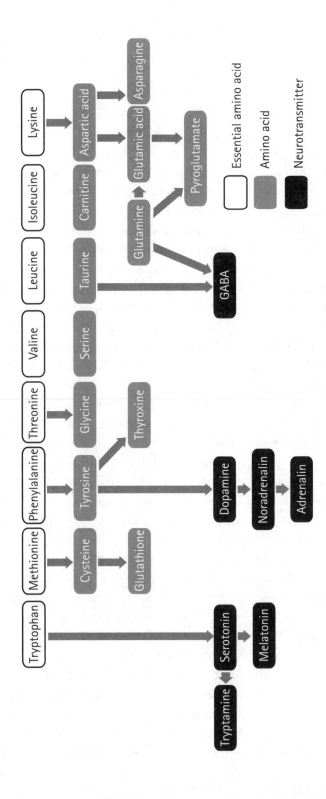

Fig 10. Family tree of key neurotransmitters

only fits into certain receptor sites—the letter boxes of the receiving cell. When the message is delivered, an electrical signal passes from one neuron to another.

Once a neurotransmitter has delivered its message, it is released from the receptor site and returns to the synapse. It can be reabsorbed or recycled by the neuron that released it, or it might be broken down and destroyed.

These neurotransmitters are made directly from amino acids taken into the body from food. There are eight essential amino acids (see Figure 10). From these eight we can make all the other amino acids our brain and body need, and from these we can make neurotransmitters. In Figure 10 you can see how the neurotransmitter *serotonin* is made from the amino acid *tryptophan*. Serotonin is known to help to improve your mood, so eating food rich in tryptophan, such as turkey, can improve your mood.

This was shown very clearly by an experiment carried out at Oxford University's psychiatry department. Eight women were given a diet devoid of tryptophan. Within eight hours, most of them started to feel more depressed. When tryptophan was added to their diet without their knowledge, their mood improved.[62]

Another example is tyrosine. Tyrosine has been well researched by the military and has been shown to improve mental and physical performance, especially under stressful circumstances. Studies by the U.S. military found that giving tyrosine to soldiers in stressful conditions of extreme cold, or intense physical activity over prolonged periods of time, shows clear improvements in both mental and physical endurance. Research from Holland demonstrates how tyrosine gives you the edge in conditions of stress. Twenty-one cadets were put through a demanding one-week military combat training course. Ten cadets were given a drink containing 2g of tyrosine a day, while the remaining 11 were given an identical drink without the tyrosine. Those on tyrosine consistently performed better, both in memorizing the task at hand and in tracking the tasks they had performed.[63]

Later on we'll see how supplementing specific amino acids such as these can help solve a wide variety of mental health problems. They work because amino acids have direct effects on neurotransmitters, as do many prescribed drugs. Amphetamines, for example, work by causing an excessive release of adrenalin. Antidepressants such as Prozac work by blocking serotonin reuptake, hence keeping more for longer in the synapse. But these drugs, as we'll see later in Chapter 22, have many undesirable side effects, and essentially work against your body's natural design, not with it.

Nutrients such as amino acids work just as well, if not better, but don't have the side effects except in massive doses, because making use of them is part of your brain and body's natural design. So, the best way to tune up your brain is to ensure you have an adequate intake of amino acids in your diet. This means eating protein.

Protein power

Protein is vital. Since almost all neurotransmitters are made from it, you can influence how you feel by giving yourself the ideal quantity and quality of protein every day. By taking this in an easily absorbed form it can be put to good use by your body and brain. The better the quality and usability of the protein you eat, the less you actually need to be optimally nourished.

The quality of a protein is determined by its balance of amino acids. Though there are 23 amino acids from which the body can build everything, from a neurotransmitter to a neuron, you actually need to eat only the eight so-called *essential* amino acids, because the body can make the rest from these. The better the balance of amino acids—expressed as a unit called an NPU, which stands for *net protein usability*—the more you can make use of the protein.

The chart on page 56 shows the top 24 individual foods and food combinations in terms of NPUs, or protein quality. Combining legumes with rice, for example, is a great way of increasing protein content. It also shows how much of a food, or food combination, you need to eat to get a 20g serving of protein. A man needs to eat the equivalent of three to four of these servings, while a woman needs to eat two to three, every day.

A typical day's allotment of protein for a man might therefore include an egg for breakfast (10g), a 200g (7oz) salmon steak for lunch (40g), and a serving of beans with dinner (20g).

For a vegetarian, a typical day's worth might be a small tub of yogurt and a heaping tablespoon of seeds on an oat-based cereal for breakfast (20g), and a 275g (10oz) serving of tofu (20g) and vegetable steam-fry, served with either a cup of quinoa (20g), or a serving of beans with rice (20g) as part of lunch or dinner. The trick for vegetarians is to eat seed foods—that is, foods that would grow if you planted them. These include seeds, nuts, beans, lentils, peas, corn, or the germ of grains such as wheat or oat. Flower foods such as broccoli or cauliflower are also relatively rich in protein.

Note that the cup measures indicated are imperial. The imperial cup is equal to approximately 1.2 U.S. customary cups.

Packed with protein: the top 24

Food	Percentage of calories as protein	How much for 20g (¾ oz)	Protein quality (NPU)
Grains/legumes			
Quinoa	16	100g (3.5oz)/1 cup dry weight	Excellent
Tofu	40	275g (10oz)/1 packet	Reasonable
Corn	4	500g (1lb 2oz)/3 cups cooked weight	Reasonable
Brown rice	5	400g (14oz)/3 cups cooked weight	Excellent
Chickpeas	22	115g (4oz)/0.66 cup cooked weight	Reasonable
Lentils	28	85g (3oz)/1 cup cooked weight	Reasonable
Fish/meat			
Tuna, canned	61	85g (3oz)/1 small can	Excellent
Cod	60	35g (1.25oz)/1 very small piece	Excellent
Salmon	50	100g (3.5oz)/1 small piece	Excellent
Sardines	49	100g (3.5oz)//1 baked	Excellent
Chicken	63	75g (2.5oz)/1 small roasted breast	Excellent
Nuts/seeds			
Sunflower seeds	15	185g (6.5oz)/1 cup	Reasonable
Pumpkin seeds	21	75g (2.5oz)/0.5 cup	Reasonable
Cashew nuts	12	115g (4oz)/1 cup	Reasonable
Almonds	13	115g (4oz)/1 cup	Reasonable
Eggs/dairy			
Eggs	34	115g (4oz)/2 medium	Excellent
Yogurt, natural	22	450g (1lb)/3 small pots	Excellent
Cottage cheese	49	125g (4.5oz)/1 small pot	Excellent
Vegetables			
Peas, frozen	26	250g (9oz)/2 cups	Reasonable

Other beans	20	200g (7oz)/2 cups	Reasonable
Broccoli	50	40g (1.5oz)/0.5 cup	Reasonable
Spinach	49	40g (1.5oz)/0.66 cup	Reasonable

Combinations

| Lentils and rice | 18 | 125g (4.5oz)/small cup dry weight | Excellent |
| Beans and rice | 15 | 125g (4.5oz)/small cup dry weight | Excellent |

Supplementing amino acids

While eating protein is the best way to start to get these essential amino acids, supplementing amino acids is the best way to guarantee you are receiving optimal amounts. This is especially relevant to some people who seem to be prone to neurotransmitter deficiencies and more dependent on certain amino acids than others. Some people who are prone to depression, for example, find that supplementing 5-hydroxy-tryptophan (5-HTP) keeps depression at bay. Tryptophan is similarly helpful, but is banned in a number of countries and so is harder to get hold of (see Chapter 15, page 150).

One of the advantages of supplementing individual amino acids is that they are more easily absorbed this way. The reason for this is that amino acids compete for absorption, so if you supplement one without eating protein-rich food at the same time, you absorb more into the bloodstream. Supplementing with fruit may be even better because the presence of carbohydrates is known to help the absorption of this amino acid.

Supplementing individual amino acids, away from food or with fruit, is best done as and when you need it. As we investigate nutritional solutions to a variety of mental health problems, I'll be recommending certain individual amino acids to help bring you back into balance.

Another option to ensure a good balance of amino acids is to supplement a powder containing the right balance of free-form amino acids. These free-form amino acids don't require digestion in the same way that protein does, so they are easily absorbed. They do, however, compete with each other, so they are not as effective as supplementing an individual amino acid.

A decent protein powder should provide the following key brain-boosting amino acids, and more, in these kinds of amounts in a daily serving:

Glutamine/glutamic acid	2,000 mg
Tyrosine	1,000 mg
GABA/taurine	1,500 mg
Tryptophan	500 mg*
Phenylalanine	1,000 mg

*Please note: the amount of tryptophan in supplements is restricted in some countries; in the U.K. it is restricted to 220 mg per serving.

Note that if you are supplementing free-form amino acids, you should be careful not to overdo it if you also choose to supplement individual amino acids. Don't exceed my recommendations for each individual amino acid. You'll find these in Part 3.

The protein powder could be added to your breakfast cereal or to a nutritious fruit shake. You can have too much protein, however, so more doesn't always mean better. Once-daily protein intake goes above 85g a day (depending on your exercise level and hence requirement) this can have negative health consequences. Breakdown products of protein, such as ammonia, are toxic to the body and stress the kidneys in their elimination. Too many amino acids mean too much acid in the blood. The body neutralises this by releasing calcium from bone. It is now well established that very high protein diets contribute to osteoporosis risk. So, make sure you get enough, not too much.

Glutamine—an amazing amino acid

Although glutamine is not one of the eight essential amino acids, it is the most abundant in the human body. There's tons of it in breast milk—five times more than any other amino acid—and hefty amounts in food. For example, there's 175 mg in a big tomato, compared to less than 10 mg for most other amino acids. Why? What does our body do with all this glutamine? It is used widely throughout the body, for example to power and heal the gut; to make glutathione, the body's most powerful antioxidant; and to boost the immune system. But most important, it is fantastically brain friendly, particularly in certain forms.

Glutamine has a few relatives, and another form of it is glutamate. In many cases, glutamate can be used instead of glutamine—but not in all, as immune cells, for instance, prefer glutamine. Beyond this, there are cousins of glutamate that work in all sorts of different ways. To illustrate how different these can be, one is the taste stimulant monosodium glutamate (MSG), which I recommend you steer clear of (see Chapter 11), while another is the powerful relaxing neurotransmitter GABA (gamma amino butyric acid). GABA is made from either glutamate or glutamine, and it turns off excess adrenalin, releasing you from anxiety and stress states. Consequently, getting enough glutamine helps chill you out.

There's another cousin of glutamine that I particularly like. It's called pyroglutamate, and is highly concentrated in the brain and spinal fluid. So powerful are its effects that there are now many slight variations of this key brain chemical being marketed as nootropic drugs for learning and memory-related problems such as Alzheimer's. Numerous studies using these drugs, one of which is piracetam, have proven that they enhance memory and mental function not only in people with pronounced memory decline, but also in those with so-called normal memory function.[64]

Pyroglutamate does three things that help improve your memory and mental alertness:

- It increases acetylcholine production.

- It boosts the number of receptors for acetylcholine.

- It improves communication between the left and right hemispheres of the brain.

In other words, it improves the brain's talking, listening, and cooperation. It is probably for these reasons that it improves learning, memory, concentration, and the speed of reflexes. It can really give you that extra mental edge.

As it's an amino acid, pyroglutamate is found in many foods, including fish, dairy products, fruit, and vegetables. Arginine pyroglutamate is the most common form found in strictly nutritional supplements, while pyroglutamate is often found in brain formulas. I take 100 mg a day as part of my daily brain-support program. If you want to take it on its own to boost memory, the optimal amount is 400 mg to 1,000 mg a day. Alternatively, if your supplement regime includes glutamine, your body may already be making its own.

SUMMARY

In summary, here are some general guidelines to help ensure you have an optimal intake of amino acids—the alphabet of mind and mood:

- Have three servings of the protein-rich foods shown above a day, if you are a man, and two if you are a woman.

- Choose good vegetable protein sources, including beans, lentils, quinoa, tofu, and seed vegetables such as peas or corn.

- If eating animal protein, choose lean meat or preferably fish, organic whenever possible.

- Consider supplementing some free-form amino acids, or individual amino acids if you have a related mental health problem. For example, increase tryptophan to boost your mood (see Chapter 15), and glutamine or pyroglutamate to give your memory a boost.

CHAPTER 7

Intelligent nutrients—
the brain's master tuners

In every great production, there are hundreds of people behind the scenes that support the main players. The same is true with your brain. These are the vitamins and minerals. One of their main roles is to help turn glucose into energy, amino acids into neurotransmitters, simple essential fats into more complex fats, like GLA or DHA and prostaglandins, and choline and serine into phospholipids. They help build and rebuild the brain and nervous system and keep everything running smoothly. They are your brain's best friends.

Knowing this, we decided to test what would happen to the intelligence of schoolchildren if given an optimal intake of vitamins and minerals. Gwillym Roberts, a schoolteacher and nutritionist from the Institute for Optimum Nutrition, and Professor David Benton, a psychologist from Swansea University, put 60 schoolchildren onto a special multivitamin and mineral supplement designed to ensure an optimal intake of key nutrients.[65] Without their knowledge, half these children were placed on a placebo.

After eight months on the supplements, the non-verbal IQs in those taking the supplements had risen by over 10 points! No changes were seen in those on the placebos. This study, published in *The Lancet* in 1988, has since been proven many times in other studies. Most have used RDA levels of nutrients, much lower than our original study, but still show increases in IQ averaging 4.5 points. But why do vitamins and minerals raise IQ?

The answer is that children, and adults, think faster and can concentrate for longer with an optimal intake of vitamins and minerals. (See Chapter 13 for more on this.)

The ultimate head start

The sooner you start optimally nourishing your brain, the better. Of course, that puts the responsibility on the mother while pregnant and breastfeeding. A 16-year study by the Medical Research Council shows just how critical optimum nutrition is in the early years. They fed 424 premature babies either a standard or an enriched milk formula containing extra protein, vitamins, and minerals. At 18 months, those fed standard milk "were doing significantly less well" then the others, and at eight years old had IQs up to 14 points lower![66]

Every one of the 50 known essential nutrients, with the exception of vitamin D, plays a major role in promoting mental health. Here are some of the key brain nutrients, the symptoms that occur in deficiency, and the best foods to eat, to help you get enough.

The B vitamins

The B-complex group of vitamins is vital for mental health. Deficiency of any one of the eight B vitamins will rapidly affect how you think and feel. This is because they are water soluble and rapidly pass out of the body. So we need a regular intake throughout the day. Also, since the brain uses a very large amount of these nutrients, a short-term deficiency will affect mental abilities.

While the deficiency symptoms of B vitamins are well known, we still do not know exactly why many of the symptoms occur. Each B vitamin has so many functions in the brain and nervous system that there are many logical explanations, but few hard proofs. Many people choose to safeguard against deficiency by taking a B-complex supplement or a multivitamin every day.

Vitamin B1 (thiamine)

Vitamin B1 helps turn glucose, the fuel for the brain, into energy. So, one of the first symptoms of deficiency is mental and physical fatigue. People low in this vitamin have poor attention spans and concentration. David Benton, one of the leading experts in nutrition and IQ, has found that low levels of thiamine correlate with poor cognitive function in young adults, and that thiamine supplementation was associated with reports of feeling more clear-headed, composed and energetic, and having faster reaction times, even in those whose thiamine status, according to the traditional criterion, was adequate.[67–68]

Vitamin B3 (niacin)

Of all the nutrients connected with mental health, niacin, or vitamin B3, is the most famous. Niacin was first discovered because deficiency was identified as the cause for pellagra, a disease in which people developed mental illness, diarrhea, and eczema. Due to the pioneering work of Abram Hoffer and Humphrey Osmond, niacin has been extensively researched as a treatment for schizophrenia and found to be highly effective in acute schizophrenia in doses of several grams (see Chapter 26). The RDA is only 18 mg! Getting enough niacin does more than stop you from developing a psychosis. In one study, 141 mg of niacin every day improved memory by more than 10 percent in both young and old people.[69] Having a high dietary intake of niacin has also been shown to cut your risk of developing dementia and age-related cognitive decline by more than half.[70]

Vitamin B5 (pantothenic acid)

Pantothenic acid, also called vitamin B5, is another potent memory booster. It is needed to make both stress hormones and the memory-boosting neurotransmitter, acetylcholine. Supplementing extra B5, particularly with choline, can sharpen your memory (see Chapter 14).

Vitamins B6, B12, and folic acid

These three, together with niacin, control a critical process in the body called methylation. This is vital in the formation of almost all the neurotransmitters. Methylation abnormalities lie behind many mental health problems, as we'll find out later in this book. A lack of B6, for example, means you won't make serotonin so efficiently, which could potentially lead to depression. B6 can help relieve stress too, while stress depletes B6.

In one study, the level of psychological distress in HIV-infected people decreased as their B6 status improved through supplementation.[71] So, if you're B6 deficient and stressed, you may be heading for depression.

In both children and adults with autism, giving large doses of vitamin B6, along with magnesium, has resulted in remarkable improvements. We've known since the 1970s that a nutritional approach can help autism, thanks to the pioneering research by the late Dr. Bernard Rimland of the Institute for Child Behavior Research in San Diego, California. He showed that vitamins B6 and C and magnesium supplements significantly improved symptoms in autistic children. In one of his early studies back in 1978, 12 out of 16 autistic children improved, then regressed when the vitamins were swapped for placebos.[72] In the decades following Dr. Rimland's study, many other researchers have also reported positive results with this approach.[73]

People with conditions including Down's syndrome, autism, ADHD, and depression have been found to have low levels of B6 and zinc—a condition in its turn associated with a proportionate increase in a substance called hydroxyhemopyrrolin-2-one (HPL). Commonly known as the mauve factor, HPL is found in the urine of patients suffering from these conditions. So supplementing B6 and zinc has been shown to return mauve levels to normal, improving clinical outcome.[74] (More on this in Chapter 26.)

Many of us are also deficient in folic acid, also known as folate. In a study at the King's College Hospital psychiatry department in London, a third of 123 patients were found to have low levels of folic acid. They were given either folic acid or placebos for six months. There was a significant improvement only in the group of people taking folic acid, which included patients with depression and schizophrenia.[48] Many other researchers have found low folate levels associated with depression[76] and manic depression.[77] Giving folic acid supplements alongside anti-depressant drugs has also been shown to enhance their anti-depressant effect, especially in women.[78]

Folic acid has been found to help people with memory problems. A study by Dr. Jane Durga from Wageningen University in the Netherlands gave a group of 818 people aged from 50 to 75 either a vitamin containing 800 micrograms of folic acid a day, or a dummy pill, for three years. On memory tests, the supplement users had scores comparable to people 5.5 years younger.[79]

It has been known for some time that folic acid deficiency is very common in patients with mental health conditions. As long ago as 1967 a consultant psychiatrist, Dr. M. Carney from Lancaster Moor Hospital, recommended that anyone with a mental health problem be checked for folic acid and B12 deficiency because they are so often found lacking.[80] Vitamin B12 is vital for a healthy nervous system as without it, neither the senses nor the brain can work properly. Deficiency has been shown to be present in as many as half of patients with dementia, with an equivalent number showing an inability to absorb it.[81–82] However, it isn't just older people who need it. Low B12 levels cause poor mental performance in adolescents too.[83]

Getting enough B6, B12, and folic acid is absolutely vital in pregnancy, both for protecting against developmental problems such as spina bifida and for general intellectual development. Children born to mothers deficient in folic acid show delayed intellectual development.[84]

These nutrients have so many critical roles to play in the brain and nervous system that ensuring you are getting optimal levels of them is a prerequisite for mental health.

Best of the rest

We've seen how vital the Bs are in keeping the brain fit. Let's take a look at the rest of the best brain-boosting nutrients.

Vitamin C

Vitamin C does much more than stop you from getting a cold. It has many roles to play in the brain too, including helping to balance neurotransmitters. While not as spectacular in effect as niacin, vitamin C has been shown to reduce the symptoms of both depression and schizophrenia.[85] A number of studies have shown that people diagnosed with mental illness may have much greater requirements for this vitamin, and are frequently deficient.[86] In one study, patients only started to excrete the same amount of vitamin C as the control group when given 1g a day—more than 10 times the RDA. Dr. Vandercamp, from the Veterans Administration Hospital in Michigan, found that schizophrenic patients could metabolise 10 times more vitamin C than people without the condition.[87] The implications of this are that people with schizophrenia need 10 times more vitamin C to obtain the same blood levels and benefits.

These studies show how unique we all are. Even a so-called well-balanced diet isn't enough for many people. That's why it's well worth supplementing your diet to enhance your mind and body.

Calcium and magnesium—nature's tranquilizers

Popping a mineral may be the last thing you'd think of doing when you're feeling anxious, edgy, and unable to relax. Calcium and magnesium can do the trick, though, by helping to relax nerve and muscle cells.

Muscle cramps are an obvious sign of magnesium deficiency. A lack of either calcium or magnesium can also make you more nervous, irritable, and aggressive. Magnesium has been used successfully to treat autistic and hyperactive children, together with other nutrients. Most of all, it helps you to sleep.

Magnesium has many roles to play in the nervous system, and researchers are starting to look more closely at the possibility that magnesium deficiency may be a cause of mental illness, including major depression and addiction. An American study of patients with severe depression found that they recovered rapidly (in less than seven days) taking 125 to 300 mg of magnesium with each meal and at bedtime. Related conditions in the participants, including headache, suicidal thoughts, anxiety, irritability, insomnia, abuse of drugs such as cocaine and alcohol, short-term memory loss and IQ loss, also improved.[88]

Ironically, when patients are put on psychotropic drugs, both calcium and magnesium levels tend to decline, which just makes matters worse.[89] Supplementing them helps to reduce the unpleasant side effects of these drugs.

Magnesium is perhaps the second most commonly deficient mineral after zinc (see page 67). Green, leafy vegetables are rich in it because it is part of the chlorophyll molecule, which makes plants green. So are nuts and seeds, particularly sesame, sunflower, and pumpkin seeds. An ideal intake is probably 500 mg a day, which is almost double what most people achieve. A tablespoon of seeds a day, plus 200 mg in a multimineral, is a good way to ensure you're getting enough.

Manganese—the forgotten mineral

With manganese, balance is all. Both too much and too little of this mineral affect the way our brain functions. Excess, found occasionally in miners inhaling dust from manganese ore, results in psychosis and nervous disorders similar to Parkinson's disease. However, this is rare because manganese is both hard to absorb and readily excreted.

Too little manganese may be a factor in schizophrenia and other psychotic problems. Even as early as 1917, manganese chloride was found to be effective for the treatment of schizophrenia. At Princeton's Brain Bio Center, Dr. Carl Pfeiffer revived the interest in these trace metals, and found that almost all patients could benefit from extra manganese and zinc.[90–91] He found that high levels of copper displace manganese and help to produce the continuous and excessive overstimulation that characterizes so many psychotic states. He also found that slight manganese deficiency is associated with insomnia, restlessness, non-productive activity, and elevated blood pressure. Clearly, one doesn't have to be psychotic to experience these common signs of deficiency. Manganese deficiency can also cause fits and convulsions (see Chapter 34).

As with many trace minerals, the difference between the amount required to prevent deficiency (defined for animals as the level at which growth and reproduction are affected) and the amount needed for optimum health vary considerably. There is no RDA for this essential mineral, although most recommend a daily intake of 2.5–5 mg. Some people need 10 times this amount![92]

Manganese is found mainly in seeds, nuts, and grains, and tropical fruit, such as bananas and pineapples. Tea is very rich in it. Because it's extremely poorly absorbed and easily excreted from the body, however, it's well worth supplementing 5 mg day, and up to 20 mg if you have a mental health problem.

Think zinc

Zinc is the most commonly deficient mineral, and the most critical nutrient for mental health. The average intake in Britain is 7.5 mg, which is half the RDA of 15 mg. This means that half the British population gets less than half the level of zinc thought to protect against deficiency. Zinc deficiency is associated with schizophrenia, depression, anxiety, anorexia, delinquency, hyperactivity, autism—in short, it's implicated in a huge range of mental health problems. Getting enough (and few of us do) is associated with improved memory. Researchers in North Dakota gave 200 seventh-grade schoolchildren zinc supplements and found that the children taking 20 mg of zinc a day, compared to those taking 10 mg (the

RDA) or a placebo, had faster and more accurate memories and better attention spans within three months.[93]

There are also many circumstances that increase one's need for zinc, quite apart from not getting enough from diet. These include stress, infections, PMS and other hormone imbalances, using the contraceptive pill, excess copper, frequent alcohol consumption, blood-sugar problems, and an inherited extra need for zinc. In the body, it is concentrated in sperm, and rapidly lost with excessive ejaculation. Zinc is found in any seed food such as nuts and seeds and the germ of grains. Meat and fish are rich sources, but none is richer than oysters: a single oyster can provide as much as 15 mg of zinc! And this is why they're recommended as an aphrodisiac—at least for men.

Major nutrients, best foods and symptoms of deficiency

Nutrient	Effects of deficiency	Food sources
Vitamin B1	Poor concentration and attention	Wholegrains, vegetables
Vitamin B3	Depression, psychosis	Wholegrains, vegetables
Vitamin B5	Poor memory, stress	Wholegrains, vegetables
Vitamin B6	Irritability, poor memory, depression, stress	Wholegrains, bananas
Folic acid	Anxiety, depression, psychosis	Green leafy vegetables
Vitamin B12	Confusion, poor memory, psychosis	Meat, fish, dairy products, eggs
Vitamin C	Depression, psychosis	Vegetables and fresh fruit
Magnesium	Irritability, insomnia, depression	Green vegetables, nuts, seeds
Manganese	Dizziness, convulsions	Nuts, seeds, tropical fruit, tea
Zinc	Confusion, blank mind, depression, loss of appetite, lack of motivation and concentration.	Oysters, nuts, seeds, fish

SUMMARY

In summary, here are some general guidelines to help ensure you have an optimal intake of vitamins and minerals to keep your brain in tune:

- Eat at least five, and ideally seven, servings of fresh fruit and vegetables a day.

- Eat nuts and seeds regularly, and choose whole foods, such as wholegrains, lentils, beans, and brown rice, rather than refined foods.

- Supplement a multivitamin and mineral that gives you at least 25 mg of all the B vitamins, 10 mcg of B12, 100 mcg of folic acid, 200 mg of magnesium, 3 mg of manganese, and 10 mg of zinc.

CHAPTER 8

Your methyl IQ—
the ultimate balancing act

One of the most important processes in the brain and body is called methylation. In essence, this is how your body keeps thousands of neurotransmitters, hormones, and other essential biochemicals in balance. This is quite a feat: there are something like a billion methylation reactions every second! So your methylation ability is a critical factor in determining your mental health, concentration, mood, and ability to deal with stress.

For example, if the fire alarm goes off at work, you'll be pumping adrenalin in 0.2 seconds—ready to act literally in a split second. But none of this would happen without methylation, as it's this process that actually manufactures the adrenalin.

To get a bit technical, the manufacturing process hinges on a small unit of organic compounds made up of three hydrogen atoms bonded to a carbon atom, which is known as a methyl group. The adrenalin is made when one of these methyl groups is added to noradrenalin, a chemical that's present in your brain and body. Methylation also helps to make the brain-friendly fats called phospholipids (see Chapter 5) and even controls gene expression, which is how the information in a gene acts to change the function of a cell. If a pregnant woman's methylation is not up to par, for example, this heightens the risk of Down's syndrome in her baby.

Methylation is linked to a number of mental states and conditions. Faulty methylation is now known to predict depression, memory loss, losing touch with reality, and even exam results. So taking the measure of your methyl IQ is important. Luckily, it's easily done by measuring the level of homocysteine, a toxic amino acid, in the blood.

The H factor

Basically, the higher your homocysteine level, the higher your risk for these and other imbalances. For example, a study of 692 Swedish schoolchildren found that their homocysteine level predicted their school grades.[94] A study of women who were tested for homocysteine levels in the blood found that a high level doubled the likelihood of depression in the participants.[95] Homocysteine is also much more likely to be high in people with Alzheimer's,[96] and even with schizophrenia.[97]

Ideally, your homocysteine level should be no higher than 7. It's easily measured by your doctor, or you can do it yourself using a home-test kit that you send off to a lab (see page 480 in Resources for details). Your homocysteine level does tend to go up with age and the absolute best level to have, if you are over 40, is not much more than your age divided by 10. So if you are 70, a homocysteine level of not more than 8 is good. If you're 40, the ideal would be below 5.

Of course, all this raises two key questions: why do some people have faulty methylation and raised homocysteine levels, and how do you lower your homocysteine level and improve your mental health? The answer to the first question lies in the combination of genes, diet and lifestyle. In fact, the discovery that inherited variations of genes predispose certain people to mental health problems is not only one of the hottest areas of research at the moment, but also holds out the very clear possibility that optimum nutrition will provide a vital breakthrough in conditions such as schizophrenia.

The reason for this is very simple. Depending on their genetic makeup, in some people certain enzymes, which are dependent on particular nutrients, don't work so well. Since you can't change the genes, the solution is to increase the specific methylating nutrients. The study of genetics is showing that we are all unique and that uniqueness means that we all have our own personal optimum nutrition.

How to improve your methyl IQ

So, the answer to the second question is that you can improve methylation, lower your homocysteine, and maximize your mental health by putting together the right combination of specific nutrients. These are:

- Vitamin B2
- Vitamin B6
- Vitamin B12
- Folic acid
- Trimethylglycine (TMG)
- Zinc.

To understand why these nutrients are so important, we need to delve into the world of homocysteine (which is also explained in more detail in Chapter 26 and is viewable as a cartoon at www.patrickholford.com/methylation).

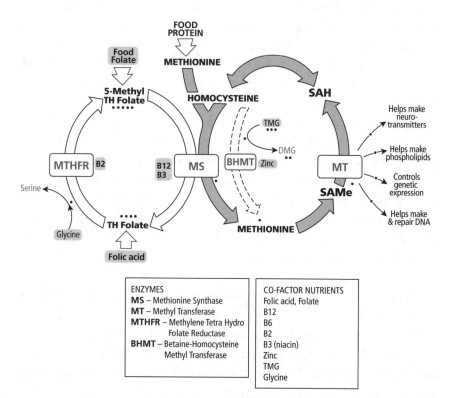

Fig 11. Nutrients needed in the methylation cycle

As an amino acid, homocysteine is actually made from dietary protein. As Figure 11 shows, if you have enough of it, along with vitamin B2, folic acid, B12, and B6—or alternatively, TMG (also called betaine) plus zinc—you can make S-adenosyl methionine (SAMe). SAMe is the clever molecule that does all the methylating by donating a methyl group (CH^3). These are shown in the diagram as tiny dots. So, the purpose of this methylation process is to pass the parcel of methyl groups to SAMe to do its work. And remember, it's this donation of methyl groups that keeps everything in balance.

So, because they help to creat SAMe, we can see why nutrients such as folic acid have proven effective in improving mental health. So far, the medical profession has cottoned on to the importance of folic acid, B6,p and B12 in this context, and there are a number of studies going on giving these nutrients in combination.

Why you need methylating nutrients

The end goal of the chemical dance that is methylation is basically to liberate methyl groups and thereby give your brain the flexibility to adapt to changing circumstances. Methyl nutrients such as TMG (trimethylglycine), which provides three methyl groups, are a classic example of the nutrients that can get us there, but there are others. The vital phospholipid phosphatidylcholine also provides three methyl groups, which may be another reason why this nutrient is considered crucial. Another way to get a methyl group is to supplement methyl-B12 or methylfolate. These are a bit more expensive than regular B12 or folic acid as supplements but worth the difference.

Of course, the best place to start is to eat more of the foods rich in these nutrients. See the chart below.

Methylation-friendly nutrients	Found in
B2	Eggs, almonds, wholegrains, soybeans, spinach, mushrooms, milk, poultry, organ meats
B6	Wholegrains, bananas
B12	Meat, fish, dairy products, eggs
Folic acid	Green leafy vegetables
Zinc	Oysters, nuts, seeds, fish
TMG	Wholegrains, spinach, beets

As far as supplements are concerned, the ideal intake does depend on your homocysteine level. This is what I recommend if your homocysteine level is under 6.

Nutrient	No risk	Low risk	High risk	Very high risk
	Below 6	6–9	9–15	Above 15
Folic acid	200 µg	400 µg	800 µg	1,000 µg
Methyl-B12	10 µg	250 µg	500 µg	1,000 µg
B6	25 mg	50 mg	75 mg	100 mg
B2	10 mg	15 mg	20 mg	50 mg
Zinc	5 mg	10 mg	15 mg	20 mg
TMG	500 mg	750 mg	1–1.5g	3–6g

But do bear in mind that this combination of nutrients is so effective at lowering your homocysteine level that you don't need to take this much of them for very long. So I advise you to retest for your homocysteine level after eight weeks, then adjust the levels you supplement accordingly.

The methyl-friendly lifestyle

It's not just about diet and supplements. There are many lifestyle factors that affect methylation, including smoking, drinking coffee, and stress, which all raise homocysteine, while alcohol in strict moderation can lower it (although large amounts are bad news), and exercise tends to improve levels.[98]

Later on in this book we'll explore further the link between homocysteine, faulty methylation, and specific mental health problems, and the evidence that large amounts of specific homocysteine-lowering nutrients can reverse these problems and maximize your mental health.

SUMMARY

In summary, here are some guidelines that apply to us all:

- Check your homocysteine level.

- If it's high (above 7), supplement specific amounts of B2, B6, B12, folic acid, zinc, and TMG. In any event take a multivitamin every day that provides at least 200 mcg folate, 10 mcg B12, 25 mg B6, 10 mg B2, and 5 mg zinc.

- Eat plenty of greens, beans, nuts, seeds, and fish/meat/eggs or dairy products for the B12 content.

- Don't smoke.

- Minimize your intake of alcohol, coffee, and caffeinated drinks.

- Minimize stress.

- Keep fit.

PART 2

Protecting Your Brain

Optimum brain nutrition isn't just about getting the right nutrients. It's also about minimizing the anti-nutrients. These include oxidants, alcohol, sugar, stimulants and stress, toxic minerals, and allergy-provoking foods: the Seven Brain Drainers.

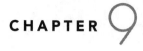

The brain agers—oxidants, alcohol, and stress

Maximizing your mental powers isn't just about what you eat. It's also about what you don't eat (and what you do drink and smoke). Your brain and nervous system are made out of essential fats, protein, and phospholipids, all of which can be damaged by oxidants—the body's own nuclear waste—as well as by alcohol and too much stress.

Oxidants: up in smoke

First we'll look at one of today's burning issues: oxidants. They're a real hazard in our fume-filled, polluted, fast-food century.

Don't fry your brain

As we saw earlier, the dry matter of the brain is 60 percent fat, and the kind of fat you eat alters the kind of fat in your brain. The worst fats you can eat are called trans fats, which these days are much in the news: some British supermarkets are even working to banish them from their own brand products. These damaged fats are found in deep-fried food and foods containing hydrogenated vegetable oils. So, if you want to minimize your exposure to trans fats, limit your intake of fried and especially deep-fried food, and don't buy foods containing hydrogenated fats. Check the list of ingredients in processed foods: if a food has the 'H' word in the ingredients, don't put it in your cart!

Why are trans fats so bad for you? After you eat them, they can be taken directly into the brain and appear in the same position as DHA in brain cells, where they mess up thinking processes. They also block the conversion of essential fats into vital brain fats such as GLA, DHA, and prostaglandins. Twice as many trans fats appear in the brains of people deficient in omega-3 fats. So a combined deficiency in omega-3 fats and an excess of trans fats is a bad scenario.

According to recent estimates, the total fat intake of an American man may be 150–250g a day (70–100g is the recommended amount), up to a quarter of which comes from trans fats. A serving of French fries or fried fish can each deliver 8g, a doughnut 12g and a bag of chips more than 4g. All these spell trouble.

As the brain is more than half fat, there is a real danger of these becoming oxidized, or going rancid. Fried food, smoking, and pollution are three main factors that introduce oxidants into the body, which cause a chain reaction of damage to the essential fats attached to phospholipids (see Figure 12) in nerve-cell membranes. As you can see in this figure, vitamin E helps protect your brain from these damaging effects.

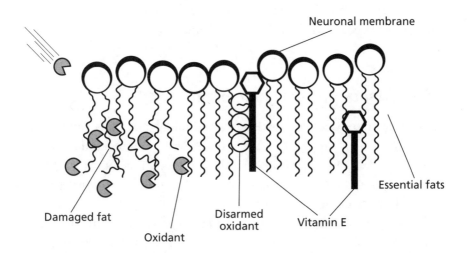

Fig 12. How oxidants damage your brain

Smoking like crazy

A single puff of a cigarette contains a trillion oxidants, which rapidly travel into your brain. It also carries high levels of the heavy metal cadmium, the gradual accumulation of which depletes zinc. And as discussed in Chapter 7, zinc has several crucial roles to play in brain development and maintenance, not least of which are the prevention of oxidation and the synthesis of serotonin and melatonin.[1] Low levels of zinc are implicated in schizophrenia, and the frequency of smoking among people with this condition has been observed to be significantly greater than in the general population.[2]

Researchers at Duke University in the U.S. have shown how nicotine withdrawal can interfere with serotonin activity and development of the brain, leading to depression in the children of women who smoke during pregnancy or in adolescent smokers.[3] Meanwhile, a study by Dr. Aiden Corvin of St. James's Hospital in Dublin found that smoking doubled the incidence of psychotic symptoms among patients with manic depression.[4]

One more thing. Smoking is a known risk factor leading to strokes—the third most common cause of death—where the brain is starved of blood because of damage to the arteries supplying it.[5]

Less avoidable are the oxidants from exhaust fumes, particularly diesel. These have an insidious effect on your body and brain. They also explain why the incidence of lung cancer among non-smokers is going up in cities.

It's no surprise to find that the risk for Alzheimer's is much higher in smokers and people who eat lots of fried and processed fats. More on this in Chapter 37.

Antioxidants protect your brain

There may not be a lot you can do to avoid many pollutants, but you can protect your brain from the inside. Antioxidants are the antidote to oxidants. If oxidants are the sparks from the fire of anything burnt, be it food, a cigarette, or gasoline, antioxidants are like fire-proof gloves that prevent the sparks from damaging your brain.

Most important for the brain is the fat-based antioxidant, vitamin E. This prevents the chain reactions of damage caused when oxidants enter the brain (see Figure 12). A U.S. study of 4,809 elderly people found that decreasing serum levels of vitamin E were consistently associated with increasing levels of poor memory.[6] Vitamin E is properly called d-alpha tocopherol, and its relatives gamma-tocopherol and tocotrienols are also important for the brain. These are only found in the better quality supplements that contain vitamin E together with mixed tocopherols. They are also present in vitamin E-rich foods, such as seeds, cold-pressed seed oils, and fish.

There are other vital antioxidants. Vitamin C, for example, helps recycle vitamin E once it has grabbed hold of an oxidant. A 22-year Swiss study has confirmed that for people aged 65 and older, higher ascorbic acid levels are associated with better memory performance.[7] Russell Matthews and colleagues of the Harvard Medical School Neurochemistry Laboratory in Boston have shown how supplementing coenzyme Q10 can increase energy production in the brain and protect it from neurotoxins.[8] Levels of coenzyme Q10 are up to 35 percent lower in the brains of schizophrenics than in the rest of the population.[9]

In fact, there are many members of the fire-fighting team. The main players are shown below, in Figure 13, which shows how the body detoxifies an oxidant from fried food.

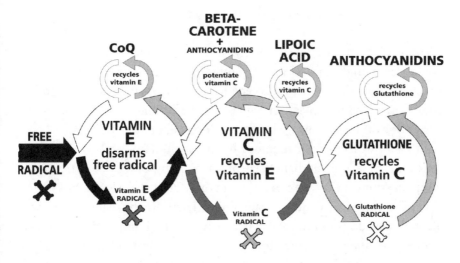

Fig 13. How antioxidants disarm an oxidant or free radical

To give yourself maximum protection, it's worth both eating foods high in these antioxidants and supplementing a good all-round antioxidant supplement. These are the foods richest in each antioxidant:

- **Beta carotene**—carrots, sweet potatoes, dried apricots, squash, watercress

- **Vitamin C**—broccoli, peppers, kiwi fruit, berries, tomatoes, citrus fruit

- **Vitamin E**—seeds and their cold-pressed oils, wheatgerm, nuts, beans, fish

- **Selenium**—oysters, Brazil nuts, seeds, molasses, tuna, mushrooms

- **Glutathione**—tuna, legumes, nuts, seeds, garlic, onions

- **Anthocyanidins**—berries, cherries, red grapes, beets, prunes

- **Lipoic acid**—red meat, potatoes, carrots, yams, beets, spinach

- **Co-enzyme Q**—sardines, mackerel, nuts, seeds, soy.

Make sure you also supplement an antioxidant formula containing all these. Eating these antioxidant-rich foods and supplementing antioxidant nutrients is your best protection against Alzheimer's and memory decline in old age. Supplementing vitamin E, for example, has been proven to prevent Alzheimer's and slow down its progression.

Alcohol pickles your brain

Alcohol is the brain's worst enemy. As soon as you start getting drunk you're damaging your brain. The brain is incapable of detoxifying alcohol, so once the liver's capacity is exceeded, alcohol starts to loosen up and disrupt normal communication signals in the brain, worsening memory. That's one of the reasons we like it—to forget about our worries.

Alcohol worsens your memory by dissolving fatty acids within brain cells and replacing the beneficial brain-building omega-3 DHA with a poor substitute, docosapentaenoic acid or DPA. It also blocks the conversion of fats into DHA and prostaglandins. These are the main reasons why alcohol consumption is associated with mental impairment. It also knocks out vitamins, so the more you drink the more nutrients you need.

While alcohol is without question a neurotoxin, evidence of lowered intelligence with moderate alcohol use, meaning one or two drinks a day, is lacking (see below). The same is not true for high alcohol consumers, whose intellectual performance is definitely impaired.

All this begs the question of how much is too much and why small amounts of alcohol might fail to affect mental performance. There are two theories. One is that smaller amounts of alcohol, which temporarily promote GABA, the brain's relaxing neurotransmitter, may keep you chilled. As you'll see later, lower stress levels are good for the brain. The other is that, if you're not getting drunk, the liver is effectively detoxifying alcohol.

Alcohol: bad news for babies and the elderly

Alcohol can cause the most damage in women who have just become pregnant. The time of greatest risk is two days before or after the moment of conception. This is because it can cause gene damage that results in the baby being born with fetal alcohol syndrome, a condition that affects growth, the nervous system, and intellectual development.

The first caution against alcohol during pregnancy comes in the Bible. In the Book of Judges in the Old Testament, the Lord advises Manoah's wife, who had become pregnant, not to "eat of anything that cometh of the vine, neither let her drink strong wine or strong drink." The Royal College of Obstetricians and Gynaecologists is less strict. It says that there is little danger below two units of alcohol a day (two small glasses of wine or one pint of beer), or 10 units a week. Not all agree. Professor Derek Bryce-Smith, whose research helped identify the dangers of toxic metal excess and mineral deficiency in relation to miscarriage and birth defect risk, believes "it is absurd to think there is a safe cut-off level." Researchers at San Diego State University, California, have recently confirmed that children prenatally exposed to alcohol can suffer from serious cognitive deficits including learning, memory, and behavioral problems, as well as alcohol-related changes in brain structure.[10] The dangers of alcohol are particularly high if a woman has a high homocysteine level (see the last chapter). Personally, I think drinking alcohol while pregnant is not worth the risk.

But what about other times of life? While a high consumption of alcohol is associated with lowered intellectual performance in tests, that doesn't hold for moderate drinkers. In fact, one study by the National Institute for Public Health in the Netherlands found less risk of poor cognitive function among those who had one or two drinks a day, compared to abstainers.[11]

While it is well known that excessive alcohol can lead to dementia, this is not the same thing as Alzheimer's disease. You may be surprised to know that the risk of Alzheimer's is higher in abstainers than in light drinkers.

Researchers at the University of Pittsburgh psychiatry department in Pennsylvania compared the performance of alcoholics with dementia versus non-alcoholics with dementia, and found a very different pattern of poor mental function, suggesting that alcohol per se wasn't causing the same kind of brain damage seen in Alzheimer's.[12] Alzheimer's patients were more impaired when it came to mental functions such as recognition memory and orientation, while the people with alcohol-triggered dementia were more impaired than control participants on abilities like free recall, although not on recognition memory. However, the results of this study are preliminary and based on small sample sizes, so they should be interpreted with caution.

This finding has been further confirmed by a recent study in which older people, from teetotallers to heavy drinkers, were given MRI scans to see whether there was a link between Alzheimer's-like damage in the brain and drinking.

The researchers, from the Erasmus Medical Center in Rotterdam, the Netherlands, scanned the brains of 1074 dementia-free people aged 60 to 90, looking for damage or evidence of stroke.[13] They also measured hippocampus size, which is a strong indicator of Alzheimer's. People were categorized according to their alcohol consumption from abstainers to very light (1 drink a week), light (up to a drink a day), moderate (1 to 4 drinks a day), and heavy (4 drinks a day) drinkers. They found that the people with the healthiest brains—meaning the least damage, the least evidence of strokes and the least hippocampal shrinking—were not the very light drinkers or abstainers, but the light or moderate drinkers. While the heavy drinkers came out worse, the abstainers and very light drinkers had smaller hippocampuses than light or moderate drinkers, but only if they carried the ApoE gene mutation. (The ApoE gene is a variation you can inherit. State of the art laboratories test for this kind of thing. Interestingly, smoking and lack of exercise are risk factors for Alzheimer's, but only in those without the ApoE4 gene.) This finding suggests that while large amounts of alcohol damage the brain, a glass of wine a day or a beer does not, and may even reduce your risk of cognitive decline.[14]

This finding has been backed by a number of studies in France that have consistently shown light to moderate alcohol drinkers as having a lower incidence of both dementia and strokes, while heavy drinkers increase their risk of developing both diseases. The moral of this story is: moderation in everything.

Why stress makes you forgetful

Have you ever noticed that you forget things when you're stressed? That's because stress increases levels of the hormone cortisol, and cortisol damages your brain. According to research by Professor Robert Sapolsky of Stanford University, two weeks of raised cortisol levels caused by stress leaves dendrites, those connections between brain cells, shriveled up.[15] Using a brain imaging technique, Douglas Bremner of Yale University, Connecticut, has shown that the part of the brain responsible for learning and memory is smaller in patients with post-traumatic stress disorder, and that this correlates with poorer memory.[16] So, if your game plan in life is to work your butt off, make a million and retire, you may retire with half a brain! That's the bad news.

The good news is that Professor Sapolsky's research showed that dendrites do grow back once cortisol levels decline. In other words, stay cool. Chapter 17 explains how to do that.

The danger of stress-triggered raised cortisol levels over long periods of time should not be underestimated. Numerous studies have linked elevated cortisol levels with impaired memory function.[17-18] It is almost certainly a major contributor to the increased incidence of memory decline in later years and Alzheimer's disease. Researchers at the La Sapienza University in Rome have shown that cortisol levels are significantly higher in Alzheimer's patients than in controls, and correlate with the severity of the disease.[19] Linda Carlson and colleagues at McGill University in Montreal have confirmed that in Alzheimer's patients, the higher the cortisol, the worse their memory.[20] They also found that the higher the levels of another stress hormone, DHEA, the better their memory.

DHEA: the anti-aging adrenal hormone

One of the more reliable indicators of adrenal exhaustion is a person's level of an adrenal hormone called DHEA, or dehydroepiandrosterone. DHEA not only helps control stress, it also maintains proper mineral balance, helps control the production of sex hormones, and builds lean body mass while reducing fat tissue. Increased levels of DHEA, nicknamed the anti-aging hormone, have many benefits associated with youth. Levels start to decline after the age of 20, especially in people who live in a state of prolonged stress. DHEA levels can be measured in blood and saliva, and low levels can be boosted by DHEA supplementation, together with stress management through diet, exercise, and lifestyle changes. Owen Wolkowitz and colleagues from the University of California, San Francisco, have shown how DHEA supplementation can dramatically improve memory and depression.[21]

Prolonged stress also disturbs blood-sugar balance and, as you'll see in the next chapter, this blunts memory and alertness, as well as potentially damaging the brain.

SUMMARY

In summary, here are a few simple steps you can take to avoid the brain agers:

- Avoid foods containing hydrogenated fats.

- Limit your intake of fried foods and processed foods.

- Eat foods rich in antioxidants—fruits, vegetables, seeds, and fish.

- Supplement an antioxidant formula containing beta carotene, vitamin C, vitamin E, selenium, glutathione, anthocyanidins, lipoic acid, and coenzyme Q10.

- Stop smoking.

- Avoid alcohol in pregnancy, and otherwise limit alcohol to the occasional beer or glass of wine.

- Do all you can to reduce your stress level (see Chapter 17).

CHAPTER 10

Sugar and stimulants make you stupid

As we learned in Chapter 3, complex carbohydrates are the best fuel for the brain, and sugar the worst. There are many reasons for this.

Not so sweet

First, the more sugar and refined carbohydrates—such as commercial cereals, cookies, muffins, cakes, and sweets—that you eat, the more you become unable to maintain even blood-sugar levels. The symptoms of blood-sugar problems, technically called hypoglycemia, are many, and include fatigue, irritability, dizziness, insomnia, excessive sweating (especially at night), poor concentration and forgetfulness, excessive thirst, depression and crying spells, digestive disturbances, and blurred vision. One of the world's experts on blood-sugar problems, Professor Gerald Reaven from Stanford University in California, estimates that 25 percent of normal, non-obese people have insulin resistance. This means their bodies don't respond properly to their own insulin, whose job is to keep your blood-sugar level even. In my experience, I would guess that the majority of people with mental health problems, from depression to schizophrenia, have blood-sugar problems as a major underlying cause.

The second reason sugar is so bad for you is that it uses up your body's stores of vitamins and minerals and provides next to none. Every teaspoon of sugar uses up B vitamins, for example, which therefore makes you more deficient. B vitamins are vital for maximizing your mental performance. About 98 percent of the chromium present in sugar cane is lost in turning it into sugar. This mineral is vital for keeping your blood-sugar level stable.

The third reason is conclusive evidence that high sugar consumption is linked to poor mental health. Researchers at the Massachusetts Institute of Technology found that the higher the intake of refined carbohydrates, the lower the IQ. In fact, the difference between the high sugar consumers and the low sugar consumers was a staggering 25 points![22] Sugar has been implicated in aggressive behavior,[23–28] anxiety,[29–30] hyperactivity and attention deficit,[31] depression,[32] eating disorders,[33] fatigue,[34] learning difficulties,[35–38] and PMS.

One study by Dr. Matti Virkkunen of the University of Helsinki in Finland investigated 69 habitual offenders for blood-sugar balance, and found that every one had a condition characterized by recurrent bouts of hypoglycemia, or abnormally low blood sugar.[39] Meanwhile, research involving 1,382 detained juvenile offenders placed on a reduced-sugar diet reported a 44 percent reduction in antisocial behavior.[40]

Sugar is, of course, everywhere, and a lot of it is lodged in foods and drinks popular among young children and adolescents. One of the worst culprits is fizzy drinks. A Norwegian study recently found a direct link between high consumption of sugar-containing soft drinks and mental distress, hyperactivity, and conduct problems among adolescents. Problems of conduct were worse among boys and girls who consumed four or more glasses of sugar-containing soft drinks per day.[41]

Dr. Carl Pfeiffer, founder of Princeton's Brain Bio Center back in the 1980s, classified blood-sugar problems as one of the five main underlying factors in schizophrenia. You can become anti-social, aggressive, fearful, phobic, psychotic, and suicidal, all by having a simple blood-sugar problem. So rule number one if you have a mental health problem, or want to optimize your mental performance, is: quit sugar and cut right back on refined carbohydrates. In practical terms, this means following a low glycemic load (GL) diet, as we saw in Chapter 3.

Glucose damages the brain

Glucose itself is not toxic, provided you can keep your blood-sugar level even. But the minute your blood-sugar levels go above the maximum threshold, which is what happens in the severest level of dysglycemia, called diabetes, glucose becomes toxic to the brain. This is why diabetics develop nerve, eye, and brain damage.

The reason this happens is that an excess of glucose, much like oxidants, damages nerve cells and stops them working properly. This happens because glucose reacts with proteins in the brain and nervous system. This reaction, called glycation, stops the protein from moving freely and membranes start to get thicker and *gunked up*, slowing down brain communication. Excesses of glucose also cause inflammation in the brain, which is the body's way of saying something's wrong.[42] The hallmark of Alzheimer's is the presence of inflamed and damaged tissue in the brain, caused, in part, by this process. (More on this in Chapter 37.)

As more and more people are becoming disglycemic, the incidence of related conditions—obesity, age-related memory loss, Alzheimer's, heart disease, and diabetes—are also on the rise. And there can be further harmful ramifications. Depression, for instance, is much more prevalent in people with diabetes.

Are you a stimulant addict?

Sugar is only one side of the coin, as far as blood-sugar problems are concerned. Stimulants and stress are the other. As you can see from the figure on page 90, if your blood-sugar level dips there are two ways to raise it. One is to eat more glucose, and the other is to increase your level of the stress hormones adrenalin and cortisol. There are two ways you can raise adrenalin and cortisol. Consume a stimulant—tea, coffee, chocolate, or cigarettes. Or react stressfully, causing an increase in your own production of adrenalin.

Knowing this, you can see how easy it is to get caught up in the vicious cycle of stress, sugar, and stimulants. It will leave you feeling tired, depressed, and stressed much of the time.

Here's how it works. Through excess sugar, stress, and stimulants you lose your blood-sugar control and wake up each morning with low blood-sugar levels and not enough adrenalin to kickstart your day. So you adopt one of two strategies:

- Either you reluctantly crawl out of bed on remote control and head for the kitchen, make yourself a strong cup of tea and coffee, light up a cigparette or have some fast-releasing sugar in the form of toast, with

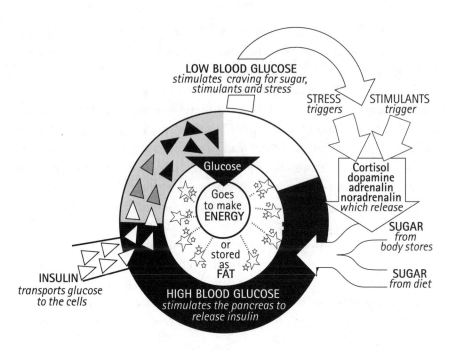

Fig 14. Blood-sugar imbalance

some sugar on it called jam. Up go your blood-sugar and adrenalin levels and you start to feel normal.

- Or you lie in bed and start to think about all the things that have gone wrong, could go wrong, will go wrong. You start to worry about everything you've got to do, haven't done, and should have done. About 10 minutes of this gets enough adrenalin pumping to get you out of bed.

If this sounds like you, you're caught in that vicious circle, with all its negative effects on your mind and mood.

Caffeine—shackled to a cup

Your morning cup of coffee or tea is addictive. Research shows that consuming as little as 100 mg of caffeine a day can lead to withdrawal symptoms when you stop, including headache, fatigue, difficulty concentrating, and drowsiness. It's worth knowing that while a small cup of instant coffee may contain less than 100 mg of caffeine, a large cup of *designer* coffee can contain as much as 500 mg—five times the addictive dose. Even more chemicals are used in manufacturing decaffeinated coffee, and in the end it still contains traces of caffeine, although usually less than 5 mg per regular cup.

The classic withdrawal effects from caffeine are fatigue, low mood, headaches, anger, and irritability. Overnight withdrawal from caffeine can induce all these, although headaches more commonly occur in regular coffee or tea drinkers after a day off it. Studies show that the energy levels of regular coffee consumers drop on withdrawal, but are usually higher after a coffee-free week. More, hand steadiness is considerably worse for those who consume 250 mg a *day*—the equivalent of two reasonably strong coffees.

A blunted mind

Here's the irony. The reason people get hooked on drinking coffee, particularly in the morning, is that it makes you feel better, more energized and alert. But, wondered Dr. Peter Rogers, a psychologist at Bristol University, does coffee actually increase your energy and mental performance, or just relieve the symptoms of withdrawal? When he researched this he found that, after that sacred cup of coffee, coffee drinkers don't feel any better than people who never drink coffee. Coffee drinkers just feel better than they did when they woke up.[43] In other words, drinking coffee relieves the symptoms of withdrawal from coffee, like any other addictive substance.

Coffee is not only addictive, it worsens mental performance. A study published in the *American Journal of Psychiatry* studied 1,500 psychology students and divided them into four categories depending on their coffee intake: abstainers, low consumers (1 cup or equivalent a day), moderate (1 to 5 cups a day) and high (5 or more cups a day). The moderate and high consumers were found to have higher levels of anxiety and depression than the abstainers, and the high consumers had the greatest incidence of stress-related medical problems, as well as lower academic performance.[44] A number of studies have shown that the ability to remember lists of words is made worse by caffeine. According to one researcher, "Caffeine may have a deleterious effect on the rapid processing of ambiguous or confusing stimuli ..." That sounds like a description of modern living!

Recipe for exhaustion

Caffeine blocks the receptors for a brain chemical called adenosine, whose function is to stop the release of the motivating neurotransmitters dopamine and adrenalin. With less adenosine activity, levels of dopamine and adrenalin increase, as do alertness and motivation. Peak concentration occurs 30–60 minutes after consumption.

The more caffeine you consume, the more the body and brain become insensitive to their own natural stimulants, dopamine and adrenalin. You then need more stimulants to feel normal, and keep pushing the body to produce more dopamine and adrenalin. The net result is adrenal exhaustion —an inability to produce these important chemicals of motivation and communication. Apathy, depression, exhaustion, and an inability to cope set in.

And be aware that coffee isn't the only source of caffeine. There's tea, and caffeine is also the active ingredient in most cola and other energy drinks such as Red Bull, which sold over 100 million cans last year. Chocolate and weak tea or green tea also contain caffeine, but much less than these drinks.

Caffeine buzzometer

Here are the caffeine levels in a number of popular products...

Product	Caffeine content
Coca-Cola Classic 350ml (12fl oz)	46 mg
Diet Coke 350ml (12fl oz)	46 mg
Red Bull (8fl oz)	80 mg
Hot cocoa 150ml (5fl oz)	10 mg
Coffee, instant 150ml (5fl oz)	40–105 mg
Espresso, cappuccino, latte (average)	30–50 mg
Coffee, filter 150ml (5fl oz)	110–150 mg
Coffee, Starbucks (grande)	500 mg*
Decaffeinated coffee 150ml (5fl oz)	0.3 mg
Tea 150ml (5fl oz)	20–100 mg
Green tea (5fl oz)	20–30 mg
Chocolate cake (1 slice)	20–30 mg
Bittersweet chocolate 28g (1oz)	5–35 mg
Pro Plus	50 mg
PEP	30 mg

*One analysis found 500 mg to be the highest level of caffeine found in a Starbucks grande coffee.

Kicking the habit

If you want to be in tip-top mental health, stay away from stimulants. This is doubly important for those with mental health problems because too much caffeine can, in some, produce symptoms that lead to a diagnosis of schizophrenia or mania. This may happen because high caffeine consumers can become both allergic to coffee and unable to detoxify caffeine. The net effect is serious disruption of both mind and mood.[45]

Here's how you can give up.

Coffee contains three stimulants—caffeine, theobromine, and theophylline. Although caffeine is the strongest, theophylline is known to disturb normal sleep patterns and theobromine has a similar effect to caffeine, although it is present in much smaller amounts in coffee. So decaffeinated coffee isn't exactly stimulant-free. As a nutritionist, I have seen many people cleared of minor health problems such as fatigue and headaches just from cutting out their two or three coffees a day. The best way to find out what effect it has on you is to quit for a trial period of two weeks. You may get withdrawal symptoms for up to three days. These reflect how addicted you've become. After that, if you begin to feel perky and your health improves, that's a good indication that you're better off without coffee. The most popular alternatives are Teeccino or Roma (made with roasted chicory and malted barley), dandelion coffee (Dandy Blend) or herb teas.

Tea is the great British addiction. A strong cup of tea contains as much caffeine as a weak cup of coffee and is certainly addictive. Tea also contains tannin, which interferes with the absorption of vital minerals such as iron and zinc. Particularly addictive is Earl Grey tea, which contains bergamot, itself a stimulant. If you're addicted to tea and can't get going without a cuppa, it may be time to stop for two weeks and see how you feel. The best-tasting alternatives are Rooibosch tea (red bush tea) with milk, and herbal or fruit teas. Drinking very weak tea from time to time, however, is unlikely to be a problem. In fact, from an overall health point of view, drinking weak or decaffeinated tea may even be beneficial due to the high polyphenol content, which acts as an antioxidant. Green tea is particularly good in this respect.

Chocolate bars are usually full of sugar, while cocoa, the active ingredient in chocolate, provides significant quantities of the stimulant theobromine and small amounts of caffeine. Theobromine is also contained in cocoa drinks like hot chocolate. As chocolate is high in sugar and stimulants, and delicious as well, it's all too easy to become a chocoholic. The best way to quit the habit is to have one month with *no* chocolate. If you crave something sweet, go for fruit or healthy sweets from health food shops that are sugar-free and don't contain chocolate. After a month you will have lost the craving.

Cola and energy drinks contain anything from 46–80 mg of caffeine per can, as we can see from the chart on page 92, which is as much as a cup of coffee. In addition, these drinks are often high in sugar and colorings and their net stimulant effect can be considerable. Check the ingredients list and stay away from drinks containing caffeine and chemical additives or colorings.

Changing any food habit can be stressful in itself, so it is best not to quit everything at one time. A good strategy is to avoid something for a month and then see how you feel. One way to greatly reduce the cravings for foods you've got hooked on is by having an excellent diet. Since all stimulants affect blood-sugar levels, you can keep yours even by always having something substantial for breakfast, such as an oat-based, not too refined cereal; unsweetened live yogurt with banana, ground sesame seeds and wheatgerm; or an egg. You can snack frequently on fresh fruit. The worst thing you can do is go for hours without eating. Eating a highly alkaline-forming diet can reduce cravings for cigarettes and alcohol. This means lots of fresh vegetables and fruit. These high-fiber foods also help to keep your blood-sugar levels even.

As we saw in Chapter 7, vitamins and minerals are important too because they help to regulate your blood-sugar level, and hence your appetite. They also minimize the withdrawal effects of stimulants and the symptoms of food allergy. The key nutrients are vitamin C, the B complex vitamins, especially vitamin B6, and the minerals calcium and magnesium. Fresh fruit and vegetables provide significant amounts of vitamin C and B vitamins, while vegetables and seeds, such as sunflower and sesame, are good sources of calcium and magnesium. For maximum effect, however, it is best to supplement these nutrients as well as eating foods rich in them. I recommend a high-strength multivitamin, plus 2,000 mg per day of vitamin C and 200 mcg of chromium.

SUMMARY

In summary, here are a few simple steps you can take to balance your blood sugar, as well as following the advice in Chapter 3:

- Avoid sugar and foods containing sugar. This means anything with added glucose, sucrose, and dextrose. Fructose is not so bad, but still best reduced. Use xylitol if you have to have sugar.

- Break your addiction to caffeine by avoiding coffee, tea, and caffeinated drinks for a month, while improving your diet. Once you are no longer craving caffeine, the occasional weak cup of tea or very occasional coffee is not a big deal.

- Break your addiction to chocolate. Once you are no longer craving it, the occasional piece of chocolate is not a problem, but choose the dark, low-sugar kind.

CHAPTER 11

Avoiding brain pollution

In the last 50 years alone, 3,500 new chemicals have been added to food. A further 3,000 have been introduced into our homes.[46] Heavy metals like lead and cadmium are so commonplace in our 21st-century environment that the average person has body levels 700 times higher than those of our ancestors.[47] Most of our food is sprayed with pesticides and herbicides. In fact, up to a gallon of them may have been sprayed on the fruit and vegetables consumed by the average person in a year.

All of these are classified as anti-nutrients—substances that interfere either with our ability to absorb or to use essential nutrients, or in some cases, promote the loss of essential nutrients from the body.

Nobody really knows how much this modern cocktail of anti-nutrients messes up our mental health. But we do know that high intakes of lead, cadmium, certain food colorings and other chemicals can have a disastrous effect on intellectual performance and behavior.

A high intake of anti-nutrients has been associated with mood swings, poor impulse control and aggressive behavior, poor attention span, depression and apathy, disturbed sleep patterns, and impaired memory and intellectual performance. If these kinds of symptoms are present, the nutritional approach to promoting mental health includes testing for high levels of anti-nutrients and, if found, removing the source and detoxifying the body. Here are some examples of anti-nutrients, their source, effects in excess on mental health, and nutritional protectors, which help to lower body levels of these unwanted substances.

Anti-nutrient	Effect	Source	Protector
Lead	Hyperactivity, aggression	Exhaust fumes	Vitamin C, Zinc
Cadmium	Aggression, confusion	Cigarettes	Vitamin C, Zinc
Mercury	Headaches, memory loss	Pesticides, fillings	Selenium
Aluminium	Associated with senility	Cookware, water	Zinc, Magnesium
Copper	Anxiety and phobia	Water	Zinc
Tartrazine	Hyperactivity	Food colorings	Zinc

Anatomy of the anti-nutrients

Now let's take a closer look at just what these culprits can do to our mental health.

Lead: one big headache

Researchers at the California Institute of Technology have been studying changes in lead concentrations throughout the world—in ocean beds, soil samples, and even snow. Their work shows that lead concentration, even in unpolluted Greenland, has risen between 500 and 1,000 times since prehistoric times. Comparisons of lead found in humans showed a similar increase. The question we must ask is, what effect is this having on us?

Children are most at risk of lead toxicity. This is especially so up to age 12, when lead can create irreversible brain damage. The most common symptoms in children are an inability to concentrate, disturbed sleep patterns, uncharacteristic aggressive outburst, fussiness about food, sinus conditions, and headaches. Adults are more likely to experience a chronic lack of physical and mental energy, together with restlessness, insomnia, irritability, confusion, anxiety, delusions, depression, disturbing dreams, neurological problems, headaches, and convulsions.

Lowering IQ

The first study to shake the status quo on lead toxicity was the Needleman study. Herbert Needleman, an associate professor of child psychiatry,

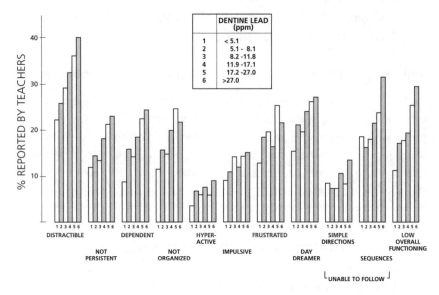

Fig 15. Classroom behavior in relation to dentine lead concentration

looked at a group of 2,146 children in first and second grade schools in Birmingham, Alabama in the U.S.. He examined lead concentrations in shed baby teeth to obtain more long-term levels than shown by a simple blood test. He then asked the schoolteachers to rate the behavior of children they had taught for at least two months. This was done using a questionnaire designed to measure the teacher's rating of children for a number of characteristics. He also ran a series of behavioral, intellectual, and physiological tests on each child before dividing the children into six groups according to their lead concentration in teeth.

As you can see, his results showed a clear relationship between lead concentrations and bad school behavior, as rated by the teachers without any knowledge of the children's lead levels. Needleman also found the average IQ for the high-lead children was 4.5 points below that of the low-lead group. Reaction time (a measure of attention capability) was also consistently worse in those with higher lead levels. EEG readings (which measure brain wave patterns) also showed clear differences, based on lead concentration. Perhaps the most interesting result was that none of the high-lead children had an IQ above 125 points (100 is average), compared to 5 percent in the low lead group.[48]

Richard Lansdown, principal psychologist at the London Hospital for Sick Children, and William Yule, psychologist at the University of London, decided to replicate the essentials of Needleman's study on London children using lead levels in the blood instead of teeth. The 160 children involved had blood-lead levels from 7 to 33 micrograms per deciliter, averaging 13.5 mcg/dl (35 mcg/dl is the 'safe' level recommended by the Lawther Report *Lead and Health*, 1980). This is similar to other national studies of mean lead levels. Again, the teachers rated the children's behavior, and IQ and other tests were made. Lansdown's results were even more striking than Needleman's. The difference in IQ score between high- and low-lead children was seven IQ points. Once again, none of the high-lead group children had IQs above 125, while in the low-lead group, 5 percent did.[49]

A further study by Dr. Gerhard Winneke, Director of the Medical Institute of Environmental Hygiene in Düsseldorf, found essentially the same results. He studied 458 children with an average blood level of 14.2mcg/dl, and found an IQ deficit of five to seven points between those with high and low lead levels.[50]

In Britain the blood levels allowed in industrial workers are 80mcg/dl for men and 40kmcg/dl for women. In the U.S. the level is 40mcg/dl regardless of sex. Yet these landmark studies from the 1980s have shown conclusively that levels of lead as low as 13mcg/dl can affect behavior and lower intelligence in children. When we consider that the average EEC lead level in the 1980s was 13mcg/dl, we must come to the appalling conclusion that lead was then damaging the minds of one in two children in the EEC. With lead-free gas now common, the situation is improving. However, this is not the end of the story.

A follow-up study of children with elevated lead levels found, 11 years later, a sevenfold increase in the odds of failure to graduate from high school, lower class standing, greater absenteeism, more reading disabilities, and deficits in vocabulary, fine motor skills, reaction time, and hand-eye coordination.[51] The toxic effects of lead on the brain will be with us for some time yet.

The important lesson from lead is that tiny changes in what we ingest can have vast consequences for our health, which, although invisible to the eye, can and has been proven by research. Banning lead in gasoline was the first campaign of the Institute for Optimum Nutrition. There are many others yet to be won.

Cadmium: peril as you puff

Cadmium is another heavy metal that is associated with disturbed mental performance and increased aggression. The most common source is in cigarettes. Cadmium levels in the blood correlate well to the number of cigarettes smoked. There is also cadmium in car exhaust fumes and small amounts in food, especially if it's refined since beneficial minerals which act as cadmium protectors are taken out in the refining process.

Aluminum: toxic intruder

Aluminum is in widespread use in food packaging and turns up in many common household products. It's in antacids, toothpaste tubes, aluminum foil, pots and pans and water. There is an association between aluminum and Alzheimer's, discussed in Chapter 37. Not all aluminum will enter the body. Only under certain circumstances will aluminum leach, for example, from a pan. Old-fashioned aluminum cookware, if used to heat something acidic like tea, tomatoes, or rhubarb, will leach particles of aluminium into the water. Also, the more zinc-deficient you are the more you absorb.

Mercury: why hatters were mad

Mercury is the reason 19th-century hatters went mad. By polishing top hats with mercury, they became overloaded with this toxic element, which disturbs brain function and makes you crazy. Mercury is very toxic indeed and small amounts reach us from contaminated foods and from tooth fillings. Of particular concern is fish caught in polluted waters.

Mercury has also been used as a constituent of thimerosal, a preservative found in diptheria and hepatitis vaccines. This practice has recently been stopped, and a good thing too. Until recently, if a child had all the shots they were meant to have at 6 months and at 12–15 months, they would have clocked up 260 mcg of mercury—a level that can cause headaches and memory loss. Meanwhile, 6.7 percent of autism in the U.K. has been attributed by parents to the MMR vaccine.[52]

In one analysis of American babies six months old, the average intake of mercury was 111.3 mcg.[53] Tiny amounts of mercury have been shown to promote abnormal methylation. Although not proven, this provides a plausible explanation as to why the MMR vaccine could trigger autism. An alternative explanation might involve the vaccine inducing measles: measles antibodies have been found in the brains of autistic children.[54-57]

Mercury is also used in a number of chemical processes, and accidents and illegal dumping have led to increased mercury levels in some areas, including the English Channel. Fish, especially larger fish like tuna, store the mercury which we then ingest. Fortunately, tuna is also high in selenium, a mercury protector. As it is, tuna contains middling to high amounts of mercury and you should limit eating it to once a month or so.

The chart below lists fish in order of best to worst, in terms of the greatest amount of omega-3 with the lowest amount of mercury. Farmed salmon may have significantly lower amounts of omega-3 compared to wild salmon because the amount of omega-3 in the fish depends to a large extent on the quality of its diet.

	Omega-3 g/100g	Mercury mg/kg	Omega-3/ mercury
Fresh wild salmon	2.7	0.05	54.0
Canned sardines	1.57	0.04	39.3
Canned and smoked salmon	1.54	0.04	38.5
Fresh mackerel	1.93	0.54	35.7
Herring (kipper)	1.31	0.04	32.8
Trout	1.15	0.06	19.2
Fresh tuna	1.5	0.4	3.8
Cod	0.25	0.11	2.3
Fresh sole	0.1	0.05	2.0
Canned tuna	0.37	0.19	1.9
Marlin	1.1	1.1	1.0
Swordfish	1.1	1.4	0.8

The copper controversy

Copper is both an essential mineral and a toxic one. It's rare to be deficient in copper, except in people with diets very high in refined foods, largely because of copper pipes. These leach small amounts of copper into water. However, if you live in a soft-water area or in a house with new copper piping that hasn't yet gotten calcified, you can be exposed to toxic levels of copper. Copper and zinc are enemies. So, if you are zinc-deficient you may not be able to get rid of excess. The birth control pill also raises copper levels.

So it's not so hard to get too much copper, which is associated with anxiety, paranoia, and schizophrenia. Consider this story. I met a headmaster of a school for problem children on holiday. We got talking about the effects of lead and other toxic metals on behavior. We decided to set up a challenge. On return, he'd send me a dozen hair samples from different students, which I would analyze and use to predict their behavior. I ran the hair mineral analyzes and found three abnormal results. One had a very high lead level. I predicted aggressive behavior, hyperactivity, and poor attention span. I was right. The child in question was the worst behaved in the school! Two others had high copper levels. I predicted anxiety. They turned out to be a schoolteacher and his wife. They had recently moved into a new house, built on the grounds of the school, with new copper pipes in a soft-water area. The wife had started to become more and more anxious and had been prescribed medication. The husband was apparently free of symptoms.

This story illustrates how easy it is to be copper toxic without knowing it. Copper excess, which can cause extreme fears, paranoia, and hallucinations, is rarely checked or tested in those with mental health problems, despite the fact that is has been often reported in people with schizophrenia.[58] The copper may be the result of drinking water passing through copper pipes, copper pots and pans, the contraceptive pill, and even copper IUDs. Or it can be the result of vitamin C, B3, or zinc deficiency, all of which are zinc antagonists. It also highlights the importance of drinking filtered or bottled water.

However, as an essential mineral with a number of different roles, copper is also important for health. One study has found that it acts as an iron antagonist, preventing iron overload.[59] Another study looking at supplementing zinc on its own in people with Alzheimer's[60] found that after just a few days of zinc supplementation, their condition actually worsened.

But the evidence is confusing. A recent study by researchers at Rush University Medical Center in Chicago, Illinois, in the U.S. found that high amounts of dietary saturated and trans fats and a total copper intake of 1.6 mg a day or more is associated with a faster rate of memory loss.[61] Copper was not found to be harmful at all in people who did not have this high-fat diet, but the combination of the two had a significant detrimental effect.

These studies show that getting the balance of copper right as well as eating a healthily balanced diet low in saturated and trans fats is crucial, as is the balance between zinc and copper. You need roughly 10 times more zinc than copper, both of which are found in whole foods such as beans, nuts and seeds. Because excess copper is a relatively common condition in places where drinking water passes through copper pipes, one of the easiest ways to minimize this possibility is to drink filtered or bottled water. A hair-mineral analysis (see below) will identify whether you have excess copper or possible zinc deficiency.

How to handle the heavies

The brain and body are constantly detoxifying and getting rid of toxic elements using a removal agent called metallothionein. If this isn't working well, possibly due to a deficiency in key nutrients and/or excess in any one of the bad guys we've examined, health problems can result. So, how do you fix it? First you need to discover which, if any, toxic minerals are affecting you.

Hair-mineral analysis: your heavy metal MOT

There's a simple way to find out if these heavy and toxic minerals are affecting you—a hair-mineral analysis. By analyzing a small amount of hair, you can be effectively screened, not only for the bad guys such as lead, cadmium, mercury, and aluminium, but also for the good guys such as magnesium, zinc, chromium, manganese, and so on. For around $60.00 it's well worth it.

One of the leading labs in London is Biolab. Having analyzed some 50,000 samples of hair, blood, and sweat (collected by placing a patch on the back), they found something worrying.[62] Every one of these toxic minerals accumulates with age, while levels of essential minerals decline. Dr. Stephen Davies, who led this study, concludes that our overexposure to toxic elements and lack of essential elements from poor diets have exceeded the human body's capacity to adapt and successfully detoxify. The lack of sufficient essential elements makes lead, cadmium, mercury, and aluminum even more toxic.[63] The combination of these factors is no doubt lowering our overall intellectual performance and emotional stability.

Detoxifying your brain

You can easily test your own mineral levels with a hair mineral analysis. Look in the Resources section on page 480 under 'Laboratory Testing'. But what do you do if you have raised levels of toxic minerals?

Once we've ingested toxic minerals they must compete with other minerals for absorption. These minerals are called antagonists and form our first line of defense. Once the mineral has been absorbed, some natural body substances latch on to it and try to take it out of the body. These are called chelators (pronounced key-lay-tors).

It is the latter principle which lies behind the administration of two drugs, penicillamine and EDTA, to treat heavy metal toxicity.

Vitamin C vs lead

One of the problems with lead poisoning is that once it is in the brain, where most damage is done, it is very difficult to remove. Neither penicillamine nor the more potent EDTA chelating drugs have much effect, because neither can readily cross the blood-brain barrier. But vitamin C can. In a study on rats with high concentrations of lead in their brains, administering EDTA resulted in an 8 percent lowering of lead, while vitamin C decreased levels by 22 percent.[64]

Vitamin C is helpful across the board, with the ability to latch on to most heavy metals in the blood and escort them out, sacrificing itself in the process. So high metal burdens call for more vitamin C. It is effective for removing lead, arsenic, and cadmium and is a most important part of any detoxification program.

Zinc vs lead and cadmium

Another substance known to lower lead is zinc, which acts as an antagonist to lead by preventing its absorption in the gut. In one study by Dr. Carl Pfeiffer at Princeton's Brain Bio Center, 2,000 mg of vitamin C and 60 mg of zinc (as zinc gluconate) were given to 22 workers at a lead battery plant, all of whom had elevated lead levels. Complete blood tests were taken at the start of the study and after 6, 12, and 24 weeks. The average blood-lead level at the start was 62.1mcg/dl. The results showed the steady decrease of lead levels over the 24-week period, although the workers were still receiving similar exposure at work. Zinc also lowers body and brain levels of cadmium. Indeed, most of us could benefit from extra zinc.

Calcium vs heavy metals

Calcium is also effective at keeping down lead levels, since lead otherwise stores more easily in our bones. Keeping calcium levels at optimum levels pushes lead out and prevents the rapid rise in toxic minerals which, according to research by Dr. Ellen O'Flaherty at the University of Cincinnati College of Medicine, goes up by 15 percent following menopause.[65] Calcium is particularly effective at keeping down cadmium and aluminium levels. Toxic elements such as lead and uranium accumulate in bone tissue over a lifetime of repeated exposure, and are released into the bloodstream as bone tissue breaks down. Bone loss can increase dramatically following menopause, which explains the rise in blood-lead levels found in O'Flaherty's research.

Selenium vs mercury

Selenium is a mercury antagonist, and normally protects us from the mercury present in most seafood. Supplementing an extra dose is always a good idea if there are signs of excess mercury. It also has a similar protective effect with arsenic and cadmium, although it is not so pronounced.

Foods that fight heavy metals

In terms of specific foods, there are a few that can help keep your brain clean. Sulphur-containing amino acids are found as the proteins in garlic, onions, and eggs. The specific amino acids are called methionine and cysteine and protect against mercury, cadmium, and lead toxicity. Alginic acid is seaweed, and pectin in apples, carrots, and citrus fruits also help chelate and remove heavy metals, thereby promoting your health. One more reason for an apple a day.

Avoid food additives

Over 200,000 tons of chemical additives are added to food each year, or approximately 10lb per person. Some of us, perhaps all of us, aren't coping well with this level of chemical onslaught.

One of these, tartrazine (E102) has been consistently linked to hyperactivity in children, yet it is still added to many popular soft drinks for children in order to color the drink yellow/orange. A closer look at this food chemical reveals something rather sinister.

Dr. Neil Ward from the University of Surrey decided to test what happens to minerals when drinks containing tartrazine were consumed. He gave children either a drink with tartrazine or an identical one without. He found that adding tartrazine to drinks increased the amount of zinc excreted in the urine, perhaps by binding to zinc in the blood and preventing it from being used by the body.[66] In this study, like many others, he also found emotional and behavioral changes in every child who drank the drink containing tartrazine. Four out of the 10 children in the study had severe reactions, three developing eczema or asthma within 45 minutes of ingestion.

Tartrazine is one of the first of over 1,000 chemical food additives to be proven to be an anti-nutrient. At this point in time we really have no idea what the combined effect of the literally hundreds of man-made chemicals have on health. My advice is to avoid foods with long lists of additives. There are a few, however, that are good for you. These are the colors E101 (vitamin B2), E160 (carotene, vitamin A); the antioxidants E300–304 (vitamin C), E306–309 (tocopherols, like vitamin E); the emulsifier E322 (lecithin); and stabilizers E375 (niacin) and E440 (pectin). Stay away from the rest.

A nutritional therapist can check for the presence of many of these anti-nutrients and devise a lifestyle, diet, and supplement program to eliminate this potential contributor to mental instability. The effect of decreasing the burden of these anti-nutrients is a greater ability to cope with the unavoidable stresses life gives us to deal with and improve mental performance.

What's wrong with MSG?

Monosodium glutamate (MSG) is a form of glutamic acid or glutamate—an amino acid that occurs naturally in food and is also made in the body by breaking down another amino acid, glutamine.

MSG (E621) is often used as a flavor enhancer, not only in Chinese restaurants but also in a wide variety of savory foods including chips, sauces, burgers, salad dressings, bouillon cubes, and gravies.

Yet recent research has proposed that too much MSG causes excessive brain-cell excitation which can lead to cell death. It has been further suggested that this could play a part in neurodegenerative diseases such as

Alzheimer's, Parkinson's, and Huntingdon's. Other studies show that an excess of MSG can cause reactions such as: difficulty in concentration, extreme mood swings, and depression. The part that dietary glutamates contribute is still controversial.

Should you avoid it?

If you know that you react to MSG you should certainly avoid it entirely. For the rest of us, it makes sense to keep intake as low as possible, since side effects are so widely reported but are far from fully understood. I recommend keeping children off foods with added MSG altogether. Of course, if you're eating mainly whole foods such as fresh fruit and vegetables, legumes, wholegrains, and high-quality proteins as I recommend, you won't be taking in much MSG anyway, as it is only added to processed food. As for the naturally occurring stuff, if you are sensitive to any added MSG, it would be worth avoiding foods that are higher in natural glutamate for a couple of weeks (see the chart below). You could then reintroduce them one by one while monitoring any symptoms to determine if you are reacting to them.

Glutamate content of foods (mg/100g)

Cow's milk	2
Eggs	23
Beef	33
Mackerel	36
Chicken	44
Potatoes	102
Corn	130
Oysters	137
Tomatoes	140
Broccoli	176
Mushrooms	180
Peas	200
Grape juice	258
Fresh tomato juice	260
Walnuts	658
Soy sauce	1,090
Parmesan cheese	1,200
Roquefort cheese	1,280

What to look for on food labels

According to the U.K.'s Food Standards Agency, added MSG must be identified on a food label as either Flavor Enhancer: mono-sodium glutamate (MSG) or Flavor enhancer: E621.

SUMMARY

In summary, here are a few simple steps you can take to avoid anti-nutrients that pollute your brain:

- Avoid foods containing chemical food additives.

- Don't smoke, and stay away from smoky places.

- Eat mineral-rich foods such as seeds and nuts.

- Drink filtered or bottled water.

- Supplement vitamin C every day, which protects you from toxic minerals.

- If you have a mental health problem, have a hair-mineral analysis (see Resources); also available through nutritional therapists.

CHAPTER 12

Brain allergies

"One man's meat is another man's poison." This is many people's experience. Some foods suit, some don't. Some days you feel good, some days you don't. Often, there is the awareness that it may be connected to what you eat, but the riddle isn't always easy to decipher.

The knowledge that allergy to foods and chemicals can adversely affect moods and behavior in susceptible individuals has been known for a very long time. Early reports, as well as the current research, have found that allergies can affect any system of the body, including the central nervous system. They can cause a diverse range of symptoms including fatigue, slowed thought processes, irritability, agitation, aggressive behavior, nervousness, anxiety, depression, schizophrenia, hyperactivity, and varied learning disabilities.[67–74] Allergic intolerance in susceptible individuals can be caused by a variety of substances, though many people have reactions to common foods and chemicals.

The most convincing evidence for this comes from a well-conducted double-blind, placebo-controlled crossover trial by Dr. Joseph Egger and his team, who studied 76 hyperactive children to find out whether diet can contribute to behavioral disorders. The results showed that 79 percent of the children tested reacted adversely to artificial food colorings and preservatives, primarily tartrazine and benzoic acid, which produced a marked deterioration in behavior. However, no child reacted to these alone. In fact, 48 different foods were found to produce symptoms among the children tested. For example, 64 percent reacted to cow's milk, 59 percent to chocolate, 49 percent to wheat, 45 percent to oranges, 39 percent to eggs, 32 percent to peanuts, and 16 percent to sugar. Interestingly enough, it was not only the children's behavior that improved after the individual dietary modifications. Most of the associated symptoms also improved considerably, such as headaches, fits, abdominal discomfort, chronic rhinitis, aches in limbs, skin rashes, and mouth ulcers.[75]

Another similar double-blind controlled food trial by Dr. Egger and his team was conducted with 88 children suffering from frequent migraines. As before, most children reacted to several foods and chemicals. However, the following foods and chemicals were found to be most prevalent: cow's milk provoked symptoms in 27 children, eggs in 24, chocolate in 22, both oranges and wheat in 21, benzoic acid in 14, and tartrazine in 12. Yet again, after dietary modification, not only their migraines improved, but also associated physical disorders such as abdominal pain, muscle aches, fits, rhinitis, recurrent mouth ulcers, asthma, eczema, and a variety of behavioral disorders.[76]

Adults are also affected by food and chemical allergy. When Dr. William Philpott, an American allergy expert, examined 250 emotionally disturbed patients for a possible presence of food or chemical allergies, he found that the highest percentage of symptoms occurred in patients diagnosed as psychotic. For example, out of 53 patients diagnosed as schizophrenic, 64 percent reacted adversely to wheat, 50 percent to cow's milk, 75 percent to tobacco, and 30 percent to petrochemical hydrocarbons. The emotional symptoms caused by allergic intolerance ranged from mild symptoms such as dizziness, blurred vision, anxiety, depression, tension, hyperactivity and speech difficulties to severe psychotic symptoms.[77]

These studies are prime examples of how problems created by allergies often produce a multitude of physical and mental symptoms and affect many body systems. They affect not just the central nervous system and brain, but also, usually, the whole body in various ways. Furthermore, these allergies are very specific to the individual, as are the symptoms they create. Therefore, any diagnosis can only be made individually by using an elimination and challenge diet.

Pinpointing the troublemakers

Here are a few examples of how an elimination and challenge diet have been used safely and effectively in treating people suffering from various mental health problems.

Study 1

Thirty patients suffering from anxiety, depression, confusion, or difficulty in concentration were tested, using a placebo-controlled trial, to discover whether individual food allergies could really produce mental symptoms in these individuals. The results showed that allergies alone, not placebos, were able to produce the following symptoms: severe depression, nervousness, feeling of anger without a particular object, loss of motivation, and severe mental blankness. The foods/chemicals that produced most severe mental reactions were wheat, milk, cane sugar, tobacco smoke, and eggs.[78]

Study 2

Ninety-six patients diagnosed as suffering from alcohol dependence, major depressive disorders, and schizophrenia were compared to 62 control subjects selected from adult hospital staff members for a possible food or chemical intolerance. The results showed that the group of patients diagnosed as depressives had the highest number of allergies: 80 percent were found to be allergic to barley and 100 percent were allergic to egg white. Over 50 percent of alcoholics tested were found to be allergic to egg white, milk, rye, and barley. Out of the group of people diagnosed as schizophrenics, 80 percent were found to be allergic to both milk and eggs. Only 9 percent of the control group were found to suffer from any allergies.[79]

Study 3

Routinely treated schizophrenics, who on admission were randomly assigned to a diet free of cereal grain and milk while on the locked ward, were discharged from the hospital in about half the time control patients assigned to a high-cereal diet were. Wheat gluten secretly added to the cereal-free diet abolished this effect, suggesting that wheat gluten may be a cause of schizophrenic symptoms in susceptible individuals.[80]

Two recent reports estimate that two in every 10 people now suffer from allergies.[81–82] The young developing nervous system is particularly vulnerable to any allergenic or toxic overload, leading frequently to various behavioral disorders such as hyperactivity and learning disabilities. A further survey estimates that at least one child in 10 may react adversely to common foods and food additives.[83]

All about allergies

If allergies are this common, it's vital that we take a closer look at them.

How food allergies affect your mind

Most food allergies provoke mental and emotional changes. This is an idea which has been resisted by conventional allergists, but it has been well proven by clinical tests, scientific analysis, and people's experiences.

We've learned that brain cells communicate through the action of neurotransmitters. This is the whole foundation of a chemical model of mental health. Yet brain cells are not unique in being able to communicate in this way. Immune cells in the digestive tract, blood, and body tissues also have receptors to many neurotransmitters. Scientists are beginning to discover there's a lot of talking going on between the brain and nervous system, the immune system, and endocrine system. In fact, there's a whole new speciality emerging in medicine called psycho-neuro-immuno-endocrinology, or PNEI for short. One of the most established links is the talking between the gut and the brain, via gut hormones and neurotransmitters. In truth, this is a highly fertile ground in medical science today as we gradually learn that the boundaries between mind and body are extremely fuzzy. Simultaneously, we are discovering a much closer connection between allergies and mental health.

One study that looked at the connection between allergies and schizophrenia and autism found that among autistic children, 87 percent had higher levels of IgG antibodies (see page 113) to gluten—which are found in wheat—and 90 percent had higher levels of these antibodies to casein, found in milk and milk products. This is significantly higher than in children without autism. Among the schizophrenic patients, the figures were also very high: 86 percent and 93 percent. Following a strict gluten/casein-free diet has resulted in dramatic improvements in patients, with some recovering completely.[84] The link between autism and wheat and milk allergy is particularly strong and I'll discuss this in more detail in Chapter 29.

To understand the connection between allergies and mental health, it's necessary to understand what an allergy is in the first place.

What is an allergy?

The classic definition of an allergy is "any idiosyncratic reaction where the immune system is clearly involved." The immune system, which is the body's defense system, has the ability to produce 'markers' for substances it doesn't like. The classic marker is an antibody called IgE (immunoglobulin type E). These attach themselves to mast cells in the body. When the offending food, called an allergen, latches onto its specific IgE antibody, the IgE molecule triggers the mast cell to release granules containing histamine and other chemicals that cause the classic symptoms of allergy—skin rashes, hay fever, rhinitis, sinusitis, asthma, eczema, and severe reactions to, for example, shellfish or peanuts, causing immediate gastrointestinal

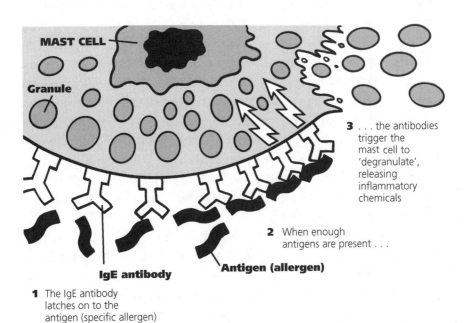

MAST CELL

Granule

3 . . . the antibodies trigger the mast cell to 'degranulate', releasing inflammatory chemicals

2 When enough antigens are present . . .

IgE antibody

Antigen (allergen)

1 The IgE antibody latches on to the antigen (specific allergen)

Fig 16. How IgE antibodies cause allergic reactions

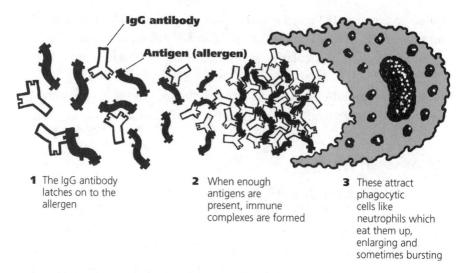

1 The IgG antibody latches on to the allergen

2 When enough antigens are present, immune complexes are formed

3 These attract phagocytic cells like neutrophils which eat them up, enlarging and sometimes bursting

Fig 17. How IgG antibodies cause allergic reactions

upsets or swelling in the face or throat. All these reactions are immediate, severe inflammatory reactions.

The emerging view now is that most allergies and intolerances are not IgE based, but involve another marker, known as IgG. According to allergy expert Dr. James Braly, "Food allergy is not rare, nor are the effects limited to the air passages, the skin, and digestive tract. Most food allergies are delayed reactions, taking anywhere from an hour to three days to show themselves, and are therefore much harder to detect. Delayed food allergy appears to be simply the inability of your digestive tract to prevent large quantities of partially digested and undigested food from entering the bloodstream." This is not a new idea. Since the 1950s, pioneering allergists such as Dr. Theron Randolph, Herbert Rinkel, Dr. Arthur Coca, and, more recently, Dr. William Philpott and Dr. Marshall Mandel, have written about delayed sensitivities causing far-reaching effects on all systems of the body, including the mind.

It is now well established that many, if not the majority, of food intolerances do not produce immediate symptoms, but have a delayed, cumulative effect. This, of course, makes them hard to detect by observation alone. I find that the majority of food-sensitive children react after two or more hours to foods. In contrast, IgE reactions are immediate, suggesting that a buildup of IgG antibodies may be a primary factor in food sensitivity.

According to Dr. Jonathan Brostoff, consultant in medical immunology at the Middlesex Hospital Medical School, certain ingested substances can cause the release of histamine, another neurotransmitter now known to have profound effects on mental health, and can also invoke classical allergic symptoms without involving IgE. These substances include lectins (in peanuts), shellfish, tomatoes, pork, alcohol, chocolate, pineapple, papaya, buckwheat, sunflower, mango, and mustard.

Allergic reactions can also occur when there is a substantial production of antibodies (mainly IgG) in response to an allergen in the blood. This results in immune complexes which the body and brain react to (see Figure 17). "It is the sheer weight of numbers that causes a problem," says Brostoff. "These immune complexes are like litter going round in the bloodstream." The litter is cleaned up by cells, principally neutrophils, which act like vacuum cleaners. But if there are too many immune complexes, the neutrophils simply can't keep up.

The top ten allergies

Most food allergies develop in reaction to the protein in food, and particularly foods we eat most frequently. Top of the list is wheat, probably because it contains a substance called gliadin, which irritates the gut wall. Gliadin is allied to gluten, a sticky protein that allows pockets to form when combined with yeast, which is how bread is made. Eating a lot of wheat products isn't good for anyone, especially if you've developed an allergy. The connections between wheat allergy, autism, and schizophrenia are well established (see Chapters 26 and 29). However, gluten sensitivity can also produce headaches and unsteadiness that go away on stopping wheat.[85]

Depression has also been linked to gluten sensitivity. A common symptom in people with a hidden food allergy is, in fact, depression that is unresponsive to antidepressant prescription drugs. Some authorities claim that clinical depression is *the* most widespread presenting symptom in untreated celiac disease, a condition in which sufferers are so sensitive to gluten from wheat and other grains that the small intestine can be damaged if they're eaten.[86]

Low brain levels of the neurotransmitters serotonin and/or noradrenalin, made from dopamine—the most commonly identified biochemical causes of depression—can also be found in food-allergic patients (and also in recovering alcoholics, as shown in Chapter 32). So simply eliminating food allergens such as gluten from the diet can result in the restoration of normal brain chemistry and potentially in relief from depression.

Oats contain much less gluten than wheat, and it is a different kind. For this reason, some people who are wheat intolerant—including some celiac patients—are not intolerant to oats. Studies of both children and adults with celiac disease have shown that most patients are able to tolerate oats without any adverse effects.[87-88] However, one study showed that small numbers of people with celiac disease react to a protein in oats called avenin, so if you have this condition you may also need to avoid oats.[89]

Dairy produce causes allergic reactions in many people. This includes cheese and yogurt. Some people can tolerate goat's or sheep's milk but not cow's milk. The symptoms are very varied but often include a blocked nose, frequent colds, bloating, indigestion, thick head, fatigue, and headaches. Other foods that can cause allergic reactions include oranges, eggs, other grains apart from wheat, yeast-containing foods, shellfish, nuts, soy, and members of the nightshade family—tomatoes, peppers, potatoes, and eggplants. Some people also develop allergies to tea and coffee, while alcohol, which irritates the gut wall and makes it more leaky, often increases allergic sensitivity to anything eaten.

Testing for allergies

If you have a history of infantile colic, eczema, asthma, ear infections, hay fever, seasonal allergies, digestive problems (especially bloating), frequent colds, or daily mood swings, or function better when you don't eat certain foods, you may have a food intolerance.

If you suspect you might have an allergy there are two courses of action. One is to avoid the suspected substances strictly for two weeks, then reintroduce them in a controlled way, recording your symptoms. This is best done under the guidance of a nutritional therapist, which is doubly important if you've ever had a severe reaction to food, such as asthma.

The other involves a relatively new blood test, developed over the last eight years, involving a method known as ELISA. This state-of-the-art method of measuring IgG sensitivity will tell you the foods you are currently eating that cause an IgG reaction, and how severe that reaction is. Ideally, it is best to also have an IgE ELISA test. This information can help a nutritional therapist devise a diet for you that avoids these allergy-provoking foods and replaces them with suitable alternatives. But then what?

Foods that invoke an immediate and pronounced IgE-type reaction may need to be avoided for life. The memory of IgE antibodies is certainly long-term, if not forever. In contrast, the cells that produce IgG antibodies have a half-life of six weeks. That means that there are half as many six weeks later. The memory of these antibodies is short-term, and, within three months there is unlikely to be any residual memory of reaction to a food that's been avoided.

Another, softer, option after a strict one-month avoidance, is to rotate foods so that an IgG-sensitive food is only eaten every four days. This reduces the buildup of allergen-antibody complexes and reduces the chances of symptoms of intolerance. Foods such as wheat and milk which are, by their nature, difficult to digest, are probably best avoided as much as possible by those who show allergic tendencies. This is especially true for wheat, since even IgG sensitivity to wheat appears to be a lifelong condition, and is possibly genetically predetermined.

Allergy or indigestion?

Digestive problems are often the underlying factor that leads someone to develop allergies. As you'll see in Chapter 29, most autistic children have digestive problems that cause allergic reactions, which in turn disturb how the brain works. Many allergy sufferers have been found to have low stomach acid, which is essential for digesting food proteins. Dr. James Braly has found zinc deficiency to be extremely common among allergy sufferers. Zinc is not only needed to digest all protein, it's also essential for the production of hydrochloric acid in the stomach. Certain foods, he says, are inherently difficult to digest, the worst being gluten in wheat and casein in dairy products. Wheat and dairy are Britain's top two allergy-provoking foods. He also suspects that many allergy sufferers may have excessively leaky digestive tracts, allowing undigested proteins to enter the bloodstream through the gut wall and cause reactions.

So, identifying and avoiding what you react to is one half of the equation. Consumption of alcohol, frequent use of aspirin, deficiency in essential fatty acids, or a gastrointestinal infection or infestation such as candidiasis are all possible contributors to leaky gut syndrome that need to be corrected to reduce intolerance to foods. Frequent use of antibiotics, which wipe out gut bacteria, paving the way for candidiasis, therefore also increase the risk of developing food intolerances.

The emerging view, shared by an increasing number of allergy specialists, is that food sensitivity is a multi-factorial phenomenon possibly involving poor nutrition, pollution, digestive problems, and overexposure to certain foods. Removing the foods may help the sufferer recover, but other factors need to be dealt with in order to have a major impact on long-term food intolerance. Due to the complex factors involved in food allergies and intolerance, it is often best to see a clinical nutritionist who can pinpoint the likely culprits from your symptoms and eating patterns, advise you on tests should they prove necessary, and help you correct digestive problems that increase your allergic potential.

At the Brain Bio Centre in London, we routinely test individuals with mental health issues for allergy. It is not at all uncommon for us to find that putting a person on the allergy-free diet they need relieves symptoms of depression, insomnia, anxiety, and even schizophrenia. So if you suffer from poor concentration, insomnia, anxiety, or other symptoms of depleted mental health, it's well worth investigating whether food allergies play a part.

SUMMARY

In summary, here's how to test for, and reduce, your allergic potential:

- Avoid wheat and dairy products strictly for two weeks and see how you feel. In any case these food groups are best not eaten frequently.

- Improve your digestion by eating plenty of fresh fruit, vegetables, seeds, and fish, which contain essential fats and zinc.

- Keep alcohol, painkillers, and antibiotics to a minimum. These damage the digestive tract.

- If you suspect you've got a food allergy, get yourself tested (see page 476). A nutritional therapist can both test what you are allergic to and devise a course of action to reduce your allergic potential.

PART 3

Improving Your IQ, Memory, and Mood

Contrary to popular belief, you can improve your IQ, boost your memory, and enhance your mood at any time of your life. In this part you will find out exactly what you need to do to maximize your mental health and performance throughout your life, stay relaxed, and get a good night's sleep.

CHAPTER 13

How to boost your intelligence

It may surprise you to know that you can boost your intelligence, and IQ score, at any age. Some people argue that your real intelligence—how smart you are—is innate, something you're born with. But the truth is that your ability to make intelligent decisions depends not only on this aspect of intelligence, but also on the clarity of your mind, how quickly you can think, your attention, how long you can concentrate, and your memory. All of these can be improved with optimum nutrition.

This should not be surprising since the brain, composed of this highly complex network of neurons, is made from what we eat. Thinking is a pattern of activity across this network. The activity, or messengers, are neurotransmitters, which are made from and directly affected by what you eat. When we learn, we actually change the wiring of the brain. When we think, we change the activity of neurotransmitters. This was the logic that made us investigate, in 1986, whether giving a person an optimal intake of nutrients used by the brain and nervous system would improve intellectual performance.

Smart supplementation

We knew already that a person's nutrient status was associated with intelligence. For instance, in 1960 a study by Dr. A.L. Kubala and colleagues had shown that increased vitamin-C status was associated with increased intelligence. Dr. Kubala used IQ as a measure. IQ stands for Intelligence Quotient and is an accepted measure of intelligence, with a score of 100, originally by definition, being average. About 5 percent of people score above 125, and less than 10 percent score below 80, which is considered to be educationally subnormal.

Dr. Kubala divided 351 students into high and low vitamin-C groups, depending on the levels in their blood. The students' IQ was then measured and found to average 113 and 109 respectively: those with higher levels of vitamin C in their blood had an average of 4.5 IQ points more.[1]

Gwillym Roberts, a headmaster and researcher at the Institute for Optimum Nutrition, and I sat down and worked out what combination of nutrients would optimally nourish the brain. We then gave these to a pilot group of students, measuring their IQ before and after. Up went their IQ, by 10 points.

To test whether these results were valid, Roberts devised a proper randomized, double-blind, placebo-controlled trial, and, together with David Benton, a psychologist from Swansea University who thought our theory was unlikely but worth testing, ran the trial. We tested a group of 60 children. Without their or our knowledge and at random, we put 30 of them on a special multivitamin and mineral supplement designed to ensure an optimal intake of key nutrients, and the other 30 on an identical placebo. This double-blind design meant that neither we nor they could bias the results through our expectations. All children had their IQ scores measured at the start of the trial, and then again after eight months.[2]

After eight months on the supplements, the non-verbal IQs in those taking the supplements had risen by an average of over 10 points! (Non-verbal IQ is that aspect of intelligence that is more fluid and susceptible to brain chemistry, while the verbal IQ is more influenced by teaching. For ease of reading, from here on IQ refers to non-verbal IQ.) Some children were getting more than 20-point improvements in IQ. No changes were seen in those on the placebos, or a control group of students who had not taken any supplements or placebos. The study was published in *The Lancet* medical journal and was the subject of a BBC *Horizon* TV documentary, the day after which every single children's multivitamin in Britain sold out.

This now-famous IQ study spawned a dozen similar studies to test if the results were real. The next big study, conducted by Stephen

Schoenthaler, professor of nutrition John Yudkin, world-famous psychologist Hans Eysenck, and Dr. Linus Pauling, involved 615 children given much lower levels of nutrients, at RDA levels. Once again, the results showed that the simple addition of a vitamin and mineral supplement could increase IQ scores by as much as 20 points, with an average increase of at least 4.5 points, this time over three months.[3]

During the press conference revealing the results of this trial, one journalist, referring to those children who had had a 20-point shift in IQ, asked if this could turn a bricklayer into a brain surgeon. He was obviously fishing for a quote. The chairman said this was entirely possible. An antagonistic journalist pointed out that the average increase was only 4.5 IQ points and asked what this would do. The spokesman said this would turn them into a journalist! The truth is that a 4.5 IQ-point shift would get many thousands of educationally subnormal children reclassified and returned to normal schools. More comprehensive nutritional programs have brought several children with IQs in the 40s back into the normal range (see Chapter 27).

But despite almost all the properly designed trials clearly showing the beneficial effect of vitamin and mineral supplements on IQ, this fact is still largely resisted by many dietitians and die-hards of the conventional nutritional establishment—although some do change their minds. At the time when our first trial was published back in 1988, John Yudkin was quoted as saying, "This is the most scandalous paper I've seen printed in *The Lancet*. The study is ludicrous meaningless nonsense."[4] Yet several years later, following a study with which he had been associated, Yudkin said: "Our studies show, we believe conclusively, that adding vitamins and minerals to the diets of children who have no obvious signs of nutrient deficiency, can nevertheless produce an increase in their IQ scores."[5]

A review of 11 trials giving multivitamins to date shows a clear IQ-boosting effect in 8 of the studies. All produced an improvement in nonverbal IQ compared to placebo. But not everybody benefits. Those trials that also measured the nutritional status of the children found that the children who respond best are those whose diet contains only low amounts of micronutrients.[6] So, the more poorly nourished a child is to start with, the more room there is for improvement. And this is borne out in our projects in primary schools, where the worst nourished children end up gaining the most IQ points when given appropriate supplementation.

And here's the rub as far as the anti-supplement brigade are concerned.

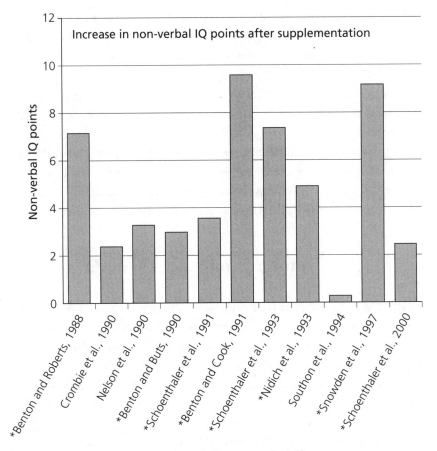

Fig 18. These are the improvement in non-verbal IQ scores versus placebo (e.g. if the placebo group had a 3-point increase and the supplemented group had a 10-point shift, the difference, shown here, is 7 points). Those marked with a * were statistically significant.

They argue that since you can get all the nutrtients you need from a well-balanced diet (meaning the RDA level of nutrients), children don't need supplements. But this argument is flawed on two big counts. First, many children simply aren't well-nourished to begin with. More importantly, we certainly cannot assume that the RDA level of nutrients is optimum nutrition for the mind. They weren't calculated on that basis and, as we have seen throughout this book, we may need more to maximize our mental performance. A study by researchers in North Dakota involving 200 teenagers illustrates the point.

They gave the children either 20 mg or 10 mg of zinc in a supplement, or a placebo. The RDA for zinc is 10 mg. Most children achieve an intake of around 7 mg from their diets anyway, so in truth these children were now receiving either around 7 mg (placebo group) or 7 + 10 mg, or 7 + 20 mg. The researchers found that only those taking 20 mg of zinc a day had faster and more accurate memories and better attention spans within three months.[7]

It's this kind of finding that shows there is much to learn about the optimum level of nutrients for IQ, but what has been learned certainly indicates that most children can benefit mentally from vitamin and mineral supplementation, especially those whose diets leave room for improvement.

Can adults bump up their IQ?

In Part 1 we saw a recent trial involving a large group of middle-aged to elderly people that found a clear improvement just by giving folic acid, one of the B vitamins. Dr. Jane Durga from Wageningen University in the Netherlands gave a group of 818 people aged 50 to 75 either a vitamin containing 800 micrograms of folic acid a day, or a placebo, for three years. On memory tests, the supplement users had scores comparable to people 5.5 years younger while on tests of cognitive speed, the folic-acid helped users perform as well as people 1.9 years younger.[8] This amount of folic acid is equivalent to eating 2.5 pounds of strawberries a day. In other words, it would appear that simply eating that mythical well-balanced diet may not be enough at any age if you want to maximize your mental performance.

How do nutrients boost IQ?

But how exactly do nutrients increase IQ scores? Wendy Snowden, a researcher from Reading University's psychology department, decided to investigate. Once again, schoolchildren were given supplements or a placebo.[9] The supplemented children showed significant increases in nonverbal IQ scores, but not verbal IQ scores, after 10 weeks. A close analysis of performances in the IQ tests showed the same error rate but the children were able to work faster and attempt more questions after the 10 weeks of supplementation. For the verbal IQ test all children completed all questions so there was no room for improvement in work rate. This suggests that the effect of the vitamin and mineral supplements is to increase the speed of processing, which is clearly a significant factor in IQ and presumably in intelligence, as well as attention span. In other words, you think faster and can concentrate for longer. Other studies, as we've seen, show improvement in memory.

Having worked with hundreds of children myself, I would say that what happens when you achieve optimum nutrition is that the act of thinking becomes more connected. You can make associations and remember things better. This means you can solve problems faster. What is also clear is that multinutrient approaches tend to work better than single nutrients. In fact, most single-nutrient trials have been ineffective in raising children's IQs. The only exceptions to date are a small effect from vitamin B1, and a larger effect from zinc, as we saw above, and folic acid.

It is highly likely that the nutrients that make the most difference are those that improve methylation (see Chapter 8)—in other words, the homocysteine-lowering nutrients. One of the most extraordinarily powerful findings is that of A.K. Borjel of the clinical chemistry department at Orebro University Hospital in Sweden. She compared the school grades, and sum of school grades, in 10 core subjects, with homocysteine levels in a group of 692 Swedish schoolchildren aged 9 to 15. Increasing homocysteine levels were strongly associated with lower grades.[10]

As we saw on page 73, the homocysteine-lowering nutrients are vitamin B2, B6, B12, folic acid, zinc, and TMG, as well as other methylating nutrients such as the 'intelligent fats' phospholipids. Optimizing your intake of all these is likely to be nutritional gold for boosting intelligence.

Brain fats

As we learned in Chapter 4, eating the right essential brain fats speeds up thinking processes in the brain. While the earlier studies we've seen in this chapter didn't supplement omega-3 fats, there's plenty of evidence that they should have. The levels of omega-3 fats at birth, especially DHA, the brain-building fat, predict intellectual development later in life.[11–12] Children with optimal intakes of omega-3s have the lowest risk of behavioral and learning problems later in life.

To date, proper controlled trials clearly show that essential fat supplements can reduce symptoms of depression and anxiety, as well as improve behavior, dyslexia, ADHD, coordination, and reading and writing difficulties. I'll discuss these trials in detail in Part 6. Other open studies, not involving placebos, have found that giving essential fat supplements improves school grades and behavior. Once again, the children with the worst diets and the greatest range of problems tend to improve the most.

The essential fats that are most important are the omega-3 fats EPA (which seems to be the key one for reversing behavioral and learning problems), and DHA, and GLA, the most potent omega-6 fat. Many of the cutting-edge researchers in this field give all three.

If you're wondering whether you can't get enough just from diet, the answer is possibly, as long as you eat fish three or more times a week. In fact, a survey we did on 37,000 adults found that those eating oily fish once a week experienced no difference in their mental health, but that those who ate oily fish twice a week had better mental health, while those who had three or more servings a week had the best mental health.

Best fish for brain fats

Amount of DHA in 100g (3½oz)

Mackerel	1,400 mg
Herring	1,000 mg
Sardine	1,000 mg
Tuna	900 mg
Anchovy	900 mg
Salmon	800 mg
Trout	500 mg

If we take DHA as an example, the ideal intake of DHA a day is probably in the order of 250 to 500 mg, or double if you have a particular mental health problem (see page 41). This is equivalent to eating 100g of fish, preferably mackerel, herring, fresh sardines, fresh or deli anchovies, or wild or organic salmon, three or four times a week. (Fresh tuna is a good source of DHA, but limit eating it to once a month because of its mercury content.) Alternatively, you can take a supplement of fish oils containing DHA. A good-quality cod liver oil supplement can provide up to 200 mg, but there are many high omega-3 fish oils on the market now; just check the DHA content. (If you're vegetarian, an option is eating flaxseeds; but this is problematic as the body finds it hard to convert the omegas in them into EPA and DHA. More on that in Chapter 4, page 40.)

The best source of all, at least for babies, is breast milk. Breast milk is naturally rich in DHA, and especially so if the mother eats fish or flaxseeds. Breast-fed babies not only have higher IQs 10 years down the road,[13] and better results in examinations, they also have fewer mental health problems.[14]

Personally, I recommend both adults and children supplementing a combination of EPA, DHA, and GLA, plus a multivitamin every day, as well as eating a well-balanced diet that includes fish three times a week. This way you're guaranteeing an optimal intake of brain-friendly nutrients.

Balancing blood sugar

Keeping an even blood-sugar level is critical to intelligence because this affects your ability to concentrate over long periods of time more than anything else. Dips in blood sugar not only lower intelligence and concentration, they can also increase aggressive behavior.[15–19] Eating slow-releasing carbohydrates and grazing, not gorging is the best way to avoid blood-sugar dips. If, on the other hand, you refuel with the wrong stuff on the move, going from one sugary snack or drink to another, then your blood-sugar level is likely to rise and fall like a roller coaster. So too will your concentration and mood. See Chapter 3 for the lowdown on what to eat to keep your blood-sugar level even.

SUMMARY

In summary, the first steps to maximizing your IQ are:

- Ensure an optimum intake of vitamins and minerals, both from diet and supplements.

- Optimize your intake of essential fats, especially omega-3 fats, by eating flaxseeds and oily fish, and/or taking fish oil supplements.

- Achieve stable and sustained blood-sugar levels.

These are the basics. But there's still plenty more that you can do to enhance your intelligence and memory (see the next chapter).

14

Enhancing your memory

If your memory isn't as good as it used to be, your concentration is flagging and your mind simply isn't as sharp, you may be another victim of a widespread epidemic of brain drain. At best, you may be failing to reach your full potential for mental health. At worst, you may be one of 4 million people now thought to be suffering from age-related memory decline. This reduces your cognitive function too young, and leaves you open to an increased risk of developing Alzheimer's disease later in life.

The good news is that mental decline is not inevitable and you can boost your memory and mental alertness at any age. Research shows clearly that healthy, well-nourished, and well-educated people show no signs of declining mental function with age. What's more, while it is true that brain cells die with age, you can also build new brain cells at any age. How? By feeding your brain, both with the right nutrients and the right information. Check yourself out on the questionnaire below to see if there's room for improvement.

❓ MEMORY CHECK

Score 1 for each *yes* answer.

☐ Is your memory deteriorating?

☐ Do you find it hard to concentrate and often get confused?

☐ Do you sometimes forget the point you're trying to make?

☐ Does it take you longer to learn things than it used to?

☐ Do you find it hard to add up numbers without writing them down?

☐ Do you often experience mental fatigue?

☐ Do you find it hard to concentrate for more than one hour?

☐ Do you sometimes meet someone you know quite well but can't remember their name?

☐ Do you often find you can remember things from the past but forget what you did yesterday?

☐ Do you ever forget what day of the week it is?

☐ Do you often misplace your keys?

☐ Do you ever go looking for something and forget what you are looking for?

☐ Do your friends and family think you're getting more forgetful now than you used to be?

☐ Do you frequently repeat yourself?

If your score is:

4 or less: Your memory and concentration are good. The advice in this chapter will help keep you mentally sharp throughout your life.

5 to 10: You are starting to suffer from brain drain. Following all the diet and supplement recommendations in this chapter will help give your memory and concentration a boost.

More than 10: You are experiencing significant memory and concentration impairment and need to do something about it. As well as following all the diet and supplement recommendations in this chapter, read Chapter 36 and see a nutritionist who can assess and help you correct the biochemical imbalances that contribute to memory decline.

How your memory works

Memories are not held in one, but several networked brain cells. These links between brain cells, hardwired by a network of interconnecting neuronal dendrites (see Figure 1b on page 11), are stimulated by learning new information. Rats put into a highly stimulating *Disneyland for rats* rapidly grow new dendrites within four days, according to research by Dr. William Greenough at the University of Illinois.[20] Stress does the opposite. As we saw in Part 2, high levels of the stress hormone, cortisol, makes dendrites shrivel up, according to Professor Robert Sapolsky of Stanford University, whose research found this effect became noticeable after as little as two weeks of stress.[21] Fortunately, dendrites do grow back once cortisol levels decline. In other words, use it or lose it—and stay cool.

Memories themselves are thought to be stored by altering the structure of a molecule called RNA within brain cells. For a memory to be made, it must enter the cell by seeing, hearing, or doing something, which accounts for the three kinds of memory—visual, auditory or kinesthetic. If a memory involves all three, it will exist in a maximum number of brain cells. That's why if you see a telephone number, repeat it to yourself

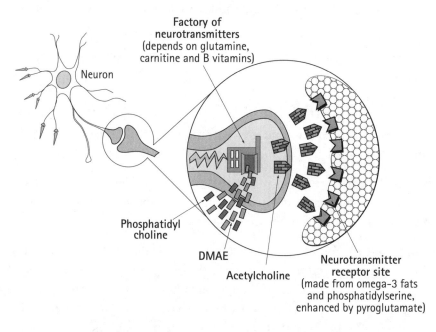

Fig 19. Acetylcholine in action: the memory molecule

aloud, and punch the numbers on the phone several times you are more likely to remember it. The brain, particularly the hippocampus region, then decides whether it's worth storing. In Alzheimer's, the hippocampus loses its ability to file memories, resulting in an inability to store new memories.

A critical question is how memories are put into storage, retrieved, and connected. The key memory molecule is the neurotransmitter acetylcholine, highly concentrated in the hippocampus. (The hippocampus is part of what's called the medial temporal lobe, which connects to other parts of the brain and is thought to be responsible for verbal memory; see Figure 20.) People with Alzheimer's, for example, show a marked deficiency in acetylcholine. Even if a memory is intact, if you don't have enough acetylcholine you can't connect one part of the memory with other parts. For example, you know the face but can't remember the name.

The hippocampus is highly sensitive to homocysteine, and methylation reactions seem to play a key part in the chemistry of memory. Increased levels of homocysteine are known to destroy cells in the brain, which is the hallmark of Alzheimer's disease, leading to increasingly poor memory. That's why keeping your homocysteine level low is the cornerstone of maximizing your memory.

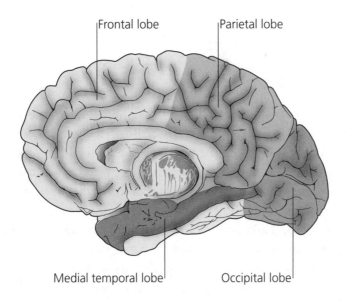

Fig 20. The anatomy of the brain

Natural mind and memory enhancers

The best way to enhance your memory and mind, and protect yourself from memory decline, is to ensure an optimal intake of not only essential vitamins, minerals, and fats, but also nine nutrients from which your body can make key brain chemicals, plus three herbs and a spice. These 13 natural mind and memory enhancers are:

- B6, B12, folic acid, and TMG—the methylators

- Phosphatidylcholine and DMAE—acetylcholine precursors

- Phosphatidylserine and pyroglutamate—receptor enhancers

- Glutamine—fuel for brain cells

- Ginkgo biloba and vinpocetine—herbal circulation improvers

- Ginseng—tonic for the mind

- Turmeric—the memory spice.

These are becoming widely available and can be found in combination in state-of-the-art brain-boosting supplements, as well as in certain foods.

The big nine nutrients

The methylators

We've already seen how important methylation is for connection in the brain, and hence memory, in Chapter 8. Also, in the last chapter, I showed you how simply supplementing folic acid, a vital methylation booster, to people aged 50 to 75 caused an extraordinary improvement in memory. So the four nutrients that are central in promoting methylation—B6, B12, and TMG, in addition to folic acid—are also key in ensuring your memory stays in shape. Later on, in Part 7, you'll see how keeping your homocysteine level low by increasing your intake of these four nutrients is the most likely way to prevent age-related memory decline. The first step is to make sure you take in enough of these nutrients, both through eating beans, nuts, seeds, and greens, and through supplementation.

Phosphatidylcholine—memory marvel

The key brain chemical for memory is acetylcholine. A deficiency in it is probably the most common cause for declining memory after high homocysteine levels. As we saw in Chapter 5, acetylcholine is derived from the nutrient phosphatidylcholine.

The richest dietary sources of phosphatidylcholine are egg yolks and fish, especially sardines. Since egg phobia set in, on the false basis that dietary cholesterol was a major cause of heart disease, the intake of choline from the average western diet has dropped dramatically. The American Medical Association says that up to seven eggs a week is fine. Phosphatidylcholine is also found in lecithin, a supplement that comes in granules and capsules. You need about 1 to 2g of phosphatidylcholine a day for maximizing mental function. Most lecithin contains about 20 percent phosphatidylcholine, so you would need 5 to 10g of lecithin a day. You can also buy High-PC lecithin, which is twice as rich in phosphatidylcholine, so you would only need 2.5–5g a day, or a heaping teaspoon. However, you don't simply make more acetylcholine by eating choline. Vitamin B5 (pantothenic acid) is essential for the formation of acetylcholine in the body, as are vitamins B1, B12, and also C. As always, nutrients work together.

In Chapter 5 we saw how recent research shows that taking choline during pregnancy can result in offspring with superbrains. This research, carried out at Duke University Medical Center in the U.S., fed pregnant rats choline halfway through their pregnancy. The infant rats whose mothers were given choline had vastly superior brains, improved learning ability, and better memory recall, all of which persisted into old age.[22] Supplementing high doses of choline has also been proven to boost memory in adults. For example, Florence Safford of Florida International University gave 41 people aged 50 to 80 choline supplements of 500 mg every day for five weeks. They reported having half as many memory lapses, such as forgetting names or losing things.[23]

Supplementing choline can help the young as well as the old. Dr. Sandra Ladd and colleagues at the West Valley College in Saratoga, California, gave 80 college students a single 25g dose of phosphatidylcholine (3.75g of choline) and found a significant improvement in memory 90 minutes later, most likely due to the improved responses of slow learners.[24] If you combine choline with other smart nutrients such as pyroglutamate, you can achieve the same memory-boosting effect at lower doses (see Chapter 36).

DMAE—naturally stimulating

DMAE (again, sardines are a rich source) is a precursor of choline that crosses much more easily from the blood into brain cells, accelerating the brain's production of acetylcholine. It reduces anxiety, stops the mind racing, improves concentration, promotes learning, and acts as a mild brain stimulant.

As we saw in Chapter 5, slight chemical variations of DMAE have been marketed under various brand names, which have helped people with learning problems, attention deficit disorder, memory, and behavior problems. In one survey by the late Dr. Bernard Rimland in California, DMAE sold under the name Deaner was found to be almost twice as effective in treating children with attention deficit disorder as the drug Ritalin, and without the side effects. The ability of DMAE to tune up your brain was also well demonstrated in a German study from 1996. When DMAE was given to a group of adults with cognitive problems, they showed improvements in brain wave patterns in parts of the brain key in memory, attention and flexibility of thinking.[25]

The ideal dose for memory enhancement is 100 to 500 mg, taken in the morning or at midday, not in the evening. (Too much can overstimulate and is therefore not recommended for those diagnosed with schizophrenia, mania, and epilepsy.) Don't expect immediate results. DMAE can take two to three weeks to work, but it's worth waiting for.

Phosphatidylserine—highly receptive

The ability of neurotransmitters to deliver messages depends on having a fully functioning docking port, or receptor site. These receptor sites are built out of phospholipids, essential fats, and protein. The predominant phospholipid is phosphatidylserine, or PS. The secret of the memory-boosting properties of PS is probably due to its key role in brain cell communication.

Supplementing PS is particularly helpful for those with learning difficulties or age-related memory decline. In one study by Dr. Thomas Crook, 149 people with age-associated memory impairment were given a daily dose of 300 mg of PS or a placebo. When tested after 12 weeks, the ability of those on the PS to match names to faces (a recognized measure of memory and mental function) improved to equal that of people 12 years younger.[26]

Pyroglutamate—master of communication

A key brain chemical in enhancing memory and mental function is the amino acid pyroglutamate. The discovery that the brain and cerebrospinal fluid contain large amounts of pyroglutamate led to its investigation as an essential brain nutrient. One extraordinary finding was that pyroglutamate promotes the flow of information between the right and left hemispheres of the brain. A study published in 1988 by Dr. H. Pilch and colleagues suggests that pyroglutamate may increase the number of acetylcholine receptors in the brain. Older mice were given piracetam, a pyroglutamate derivative, for two weeks. The researchers found that these older mice had a 30–40 percent higher density of receptors than before.[27] This suggests that pyroglutamate-like molecules do not only maximize mental performance but may also have a regenerative effect on the nervous system.

Pyroglutamate improves memory and mental alertness by:

- Increasing acetylcholine production.

- Boosting the number of receptors for acetylcholine.

- Improving communication between the left and right hemispheres of the brain.

So powerful are the effects of pyroglutamate that there are now many slight variations of this key brain chemical being marketed as drugs for learning and memory-related problems. Numerous studies using these *smart drugs* have proven to enhance memory and mental function, not only in those with pronounced memory decline but also in people with so-called normal memory function.[28]

Researchers at the University of Catania, Sicily, tested 40 patients with age-related memory decline. Twenty were given pyroglutamate and 20 a placebo. After two months, various memory tests revealed that those on pyroglutamate had significantly improving memory compared to those on the placebo.[29]

Pyroglutamate is found in many foods, including fish, dairy products, fruit, and vegetables. The most common supplemental form is arginine pyroglutamate. You need about 400–1,000 mg a day for a mind-enhancing effect.

Glutamine—amazing brain fuel

While acetylcholine is the major player as far as memory is concerned, many neurotransmitters are also involved. Some stimulate mental processes, while others prevent information overload. For example, the stimulating neurotransmitter glutamate helps forge links between memories, but too much can literally overexcite neurons to death. This is how MSG (monosodium glutamate) turns up the volume on tastes, but can be a bad thing in large quantities. Pyroglutamate greatly enhances learning, while GABA, a close relative of glutamate, calms down the nervous system. The right balance of these neurotransmitters is important for learning, memory, and mental function in general. So supplementing glutamine, an amino acid from which the brain can build and balance these neurotransmitters, can help promote memory.

Glutamine is the most abundant amino acid in the cerebrospinal fluid that surrounds the brain. Glutamine can be used directly as fuel for the brain and has been shown to enhance mood and mental performance and decrease addictive tendencies.[30] In studies designed to test whether glutamine proved safe in large doses, researchers from Boston Women's Hospital, Massachusetts, gave healthy volunteers between 40 and 60g a day. Not only was it shown to be safe, but one of the side effects was enhanced ability to solve problems on continuous performance tests. This study was only five days long, showing that glutamine has an immediate effect, and possibly a greater effect over time.[31] In another study, this time on bone-marrow-transplant patients, large amounts of glutamine were reported to make patients more "vigorous, less angry, and fatigued."[32]

Glutamine is an important nutrient for the brain and there is good logic to adding 5–10g, which can be bought as a powder, to your daily supplement program. This equates to 1 to 2 heaping teaspoons a day.

Another amino acid, carnitine, can be used directly by the brain as fuel. Acetyl-l-carnitine, often abbreviated to ALC , is an especially useful form of this amino acid, since the *acetyl* part helps to make acetylcholine—the brain's memory neurotransmitter. Together with an antioxidant called alpha lipoic acid, acetyl-l-carnitine can reverse aging and promote memory in animals, according to research by Professor Bruce Ames at the University of California, Berkeley.[33] Not only did the rats in this study have improved memory after only a month on these supplements, they also become more active.

You need between 250 and 1,500 mg of ALC a day to get any benefit. Unfortunately, it is very expensive and is perhaps not my smart nutrient of choice for this reason. It's best to take it sometime before or after eating to maximize absorption.

Best of the rest

Ginkgo biloba: ancient wisdom

Ginkgo biloba is an herbal remedy that has been used for memory enhancement in the East for thousands of years and comes from one of the oldest species of tree known. Research has shown that it improves short-term and age-related memory loss, slow thinking, depression, and circulation, and improves blood flow to the brain. A review of 10 studies testing ginkgo's effects on people with circulation problems, carried out at the University of Limburg in the Netherlands, found significant improvement in memory, concentration, energy, and mood.[34] A more comprehensive double-blind, placebo-controlled trial carried out in France found remarkable improvement in speed of cognitive processing of 60- to 80-year-olds, almost comparable to that of healthy young people, when given 320 mg a day.[35]

Ginkgo contains two phytochemicals called ginkgo flavone glycosides and terpene lactones which give it its remarkable healing properties. It usually comes in capsule form, and you should look for a brand that shows the flavonoid concentration, which determines strength. The recommended flavonoid concentration is 24 percent and you should take 30–50 mg of such a supplement, three times a day. You need to try ginkgo for at least three months before evaluating the results.

Vinpocetine: secret of the periwinkle

Vinpocetine, much like ginkgo, is an herb that improves blood flow and circulation, thus helping to deliver oxygen to the brain. Vinpocetine is actually an extract from the periwinkle plant (*Vinca minor*).

Research carried out at the University of Surrey gave 203 people with memory problems either a placebo or vinpocetine. This and other studies have shown that those on vinpocetine experience a significant improvement in their cognitive performance.[36-37] Remarkably, improvements in concentration, memory recall, and learning have been reported after just one dose. One double-blind crossover study showed a significant improvement in memory after just one hour of taking 40 mg of vinpocetine.[38]

Vinpocetine is recommended for those who've noticed a decline in memory, concentration, learning speed, neuromuscular coordination, and reaction time, or deficits in hearing or vision.

However, research shows that vinpocetine is particularly protective in cases where blood flow to the brain is diminished, usually by cerebral atherosclerosis (a condition in which a buildup of plaque clogs the arteries that supply oxygen to the brain) occurs, as well as during mini-strokes or situations where the blood supply to the brain is temporarily shut off. Like ginkgo, it may also help people with tinnitus, which can be caused by such circulation problems.

The secrets of vinpocetine's success in enhancing mind and memory are many. Firstly, it definitely improves circulation in the brain, helping to deliver nutrients more effectively. Studies show that it widens blood vessels in the brain. Because of this action, red blood cells are better able to pass through narrow passages, resulting in better oxygen delivery. Vinpocetine also inhibits platelet aggregation, stopping blood cells from clumping together and clogging the blood vessels.

Brain cells not only need a constant, good supply of oxygen. They also need energy, and vinpocetine has been shown to enhance energy production in brain cells.

By speeding up the transport of glucose and oxygen to the brain and their use once they get there, vinpocetine may reduce the effects of both strokes and the less dramatic mini-strokes that can lead to dementia.

Finally, vinpocetine has been found to stimulate noradrenergic neurons in an area of the brain called the *locus coeruleus*. These neurons affect the function of the cerebral cortex—the part of the brain we use to think, plan, and act. The number of these neurons declines with age, impairing concentration, alertness, and the speed with which we process information.

You need about 10–40 mg of vinpocetine a day for these positive effects. To date, no negative effects have been reported.

Ginseng—mind tonic

Ginseng is one of the most widely used and researched energy-promoting herbs, and there's no doubt it works in this context. The active ingredients are called ginsenosides, and there are many of them, each with specific effects.

Can ginseng boost mental acuity, though? In 1988, German academic E. Ploss published a summary and analysis of studies on the clinical use of Asian ginseng, which was followed in 1990 by a review by Professors Ulrich Sonnenborn and Yvonne Proppert. These articles surveyed a total of 37 experiments done betweeen 1968 and 1990, involving 2,562 people in all, with treatments averaging 2–3 months. In 11 of the studies the participants showed an improvement in intellectual performance. All showed a near-absence of side effects.

More recent double-blind, controlled trials on ginseng, or ginseng plus ginkgo biloba versus placebos, have proven measurable benefits for energy and memory in both young and old people.[39] Researchers at the Human Cognitive Neuroscience Unit at the University of Northumbria in Newcastle have run three trials, all finding benefit, and are now investigating the herb's precise effect on mental performance.[40]

As with any herb, the dose is critical and ginseng can vary greatly in quality. Good-quality ginseng will state that it is standardized to contain 4–7 percent ginsenosides. The recommended dose of such a standardized extract is 100–200 mg a day.

Turmeric—spice up your memory

Turmeric, the bright yellow spice found in most curry powders, does much more than add zing to food. It reduces joint pain, boosts your immune system, and has even been shown to have a potential effect on age-related memory loss.

The spice contains the active ingredient curcumin, which has a variety of powerful anti-inflammatory actions. It's also a potent antioxidant. In 1995 a patent was filed for turmeric as a new discovery for the treatment of inflammation, but this was rejected after the Indian government challenged it, on the grounds that turmeric had been used for that very purpose for many years in India!

How does turmeric help with memory? Recent exciting research from the University of California and the Veterans Affairs Geriatric Research,

Education and Clinical Center in Los Angeles has found that curcumin may be capable of breaking up the protein plaques that show up in the brains of Alzheimer's patients. The curcumin was able to reduce deposits of the beta-amyloid proteins that make up the plaques in the brains of elderly lab mice that ate curcumin as part of their diets.

When the researchers added low doses of curcumin to human beta-amyloid proteins in a test tube, the curcumin kept the proteins from clumping and blocked the formation of the plaques. Study co-author Dr. Gregory Cole said, "The new findings suggest that curcumin could be capable of both treating Alzheimer's and lowering a person's risk of developing the disease."[41]

Don't forget B vitamins and zinc

While I've already extolled the virtues of B vitamins, there are three that need special mention in relation to memory. Niacin, or vitamin B3, is particularly good for memory enhancement. In one study, 141 mg of niacin was given daily to a group of subjects of various ages. Memory was improved by 10–40 percent in all age groups.[42] B5 (pantothenic acid) is essential for the brain to make acetylcholine—it adds on the acetyl part. It is also essential for the formation of steroid hormones, including the stress hormone cortisol, so is particularly important for people under stress.[43] An optimal intake is probably as much as 200 mg, although some people respond better to 500 mg. Compare this with the RDA, which is just 6 mg in Europe!

B12, which as we've seen is vital for methylation, has also been shown to accelerate learning in rats[44] and is very important for the health of brain cells. B vitamins work together in many ways to help the brain make and use neurotransmitters. It is important to remember that B vitamins should be taken together, so if you wish to concentrate on a specific B vitamin, take this in conjunction with a B complex or multivitamin.

As we saw in Chapter 7, zinc is another brain-friendly nutrient thought to be involved in memory. One theory is that memories are encoded by changing protein molecules in the brain, involving RNA, which is the master builder of proteins in the body. RNA is itself highly dependent on zinc. Deficiencies of zinc are well known to lead to an inability to recall dreams. Children with serious learning difficulties often have low zinc levels, and low zinc is also thought to be involved in the severe memory loss of dementia. As you'll see later in this book, correcting low zinc levels can also have remarkable results for people with depression and schizophrenia. The chances are you are low in zinc because it is the mineral in which we're generally most deficient. The RDA is 15 mg, more if you're pregnant or breastfeeding. Yet, according to government surveys, the average intake is 7.6 mg a day. That means that almost half the British population achieves less than half the recommended intake.

Seeds and seed foods are rich in zinc. Why seeds? Basically, if you can plant it and it grows it's zinc-rich, because zinc is vital for the growth of both plants and animals. This means that seeds, beans, peas, and lentils are all rich in zinc. So are nuts, meat, and fish, and especially oysters. Eating these foods, as well as supplementing 10 mg of zinc every day, is the best way to ensure optimal amounts of this essential nutrient.

The synergy effect

The effects of enhancing mental performance through supplementation of smart nutrients such as phosphatidylcholine, pantothenic acid, DMAE, and pyroglutamate are likely to be far greater when taken in combination than individually. For example, a team of researchers led by Raymond Bartus gave choline and piracetam, a pyroglutamate derivative (see page 135), to some old lab rats with age-related memory decline, and piracetam alone to others.[45] They found that rats given the combination showed better memory retention than those that took piracetam alone. Results also showed that half the dose was needed when piracetam and choline were combined. Dr. S. Ferris and associates at New York University School of Medicine then carried out a study on humans. These researchers, too, found dramatic clinical improvements, way beyond those of people who were given either choline or piracetam separately.[46]

Since nutrients are more powerful in combination, my daily brain plan, in addition to a healthy diet and basic supplement program, consists of taking a teaspoon of hiPC lecithin every day, plus a combination of the following mind- and memory-enhancing nutrients, which can be found in combination supplements.

Nutrient	Daily amount
Phosphatidylcholine	250–400 mg
DMAE	200–300 mg
Phosphatidylserine	20–45 mg
Arginine pyroglutamate	300–450 mg

| Ginkgo | 200–300 mg |
| Vinpocetine | 10–20 mg |

Plus B vitamins including:

Niacin (B3)	10–15 mg
B12	10–30 mcg
Pantothenic acid	200–300 mg
B6	25–50 mg
Folic acid	200–400 mcg

If you are over 50 or suffering from age-related memory decline I recommend you add the following every day:

Phosphatidylserine	100 mg
DHA	250 mg
TMG	1,000 mg
Glutamine powder	5,000 mg (one heaping teaspoon)

SUMMARY

In summary, here are some important tips to enhance your memory, in addition to the diet and supplement recommendations in Part 1:

- Add a heaping teaspoon of lecithin high in phosphatidyl-choline to your cereal each morning, 2 teaspoons of regular lecithin, or supplement the phospholipids phosphatidylserine and phosphatidylcholine.

- Supplement a brain nutrient formula containing the nutrients and herbs listed above, and a methylation nutrient complex if your homocysteine level is high.

- Learn something new every day. Keep your brain active. If you don't use it, you lose it.

The nutrients above are your first line of defense against memory decline. There are some other smart nutrients, drugs, and hormones that have proven memory-boosting effects. These are discussed in Part 7, "Mental Health in Old Age," because they are most effective later in life and for reversing more serious memory deficit diseases such as Alzheimer's.

CHAPTER 15

Beating the blues

Depression isn't a disease that you've either got or you haven't. We are all somewhere along a sliding scale that ranges from generally happy to completely depressed. Officially, 3 million people in Britain, or one in 20, are depressed, with three times as many women suffering as men. They swallow 20 million antidepressants every week, take 80 million days off work each year because of it, and cost the nation between $4.9 billion and $8.2 billion.

But many more people feel blue a lot of the time. The ONUK survey, carried out by the Institute for Optimum Nutrition and involving 37,000 people in Britain, found that as many as one in three people say they sometimes or frequently feel depressed and suffer from low moods.[47] Perhaps you are one of them. This number goes up in the winter as millions suffer from SAD—seasonal affective disorder, commonly known as the winter blues.

A small proportion of people may slide into deeper depression, and cry uncontrollably, lose their appetite, or have suicidal thoughts. People under this kind of pressure are more likely to go to their doctor to seek help, where they may be diagnosed with clinical depression, a subject I'll go into in more detail in Part 5.

Many of us sell ourselves short on mood. We may be consistently quite low, but would never consider ourselves depressed or go to the doctor for treatment. Unless you feel relatively consistently happy and motivated the odds are you can improve how you feel, just as the last two chapters explained how you can improve how you think. Check yourself out on the questionnaire below to see if there's room for improvement.

❓ MOOD CHECK

Score 1 for each *yes* answer.

☐ Do you often feel downhearted or sad?

☐ Do you often feel worse in the morning?

☐ Do you find it difficult to face the day?

☐ Do you sometimes have crying spells, or feel like it?

☐ Do you have trouble falling asleep, or sleeping through the night?

☐ Is your appetite, or desire to eat, poor?

☐ Are you losing weight without trying?

☐ Do you feel unattractive and unlovable?

☐ Do you shun company and prefer to be alone?

☐ Do you often feel fearful?

☐ Are you often irritable or angry?

☐ Do you find it difficult to make decisions?

☐ Is it an effort to motivate yourself to do the things you used to do?

☐ Do you feel hopeless about the future?

☐ Do you feel less enjoyment from activities that once gave you pleasure?

If your score is:

Below 5: You are basically normal, even if you do occasionally feel a bit blue. Following the advice in this chapter will help keep your mood good and balanced.

5–10: Your mood needs a boost. The advice in this chapter will help improve how you feel.

10 or more: You are depressed and could do with some help. As well as following the advice in this chapter, read Chapter 23 and consider seeing both a clinical nutritionist and a psychotherapist.

Depression: anger without enthusiasm?

If your mood is often low there are two avenues to explore—your mind frame and your chemistry. Many people taking antidepressants really need to deal with something that isn't working in their life. For example, depression is often anger, without enthusiasm. Ask yourself honestly whether you are angry about something. Make a list. Maybe there's a relationship that didn't work out, a job that's selling you short, a dream that didn't come true. Much of grief is often anger, but if you were brought up unable to express anger, you may be bottling it up inside in the form of depression. You may be depressed because you have unfinished business.

Many people become depressed because they are betraying themselves. Ask yourself in what way you are betraying yourself, not living your life true to who you are or who you could be. Does your work, your relationship, your life give you the opportunity to express yourself and your true feelings?

If all this is ringing big bells, you may benefit greatly from seeing a psychotherapist or counselor or doing a life-enhancing course. My favorites are listed in the Useful Addresses section on page 484. You may also benefit from tuning up your brain and neurotransmitters because your mood and motivation isn't only in your mind, it's in the chemistry of your mind.

Anatomy of low mood and motivation

One of the greatest unrecognized truths is that ensuring optimum nutrition for your mind not only improves mood, but gives you the energy and motivation to make changes in your life. Few psychotherapists recognize how much better their results would be if they helped their clients tune up their brain biochemistry.

These are the common imbalances connected to nutrition that can worsen your mood and motivation:

- Blood-sugar imbalances (often associated with excessive sugar and stimulant intake)

- Deficiencies of nutrients (vitamins B6, B12, folic acid, C, zinc, magnesium, chromium, essential fatty acids)

- Deficiencies of tryptophan and tyrosine (precursors of neurotransmitters)

- Allergies and sensitivities.

One factor that underlies most depression is poor control of blood-glucose levels. Keeping blood-sugar levels more even can be achieved by eating small regular meals of natural, unprocessed foods, including protein and fiber at each one, and taking a combination of B vitamins and the mineral chromium. All this is explained in Chapter 3.

The most promising nutrients for improving mood are vitamins B6, B12, and folic acid; the minerals zinc, chromium, and magnesium; and essential fatty acids (EFAs). The first three are involved in the vital biochemical process known as methylation, which is critical for balancing the neurotransmitters dopamine and adrenalin. The most powerful methylating nutrient is called SAMe and it's also well proven as an antidepressant (see page 157). Vitamin B6 and zinc are also needed to correct a common biochemical imbalance that can promote low moods, called pyroluria (more on this in Chapter 26). Giving vitamin C in large amounts has also been proven to enhance recovery from depression.[48]

Chemical blues

There are often two sides to feeling blue—feeling miserable, and feeling apathetic and unmotivated. The most prevalent theory for the cause of these imbalances is a brain imbalance in two families of neurotransmitters, the molecules of emotion. These are:

- Serotonin, which influences your mood

- Adrenalin and noradrenalin, made from dopamine, which influence your motivation.

All the major antidepressant drugs are designed to influence the balance and function of these neurotransmitters. These include serotonin reuptake inhibitors (SSRIs) such as Prozac, Lustral, and Seroxat, which are designed to keep serotonin in circulation; adrenalin reuptake inhibitors such as Edronax; a noradrenalin reuptake inhibitor (NARI), designed to keep adrenalin in circulation; monoamine oxidase inhibitors, which help maintain adrenalin and dopamine levels; and the tricyclic antidepressants such as amitriptyline which also prevent adrenalin breakdown. As the patents for the major SSRI drugs are running out, a new family of antidepressants is being heavily promoted: the serotonin and noradrenalin reuptake inhibitiors (SNRIs), marketed under brand names such as Effexor and Cymbalta. We have no guarantees that they will be more effective or safer than the others. Meanwhile, all of these neurotransmitters are directly influenced by nutrition.[49]

The major focus of attention has been on noradrenalin/adrenalin and serotonin. To test the theory that serotonin primarily controlled mood, and adrenalin and noradrenalin control motivation, Antonella Dubini from the Pharmacia and Upjohn Medical Department in Milan, Italy, gave 203 people suffering from low mood and motivation either an SSRI drug, promoting serotonin, or a NARI drug, promoting noradrenalin. Sure enough, the former was more effective at improving mood, while the latter was more effective at improving motivation.[50]

If this theory is correct, that low mood is often a serotonin-deficiency symptom, and that low motivation is an adrenalin/noradrenalin-deficiency symptom, then that begs two questions. Why are some people deficient and which nutrients would correct these deficiencies?

I believe that, for many people, the pace of life and the speed at which we are having to adapt and change is stressing us out. The brain responds by producing more and more adrenalin and serotonin in response to our too frequent ups and downs, stresses and strains. This is akin to the body producing more and more insulin to even out frequently fluctuating blood-sugar levels. This increases our need for the building blocks, the nutrients from which we make these mood-enhancing neurotransmitters. So we end up suboptimally nourished in the nutrients from which we make these neurotransmitters—partly because our diets are inadequate and partly because our demand for these nutrients is higher. Just as the stress of pollution increases our need for vitamin C, the stress of life increases our demand for tryptophan.

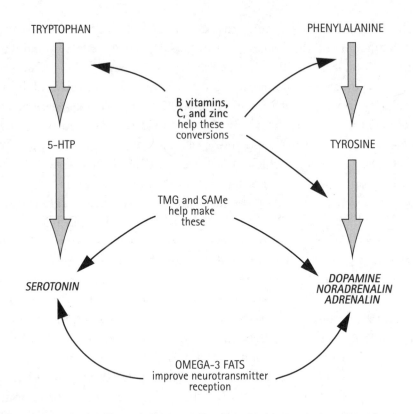

Fig 21. Nutrients that make mood-enhancing neurotransmitters

The figure above shows those nutrients that are needed for the brain and body to make enough serotonin, adrenalin, and noradrenalin.

Depression in women

Women are three times as prone to low moods as men. Many theories as to why this is have been proposed, some psychological, some social, but the truth is that women and men are biochemically very different. The research of Mirko Diksic and colleagues at McGill University in Montreal, Canada, demonstrates this. They developed a technique using PET neuro-imaging to measure the rate at which we make serotonin in the brain.[51] What they found was that men's average synthesis rate of serotonin was 52 percent higher than women. This, and other research, has clearly shown that women are more prone to low serotonin. They also react differently. In women, low serotonin is associated with depression and anxiety, while in men, low serotonin is related to aggression and alcoholism. One possibility is our social conditioning: men *act out* their moods, while women are more conditioned to *act in* their moods. Another example of depression being the flip side of anger.

What has been learned about serotonin in the last few years is that there are six main reasons for deficiency, in addition to a lack of tryptophan:

- Not enough estrogen (in women)

- Not enough testosterone (in men)

- Not enough light

- Not enough exercise

- Too much stress, especially in women

- Not enough co-factor vitamins and minerals

- Blood-sugar imbalances.

If you are suffering from low mood, feel tense and irritable, are low in energy, tend to comfort eat, have sleeping problems and a reduced interest in sex, and the above apply to you, the chances are you are short on serotonin.

Low estrogen means low serotonin and low moods.[52-53] This is because estrogen blocks the breakdown of serotonin. This may largely explain why women are more prone to depression premenstrually and in menopause and thereafter. Low testosterone has a similar effect in men (see Chapter 16.)

Light stimulates estrogen and most of us don't get enough of it. The difference in light exposure outside and inside is massive. Most of us spend 23 out of 24 hours a day indoors, exposed to an average of 100 units (called lux) of light. That's compared to 20,000 lux on a sunny day and 7,000 lux on an overcast day. Now, more than ever before, many of us rarely expose ourselves to direct sunlight, and certainly not enough to maximize serotonin production. Of course, light deficiency is worse in the winter.

Stress also rapidly reduces serotonin levels. Physical exercise improves stress response, and therefore reduces stress-induced depletion of serotonin.

Each of these reasons for serotonin depletion affects women more than men. Men produce serotonin twice as fast as women, allowing them to rebalance from any of these serotonin depleters, without prolonged blues, provided there's enough tryptophan in their diet.

Now we need to take a closer look at both serotonin and tryptophan.

The blues busters

Is depression a tryptophan deficiency?

Antidepressant drugs like Prozac work by stopping the body from breaking down the neurotransmitter serotonin, therefore keeping more circulating in the brain. The trouble is that these kinds of drugs induce unpleasant side effects in about a quarter of those who take them and severe reactions in a minority, the most worrying of which is an increased risk of suicide (see Chapter 22). The natural alternative is to eat your way to happiness by choosing foods from which the body makes serotonin.

Serotonin is made from a constituent of protein, the amino acid tryptophan. Dr. Philip Cowen from Oxford University's psychiatry department wondered what would happen if you deprived people of tryptophan. He gave 15 volunteers who had a history of depression, but were currently fine, a nutritionally balanced drink that excluded tryptophan. Within seven hours 10 out of 15 noticed a worsening of their mood and started to show signs of depression. On being given the same drink, but this time with tryptophan added, their mood improved.[54] Fish, turkey, chicken, cheese, beans, tofu, oats, and eggs are particularly rich in tryptophan.

Supplementing tryptophan is already well proven to improve mood. Donald Ecclestone, professor of medicine at the Royal Victoria Infirmary in Newcastle in the U.K. reviewed the available studies and concluded that supplementing tryptophan leads to an increase in the synthesis of serotonin in the brain, improving mood as well as some antidepressant drugs. You need 1g for low mood, and up to 3g a day for actual depression, taken either on an empty stomach or preferably with a carbohydrate food such as fruit, since carbohydrates help its absorption. Tryptophan promotes sleep, so it's best taken before bed.

As well as supplementing tryptophan, make sure your diet gives you at least 1g a day by eating any two of the following meals, each giving 500 mg of tryptophan.

Five ways to eat 500 mg of tryptophan

Oatmeal, soy milk and two scrambled eggs
Baked potato with cottage cheese and tuna salad
Chicken breast, potatoes *au gratin*, and green beans
Wholewheat spaghetti with bean, tofu, or meat sauce
Salmon filet, quinoa and lentil pilaf, and green salad with yogurt dressing

---

However, ironically, eating a meal containing tryptophan doesn't raise bain levels of tryptophan as high as eating a carbohydrate meal does. This anomaly was discovered by Professor Richard Wurtman at the Massachusetts Institute of Technology. He fed people standard American high-protein breakfasts versus high-carbohydrate breakfasts and found that only the latter caused increases in brain serotonin levels, despite containing no tryptophan![55] The reason for this anomaly is that tryptophan in the bloodstream competes very badly with all the other amino acids in protein, so little gets across into the brain. However, when you eat a carbohydrate food such as a banana, this causes insulin to be released into the bloodstream, from which it carries tryptophan into the brain.

This may be why depressed people instinctly crave sweet foods to give them a lift. This causes a surge of insulin, which carries tryptophan into the brain, causing serotonin levels to rise! So, if you find sugar gives you a mood lift, you are probably low in serotonin. The trouble is, most carbohydrate snacks are high in refined sugar and fat, and make you fat, which is depressing. The solution is to supplement tryptophan with carbohydrate. This not only improves your mood, but also will reduce your appetite, especially for sugary foods. That's why tryptophan can also help you lose weight. Tryptophan's link with carbohydrate also explains why some people feel more depressed on a high-protein diet, and why most feel a boost in mood on a low-GL diet, which emphasizes eating the very best carbohydrates for blood-sugar balance. In our own research, one in two people on the Holford Low-GL Diet report fewer feelings of depression and more stable mood.[56]

The tryptophan controversy

So why don't we supplement tryptophan? Thousands of people did, up to 1989, with tremendous results both for depression and for promoting sleep (see Chapter 18). And, in doses of 1,000–3,000 mg, it worked. Tryptophan is an important building block not just for serotonin but also for melatonin (the sleep hormone). Taken one hour before bedtime, it promotes sleep. And 1,000 mg taken once in the morning and once in the evening (in between meals, with a carbohydrate snack such as fruit) helps relieve depression.

But in 1989, disaster struck. Hundreds of people taking tryptophan supplements mysteriously developed a condition called eosinophilia-myalgia syndrome (EMS), resulting in 37 deaths. Tryptophan was immediately withdrawn from the market. A long and thorough investigation determined that the culprit was a contaminated or altered tryptophan molecule that contained something called *peak x*. The contamination occurred when a Japanese company used a new production technology that involved genetically altering a yeast to produce tryptophan. It was one of the first blunders of genetic modification, resulting in unexpected deaths. The mystery was solved.

Despite this finding, tryptophan remained banned in the U.S. and many other countries. Five years ago at ION, we started searching through every reported case of EMS and proved to the British government that they could all be linked to the contaminated batch of tryptophan—thus showing that the pure amino acid tryptophan is not at all toxic. In fact, despite the ban on tryptophan supplements, drug companies in the U.K. and the U.S. have continued to sell prescription forms of tryptophan and no cases of EMS have been reported.

In November last year, thanks to the ION report, the British government rescinded the ban on tryptophan in the U.K. Quite rightly, the requirement for the removal of the ban was that companies could only sell pure, pharmaceutical-grade tryptophan. The same applies in the U.S.. However, you probably won't see tryptophan supplements on the shelves at your health food store. That's because of insurance. Even though tryptophan itself is remarkably safe and effective, its tarnished history classifies it as a high insurance risk and most liability insurance policies won't cover it.

Another way to serotonin: 5-HTP

While supplementing tryptophan itself has proven an effective blues buster, even more effective is a derivative of tryptophan that is one step closer to serotonin. This is called 5-hydroxytryptophan, or 5-HTP for short, and is derived from an African plant called griffonia. The first study proving the mood-boosting power of 5-HTP was done in the 1970s in Japan, under the direction of Professor Isamu Sano of the Osaka University Medical School.[57] He gave 107 patients 50–300 mg of 5-HTP per day, and within two weeks, more than half experienced improvements in their symptoms. By the end of the four weeks of the study, nearly three-quarters of the patients reported either complete relief or significant improvement, with no side effects. This study was repeated by other researchers who also found that 69 percent of patients improved their mood.[58]

To date there have been 27 studies of 5-HTP, involving 990 people, most of which have proved positive.[59] So how does 5-HTP compare with antidepressants? Eleven of the trials were double-blind placebo controlled, and six of those measured depression using the Hamilton Rating Scale, which is one of the most widely used psychological tests for depression. SSRI antidepressant drugs generally produce around a 15 percent improvement using this test. The 5-HTP studies differed in design, so you cannot just add up the scores to get an average, but the improvement shown in them rated 13, 30, 34, 39, 40, 56, and 61 percent. It doesn't take a scientist to realize these results are a lot better than the average for antidepressant drugs, with a fraction of the side effects.

One double-blind trial, for example, headed by Dr. Walter Poldinger at Basel University in Switzerland, gave 34 depressed volunteers either the SSRI antidepressant fluvoxamine, or 300 mg of 5-HTP. Each patient was assessed for their degree of depression using the Hamilton Rating Scale, plus their own subjective self-assessment. At the end of the six weeks, both groups of patients had had a significant improvement in their depression. However, those taking 5-HTP had a greater improvement in each of the four criteria assessed—depression, anxiety, insomnia, and physical symptoms, as well as the patient's self-assessment.[60]

While previous studies had shown 5-HTP to be as effective as the tricyclic antidepressant imipramine,[61] in this study 5-HTP had outperformed an SSRI antidepressant. Given that 5-HTP is less expensive and has significantly fewer side effects, it is extraordinary that psychiatrists, despite plenty of scientific evidence that it helps restore normal mood and normal serotonin levels, virtually never prescribe it.[62]

What about potential down sides? Since in some sensitive people, antidepressant drugs can induce an overload of serotonin called serotonin syndrome—characterized by feeling overheated, with high blood pressure, twitching, cramping, dizziness, and disorientation—some concern has been expressed about the possibility of increasing the odds of developing serotonin syndrome with the combination of 5-HTP and an SSRI drug. However, a recent review on the safety of 5-HTP concludes that "serotonin syndrome has not been reported in humans in association with 5-HTP, either as monotherapy [on its own] or in combination with other medications."[63] Even so, I don't recommend you supplement this nutrient if you are currently taking SSRI medication.

The recommended dosage of this natural supplement, available in any health food store, is 50–100 mg of 5-HTP, twice a day, for depression. In studies, amounts above 300 mg a day are not generally more effective. Some supplements also provide various vitamins and minerals such as vitamin B3, B6, and folic acid, which may be even more effective because these nutrients help to turn 5-HTP into serotonin. A small percentage of people, less than 5 percent, experience nausea on 5-HTP, especially the first time they take it. This is because 5-HTP can be converted into serotonin in the gut, as well as in the brain. Since there are serotonin receptors in the gut, which don't normally expect to get the real thing so easily, they can overreact if the amount is too high, and nausea can result. If so, just lower the dose. Your body soon adjusts. This effect can be minimized, and the absorption of 5-HTP greatly maximized, by taking your 5-HTP supplement with a carbohydrate food such as an oatmeal cookie or a piece of fruit.

If you get very sleepy on 5-HTP, you probably don't need it. The same applies with tryptophan. 5-HTP is best absorbed on an empty stomach.

Is apathy a tyrosine deficiency?

Another neurotransmitter deficiency associated with depression and lack of motivation is adrenalin and its brother, noradrenalin. As you can see in Figure 22, adrenalin and noradrenalin are made from a neurotransmitter called dopamine, which is made from the amino acid tyrosine, which is itself made from the amino acid phenylalanine. Now that we understand the family tree of adrenalin, it is logical to assume that, if drugs that block the breakdown of these neurotransmitters do elevate mood, albeit with undesirable side effects, then supplementing the amino acid phenylalanine or tyrosine might work too. And it does.

In a double-blind study by Helmut Beckmann and colleagues at the University of Wurzburg, Germany, 150–200 mg of the amino acid phenylalanine, or the antidepressant drug imipramine, were administered to 40 depressed patients for one month. Both groups had the same degree of positive results—less depression, anxiety, and sleep disturbance.[64] A group of researchers at the Rush Medical Center, Chicago, screened depressed patients by testing phenythylamine in the blood; low levels mean you need more phenylalanine. They then gave 40 depressed patients supplements of phenylalanine, and 31 of them improved.[65]

Tyrosine has been shown to work well in those with dopamine-

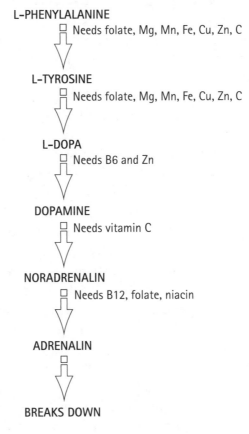

Fig 22. The catecholamine pathway

dependent depression. In a pilot study administering 3,200 mg tyrosine a day to 12 patients at the Hopital du Vinatier, France, a significant improvement in mood and sleep was observed on the very first day.[66]

The military has long known that tyrosine improves mental and physical performance under stress. Recent research from the Netherlands demonstrates how tyrosine gives you the edge in conditions of stress. Twenty-one cadets were put through a demanding one-week military combat training course. Ten cadets were given a drink containing 2g of tyrosine a day, while the remaining 11 were given an identical drink without the tyrosine. Those on tyrosine consistently performed better, both in memorizing the task at hand and in tracking the tasks they had performed.[67]

However, giving people a tyrosine and phenylalanine-free diet doesn't induce depression in the same way taking tryptophan out can do.[68] This suggests that tyrosine or phenylalanine deficiency is unlikely to be a common cause of depression. So, these amino acids on their own are not as potent as 5-HTP.

Of course, the big question is, how do you know what's going to work for you? A more scientific approach would be to check whether depressed patients actually had an imbalance in their neurotransmitters, and if so, exactly which were low so they could be given a boost. But that is not what happens. Instead, the diagnosis of depression is based solely on a checklist of psychological symptoms, which doesn't tell you anything about what is going on with brain or indeed body chemistry.

In fact, it has taken a nutritionally minded doctor to take this obvious scientific step. Professor Tapan Audhya from New York University Medical Center in the U.S. first showed that the level of serotonin found in platelets, tiny disclike bodies in the blood, correlates with the level of these neurotransmitters in the brain.[69] Next he investigated whether people with depression do actually have abnormal levels of platelet serotonin by measuring platelet levels in 52 normal and 74 depressed volunteers. The difference was striking. In 73 percent of the people suffering from depression, serotonin levels were barely a fifth of those in the participants who weren't depressed.[70]

Knowing that this neurotransmitter is made directly from amino acids found in food, Audhya then gave his patients 5-hydroxytryptophan (5-HTP), the amino acid from which serotonin is made. This corrected the deficiency and resulted in major and rapid relief from depression.[71] In two-thirds of them, noradrenalin levels were also very low and these people did respond to tyrosine supplementation.

When it comes to treating depression or any other chronic condition, nutrition is a real alternative because it is based on finding out what is actually going on in the patient's system and then sorting out any specific imbalances. That makes a lot more sense, and is far more scientific, than giving millions of people precisely the same chemical regardless of what is actually wrong with them. So in addition to the Hamilton Rating Scale, anyone trying to find out the root cause of depression needs to take blood and urine tests to discover:

- Serotonin and noradrenalin levels—do they need boosting?

- Your homocysteine level—is it too high?

- Essential fats—are your levels high enough?

- Blood-sugar balance—is yours within the healthy range?

B vitamins that boost mood

The best results of all are usually achieved by supplementing the right balance of all the amino acids we've looked at—5-HTP, phenylalanine, and tyrosine—depending on a person's imbalances, together with the B vitamins that help turn them into neurotransmitters, which are B6, B12, and folic acid. These three B vitamins are the catalysts that help balance the brain's neurotransmitters—and there's plenty of evidence that deficiency in vitamin B12, and especially in folic acid, can lead to depression, which I'll be discussing in detail in Part 5. The best way to know if you are getting enough for your mood is to measure your homocysteine level (see Chapter 8), as this will determine your ideal amount of these B vitamins. A good starting point is to make sure that your diet contains the foods listed in Chapter 8 and that your daily supplement program contains at least 400 mcg of folic acid, 10 mcg of B12, and 20 mg of B6.

SAMe and TMG: the master tuners

We have already encountered these two strange-sounding nutrients; now let's see how they affect depression. SAMe (s-adenosyl methionine) and TMG (trimethylglycine) are both amino acids that are vital for methylation. They help to keep the brain and nervous system well tuned by donating methyl groups. For example, noradrenalin turns into adrenalin by having a methyl group added. This process of adding on methyl groups, and sometimes taking them away, is critical to keeping the brain in balance, and it's this balancing act that the B vitamins B6, B12, and folic acid support. In fact, as you'll see in Chapter 25, many people with schizophrenia go crazy because their brains don't do this properly. These nutrients, plus B vitamins, can make all the difference.

SAMe is one of the most comprehensively studied natural antidepressants. Over 100 placebo-controlled, double-blind studies show that SAMe is equal to or superior to antidepressants, and works faster, most often within a few days (most pharmaceutical antidepressants may take three to six weeks to take effect) and with few side effects.[72–74] (As with all antidepressants, there is a small risk of a rapid switch to mania in bipolar disorder with SAMe, so it should be used under supervision in these cases.)

Instead of side effects, SAMe has side benefits, including being an effective treatment for degenerative joint disease, fibromyalgia, and liver problems. According to one comprehensive review of all the studies, 92 percent of depressive patients responded to SAMe, compared with 85 percent for the medications.[75]

You need 200–600 mg a day, but the trouble is it's been classified as a medicine in the European Union, which effectively means it's banned and no longer available in health food stores. You can get it in other countries, or for your own use on the Internet. SAMe is quite expensive and not very stable, so make sure you get it in the form of butanedisulfonate, which is more stable. Buy it and keep it refrigerated.

An alternative that is much more stable and less costly is TMG. In the body it turns into SAMe, but you need to supplement three times as much. Try supplementing 600–2,000 mg a day, again on an empty stomach or with fruit. Together with B6, B12, and folic acid, your body can then make its own SAMe.

Mood-boosting fats

We've already encountered omega-3 fish oils. They are not just essential for building and rebuilding your brain—they're also very much part of the equation for happiness. The higher your blood levels of omega-3 fats, the higher your levels of serotonin are likely to be. The reason for this is that omega-3 fats help build receptor sites, as well as improve reception. According to Dr. J.R. Hibbeln, who discovered that fisheaters are less prone to depression, "It's like building more serotonin factories, instead of just increasing the efficiency of the serotonin you have."[76] A recent survey is Norway found the same thing. Those who consumed cod liver oil had the lowest incidence of depression, and the longer a person had been taking it the less likely they were to be depressed.[77]

There have been six double-blind, placebo-controlled trials to date giving fish oils rich in omega-3s to depressed people. In five of them, the findings showed significant improvement.[78] The first trial by Dr. Andrew Stoll from Harvard Medical School, published in *The Archives of General Psychiatry*, gave 40 depressed patients either omega-3 supplements or a placebo and found a highly significant improvement in the patients on supplements. In the next, published in the *American Journal of Psychiatry*, 20 people suffering from severe depression, who were already on antidepressants but still depressed, were given either a highly concentrated form of omega-3 fat, ethyl-EPA, or a placebo. By the third week the depressed patients taking ethyl-EPA were showing major improvement in their mood, while those on the placebo were not.[79]

Frangou study

The latest trial, by Dr. Sophia Frangou from the Institute of Psychiatry in London, gave a concentrated form of EPA or a placebo to 26 depressed people with bipolar disorder (also known as manic depression) and again found a significant improvement in those taking the EPA.[80] In the studies that used the Hamilton Rating Scale, including one recent open trial that did not involve the use of placebos, the average improvement in depression was approximately double that shown by antidepressant drugs, without the side effects.

So how do the omega-3s do it? It may be because these essential fatty acids help to build your brain's neuronal connections as well as the receptor sites for neurotransmitters. So the more omega-3s in your blood, the more serotonin you are likely to make, and the more responsive you become to its effects.

In this context it's EPA, rather than DHA, that seems to be the most potent mood-boosting omega 3, with amounts of 1,000 mg or more proving most effective. This means supplementing the equivalent of two high-EPA 1g fish oil capsules a day, and eating oily fish three times a week.

Marvelous minerals

Omega-3 fats are not the only nutrients found to be lacking in people suffering from depression. The minerals chromium and magnesium have also been found to be very low in depressed people, and studies looking at supplementing these two minerals to help relieve depression have shown some excellent results. As you'll see, chromium is most helpful for people with atypical depression. This describes a set of symptoms that include feeling tired a lot of the time, needing a lot of sleep, gaining weight, craving carbohydrates, and experiencing fluctuating moods and emotional sensitivity. If this sounds like you, read Chapter 23 to discover chromium's amazing mood-boosting effects.

Let there be light

If you are particularly prone to the winter blues, technically known as Seasonal Affective Disorder (SAD), all the above will help, but there's one more nutrient you'll need: light. The main reason for feeling blue in the winter, according to research from the Baker Heart Research Institute in Melbourne, Australia, published in *The Lancet*, is that serotonin levels in the brain are lowest in winter and that the amount of serotonin our brains produce is directly related to how much daylight we are exposed to.[81] So, with shorter days and less light, people with SAD can really suffer. Some people, especially women, are prone to low levels of serotonin anyway, and a relative lack of light can tip them over the edge into full-blown depression.

For these people, the symptoms of SAD usually recur regularly each winter and may include sleep problems, lethargy, overeating, social problems, anxiety, loss of libido, and mood changes. Most sufferers show signs of a weakened immune system during the winter, and are more vulnerable to infections and other illnesses.

So, how do you get more winter light without heading to the Southern Hemisphere? All it involves is buying a 60-watt light bulb. Then do the exercise described on the following page.

Light exercise

Here's a simple exercise you can do with a regular light bulb to increase your serotonin levels.

- Sit down in a quiet place, on the floor or on a chair. It is best to choose a place that you can completely darken. If not, you will need a blindfold.

- Place a table lamp with a 60-watt opaque (not clear) bulb, preferably with no writing on it, 3 feet away and directly in line with your line of vision.

- Make sure you can turn the light on and off without moving your head position.

- Turn the light on and look directly at the bulb for one minute, no longer. (You'll need a timer for this.)

- After one minute, turn the light off, close your eyes (put on your blindfold if the room is not completely dark) and focus on the after-image, the phosphene, without moving your head, until it completely vanishes. This usually takes three to four minutes.

- This exercise is best done at dusk, effectively extending daylight hours.

It is also well worth investing in full-spectrum lighting. Full-spectrum light bulbs have the same quality of light as the sun, determined by the spread of different wavelengths. That's why sunlight, and full-spectrum lighting, appears much whiter than a normal artificial light, which is yellower. Compared to ordinary bulbs, full-spectrum bulbs, although more expensive to start with, last 10 times longer and use a quarter of the electricity. (See the Product and Supplement Directory on page 486.)

Melatonin, another tryptophan-derived brain chemical, helps balance the brain in the absence of light. Supplementing melatonin has also proven helpful for those with SAD.

Move to boost your mood

Exercise plays a key part in beating the blues. In fact, it turns out to be as effective as taking antidepressants. A number of studies in which people exercised for 30–60 minutes 3–5 times a week found a drop of around 5 points in their Hamilton Rating Scale—more than double what you'd expect from antidepressants alone.[82] In an Australian study published in 2005 and involving 60 adults over the age of 60, half took up high-intensity exercise three days a week, while the other half did low-intensity exercise. Of those doing high-intensity exercise, 61 percent halved their score on the Hamilton Rating Scale, while only 29 percent of those doing low-intensity exercise halved their score.[83]

And if you exercise in bright light, you get a double dose of natural antidepressant, as a number of studies using full-spectrum lighting (versus normal room lighting) have shown. In one study published in 2004, a third of depressed volunteers who exercised in full-spectrum lighting experienced a major improvement (a 50 percent or more decrease on the Hamilton Rating Scale).[84] Other studies from 2005 have also found a definitive improvement, even among those not specifically prone to SAD.[85] The effect could be due to the direct effect of light on raising serotonin.[86]

Good-mood foods and supplements

If you want to eat your way to happiness, the key is to follow a diet that keeps your blood-sugar level even and provides plenty of tryptophan, phenylalanine, B vitamins, and omega-3 fats. It's also worth supplementing these nutrients, and they can be found together in some supplements.

SUMMARY

In summary, what this means, in addition to the basics outlined in Part 1 including omega-3 fats, is supplementing:

- 2g of phenylalanine or tyrosine, or 1g of both.

- 1.5g of tryptophan or 150 mg of 5-HTP.

- A good multivitamin providing all the B vitamins, including 20 mg of B6, 10 mcg of B12, and 400 mcg of folic acid, plus 100 mg of magnesium and 40 mcg of chromium.

- Either 200 mg of SAMe or 600 mg of TMG.

▶

All these can be found together in some supplements. Combinations are the most effective, but if you choose to take them separately, phenylalanine or tyrosine are best taken in the morning, before breakfast, because they increase motivation. Tryptophan and 5-HTP are best taken in the evening because they help promote a good night's sleep. All these amino acids are best absorbed away from main meals, but with a small amount of carbohydrate, such as a piece of fruit or an oatmeal cookie.

However, there are other causes for low moods, and other cures for depression. These include hormonal imbalances, which are discussed in the next chapter, and can be helped by herbs such as St. John's wort. These are also discussed more fully in Chapter 23, which explores nutritional solutions to chronic depression, rather than low moods.

CHAPTER 16

Balancing out hormonal mood swings

A common reason for mood swings is a hormone imbalance. This doesn't just affect women and it isn't only related to pre-menstrual syndrome. Hormones are little different from neurotransmitters. They are both chemicals of communication that tell the body and brain cells how to behave. If out of balance, your mood goes out of balance too.

Here are the common imbalances that wreak havoc on how you feel:

- **Estrogen and progesterone deficiency** in menopause, for example, can cause depression.

- **Testosterone deficiency** in both men and women can cause depression, loss of motivation, and sex drive.

- **Testosterone excess** can lead to hyperactivity and aggression.

- **DHEA deficiency** can lead to depression and loss of motivation.

- **High estrogen and low progesterone** can lead to pre-menstrual syndrome, with cyclic depression and anxiety.

- **Melatonin** deficiency can lead to depression and insomnia (see Chapter 18).

- **Deficiency of thyroxine**, the hormone of the thyroid gland, can cause depression and lack of motivation (see Chapter 23), while excess can lead to hyperactivity and even mania.

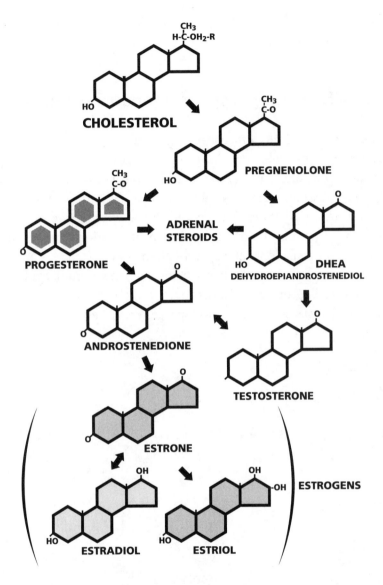

Fig 23. The family tree of steroid hormones

All of these hormones are produced in both men and women. Unlike the neurotransmitters we've spoken about already, which are made from protein, these hormones, with the exception of melatonin and thyroxine, are made from fat (stearic acid) and are thus called steroid hormones.

That's why people on very low fat diets often develop hormonal imbalances. We need essential fats for the body to make its own cholesterol, from which it can make all these hormones. Figure 23 shows the family tree of all these hormones.

Banishing the premenstrual blues

More than a third of all menstruating women suffer from premenstrual syndrome (PMS), with 10 percent suffering severely. Common symptoms include depression, anxiety, irritability, fluid retention, mood swings, bloating, breast tenderness, weight gain, acne, fatigue, sweet cravings, and forgetfulness, most often experienced in the week before menstruation and stopping within hours of the start of the period. Some women get symptoms at ovulation, halfway through their cycle.

As you can see from the figure below, these two times, ovulation and the days leading up to menstruation, are the times when there are the greatest changes in estrogen and progesterone levels. It's the balance

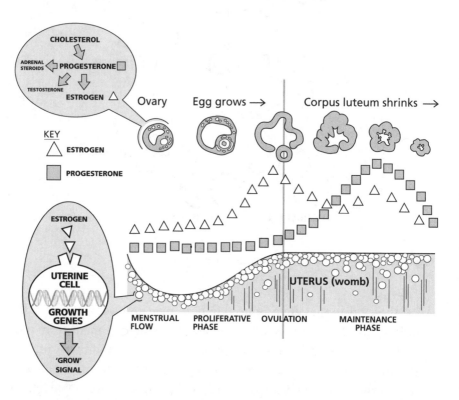

Figure 24. Hormone levels in a normal menstrual cycle

between these hormones that is thought to be mainly responsible for the symptoms of PMS. The less adaptive capacity you've got, the worse you respond to these hormonal changes and others, such as the drop-off in estrogen and progesterone at menopause and the equivalent drop-off in testosterone at the male menopause. Yes, men have a menopause too—it's called andropause.

If you're deficient in vitamins, lacking in essential fats, and have poor blood-sugar control, you are likely to suffer with mood swings when your hormones go up and down. Stress is also a big factor which can upset hormonal balance. So the first tip to banishing those monthly blues is to follow the advice in Parts 1 and 2 of this book.

There are also different kinds of PMS. Some women get breast tenderness and water retention, some don't. Some get food cravings, some don't. Breast tenderness, probably a symptom of water retention, can be helped by supplementing 300 mg of magnesium a day, plus 100 mg of vitamin B6, which is a natural diuretic. It is also wise to avoid salt, although there is one high in magnesium and potassium, and low-sodium salt called Solo, which is OK.

Women suffering from PMS often crave high-sugar, high-calorie foods. These are almost certainly linked to hypoglycemia, so stabilize blood-sugar levels by avoiding sugar and stimulants throughout the month and grazing on slow-releasing carbohydrates, with some protein. They may also be connected to serotonin deficiency, corrected by increasing your intake of tryptophan or 5-HTP.

An overload of estrogen?

An estimated 75 percent of PMS sufferers have high estrogen levels in relation to progesterone. This may be partly due to our exposure to so many estrogen-mimicking chemicals, found in anything from detergents, plastics, and pesticides, and to stress, which raises estrogen levels. The antidote is optimum nutrition, with the right supplements. One study found that taking B6 in the range of 200–800 mg reduced blood estrogen, increased progesterone, and reduced symptoms in a clinical trial.[87] A simple saliva test can help identify whether you are estrogen dominant.

Following all the recommendations in this book, including eating organically grown produce, reducing consumption of high-fat meat and dairy produce, and eating foods rich in phytoestrogens such as beans and lentils, especially soy, can help balance excess estrogen. Paradoxical as it sounds, phytoestrogens lower excessive estrogen signals in the body, and raise very low levels, as found in menopause. They do this by blocking the estrogen receptors, thereby preventing all those harmful estrogen-mimicking chemicals from wreaking havoc. They are very weak estrogens themselves, so they have little impact on overloading or imbalancing the system. These plant-based phytoestrogens are best thought of as hormone regulators.

Too much estrogen has many effects in the body that could explain an increased risk of mood swings and depression. High levels of the stress hormone cortisol are associated with depression and anxiety. Estrogen stops the body breaking down cortisol, hence prolonging its effects. This may explain why women tend to be more greatly affected by stress and traumatic events. Estrogen increases copper levels, and high copper can deplete the body of zinc, while both high copper and low zinc are associated with depression. Zinc also helps vitamin B6 to work, so make sure you supplement at least 15 mg a day if you suffer from PMS.

The four most important nutrients for banishing PMS-related mood swings are vitamin B6, zinc, magnesium, and essential fats. Each have been proven to reduce symptoms of PMS on their own, but they are much more powerful in combination. Researchers at St. Thomas's Hospital in London gave 630 women up to 200 mg of vitamin B6 as long ago as 1976 and found up to 88 percent had a significant improvement in their PMS.[88]

PMS sufferers have been shown to have significantly lower magnesium levels than women who do not have PMS,[89] and French researchers who gave 192 women up to 6g of magnesium daily for the week before and the first two days of their period achieved amazing results—nervous tension was relieved in 89 percent, weight gain in 95 percent, breast tenderness in 96 percent, and headaches in 43 percent of sufferers.[90]

The key, though, may be evening primrose oil (EPO). Numerous studies, including one large open study on women for whom other kinds of PMS therapy had failed, and several double-blind, placebo-controlled trials, have all demonstrated that EPO is a highly effective treatment for the depression and irritability, the breast pain and tenderness, and the fluid retention associated with PMS.[91] Nutrients known to increase the utilization and effectiveness of EPO include, you guessed it, vitamin B6, zinc, and magnesium. So the clinical success obtained with some of these nutrients may in part relate to their effects on EPO (i.e. essential fat) metabolism.

Women with PMS are often deficient in these nutrients, which can help banish mood swings and depression, not only premenstrually, but also during menopause. Some women do benefit from natural progesterone, given as a transdermal skin cream, but I don't recommend this for premenstrual women unless these diet and supplement recommendations haven't worked and a hormone test confirms progesterone deficiency. This can occur because a woman isn't ovulating. When the egg isn't released from the ovum, the ovum no longer produces progesterone in the second half of the cycle, which leads to relative estrogen dominance.

There is a very worrying trend in medicine to treat PMS with antidepressant drugs. While this can help, demonstrating the importance of adequate serotonin in relation to all mood-related problems, in my experience the optimum nutrition approach works better, without the associated risks inherent with these drugs (see Chapter 22). In fact, I have never seen a PMS sufferer who didn't improve dramatically with the right diet and supplements.

Preventing menopausal mood swings and depression

Mental health problems during the menopausal phase are exceedingly common. The most widespread are depression, anxiety, insomnia, and worsening memory. In one survey, 45 percent of women experienced minor depressive symptoms during menopause, while 27 percent complained of nervousness or irritability.

The same nutrients—B6, zinc, magnesium, and essential fats—all greatly help to reduce menopausal symptoms and allow the body to better adapt to changing hormonal levels. Serotonin deficiency is also very common in menopausal women, who often benefit greatly from additional tryptophan or 5-HTP (see Chapter 15).

Menopausal depression and worsening mental acuity can occur due to estrogen and progesterone deficiency. According to John Lee, a doctor from California who pioneered research using natural progesterone, mood, mental clarity, and concentration frequently improve with the use of transdermal progesterone skin creams. Most conventional HRT includes synthetic progestins, sometimes called progestogens. These not only don't work so well, they've been linked to increasing risk of breast cancer.[92]

The good thing about natural progesterone is that the body can also make estrogen from it (follow the arrows in Figure 22). However, that being said, some women find greater relief with both estrogen and natural progesterone therapy. The combination of the two prevents the cancer risks associated with unopposed estrogen.

Andropause and depression in men

The effects of testosterone deficiency are not unlike the effects of estrogen and progesterone deficiency. Around a third of men in the 40–69 age group complain of a range of symptoms that commonly include, in order of importance, loss of libido, erectile dysfunction (inability to get or maintain an erection), depression, and worsening memory and concentration. These are the classic symptoms of andropause.

Despite years of research, pioneered in Britain by Dr. Malcolm Carruthers, who wrote *The Testosterone Revolution*, many doctors still deny the existence of male menopause. However, these symptoms, especially depression, should be taken seriously. Depression in men is harder to diagnose since men tend to get angry rather than sad. They are also more likely to commit suicide. Andropause can be helped by supplementing the hormone testosterone.

If the symptoms above do sound like you, it is well worth having your testosterone levels measured. If low, meaning below 12 nmol/l, then you may benefit from testosterone replacement therapy. However, symptoms are as important, if not more so, than testosterone levels in the blood. This is because most testosterone in the blood is not *free*, but bound and unavailable. The free testosterone is much harder to measure. Salivary testosterone levels may be a better indicator, backed up by symptoms. You can both test your symptoms and get a salivary testosterone test by visiting www.andropause.com. The salivary test also measures your DHEA levels (see page 171). These tests are also available through clinical nutritionists.

If you do have low testosterone, extra supplementing can really help.

Dr. Elizabeth Barrett-Connor studied 680 men aged between 50 and 89 and found a direct relationship between testosterone levels and mood.[93] In the U.K., Dr. Carruthers has treated 1,500 men and found a consistent elevation in mood once testosterone levels become normal.

From a nutritional point of view, make sure you are eating adequate protein and complex carbohydrates. Essential fats are required for healthy sperm and prostate function, antioxidant nutrients protect testosterone from being destroyed, and zinc helps everything to do with male sexual health and hormonal balance. So make sure you are getting enough of all these nutrients.

DHEA deficiency and adrenal exhaustion

Sometimes mood swings and depression can be a result of too much stress and adrenal exhaustion. The adrenal glands, on top of the kidneys, produce a number of hormones—cortisol, adrenalin, noradrenalin, and DHEA. Prolonged stress can result in an inability to produce sufficient amounts of these motivating molecules. DHEA levels are frequently low in both anxious and depressed people, and have been associated with aggressive and cynical attitudes and loss of enjoyment of life. Without sufficient adrenal hormones, especially DHEA, you lose your get up and go and ability to cope with the normal stresses of life, becoming more anxious, on edge, and depressed. Of course, the answer is to decrease stress, but how do you get your adrenal function up to scratch?

The answer can be to supplement DHEA. A study at the University of California psychiatry department in 1997 gave depressed, middle-aged and elderly people 30–90 mg of DHEA and found a clear improvement in their mood.[94]

I never recommend DHEA, from which the body can make other adrenal hormones (follow the arrows in Figure 23), without first running a saliva test to determine whether you have low levels of this hormone. If they are low, I recommend 25 mg a day for women and 50 mg a day for men until these levels are normalized. DHEA isn't available over the counter in Britain but is in the U.S.. You and I can buy it by mail order for our own use. A nutritional therapist can both determine your DHEA levels and let you know how you can order this supplement.

SUMMARY

If you do suffer from mood swings and depression and basic changes to your diet, including supplements, haven't helped, you can check for hormonal imbalances quite simply. A simple saliva test can measure your estrogen, progesterone, testosterone, and DHEA levels. These tests are available through clinical nutritionists who can then advise you about how to bring your hormones back into balance.

In the meantime, here are a few things you can do for yourself:

- Ensure your diet is giving your plenty of essential fats and supplement 200 mg of GLA (either a borage oil 1,000 mg supplement a day, or 4 evening primrose oil 500 mg supplements).

- Supplement 100 mg of vitamin B6, 20 mg of zinc, and 300 mg of magnesium.

- Eat little and often, choosing complex carbohydrate foods, combined with protein.

- Try adding 100 mg of 5-HTP if all the above don't help.

CHAPTER 17

Unwinding stress and anxiety with natural relaxants

For many people, anxiety and the blues are inextricably connected, and feeling stressed, anxious, and irritable sometimes seems to be a hallmark of 21st-century living. The ONUK survey of 37,000 people in Britain found that 82 percent reported often becoming quickly impatient, while 64 percent said they often become anxious or tense easily, and 38 percent said they often feel nervous or hyperactive. Feelings and symptoms of stress affect most of us. These include headaches, muscle tension, dry mouth, excessive perspiration, pounding heart, insomnia, and fatigue.

In the long run, stress and anxiety age you. This is because they put the body into emergency mode, known as the fight-or-flight syndrome, in which the body's energy is channeled away from maintenance and repair, and towards reacting physically to a stressful event. Adrenalin and cortisol start pumping, blood-sugar levels go up, pupils dilate to let in more light, we huff and puff to take in more oxygen—all of which are physiological reactions designed to prepare you for fight or flight. But, unlike our ancestors, we don't (often) fight or take flight. The most we do is toot the car horn, raise our voice, or bottle it up inside.

Most people, when faced with an intense or constant feeling of anxiety, will either self-medicate with alcohol or marijuana, or see their doctor, possibly to be given a prescription for a tranquilizer. In one week in Britain, we pop 10 million tranquilizers, puff 10 million joints and drink 120 million alcoholic drinks.

GABA: the antidote to anxiety

The choice of these three drugs—alcohol, marijuana, and tranquilizers—is no coincidence. They all promote the neurotransmitter GABA, which is the brain's peacemaker, helping to turn off excess adrenalin and calm you down.

That's why that beer or glass of wine makes you feel sociable, relaxed, happy, and less serious, at least for an hour as GABA levels rise. But after an hour or so GABA starts to fall and you feel irritable and disconnected, so you have another one, and another one. The trouble is that after a session of drinking, GABA levels become very suppressed, leaving you grumpy and irritable. So most of us avoid this by drinking in the evening and going to sleep under the influence. What we don't realize is that alcohol also disturbs the normal cycle of dreaming, and it's dreaming that regenerates the mind. So, when you wake up in the morning, you're mentally tired, grumpy, and irritable because of the low GABA, dehydrated, and feeling sluggish as your body detoxifies the alcohol from the night before. The net effect is that alcohol, in the long run, makes you more anxious, not less. The same is essentially true for marijuana which, if habitually smoked, reduces drive and motivation.

1.5 million people in Britain are addicted to tranquilizers

The most common anti-anxiety drugs are the benzodiazepine tranquilizers, such as Valium (diazepam), Librium, and Ativan. These are highly effective at reducing anxiety in the short term, but highly addictive in as little as four weeks. For this reason doctors are strongly advised not to prescribe these for more than four weeks.

Despite this, a poll carried out by *Panorama* found that 3 percent of people polled, equivalent to one and a half million people nationally, have been on tranquilizers for more than four months. Of these, 28 percent had been on them for more than 10 years![95]

These tranquilizers are more addictive than heroin, and coming off them is no joke. Withdrawal can lead to insomnia, anxiety, irritability, sweating, blurred vision, diarrhea, tremors, mental impairment, and headaches. Abrupt withdrawal from high doses can lead to seizures or even death.

The sad truth is that tranquilizers, much like alcohol, increase anxiety and depression in the long run, as well as being addictive. With tranquilizers, however, the reason is slightly different. Tranquilizers open up the brain's receptor sites for GABA, making the brain more sensitive to its effects. So you feel more relaxed, less anxious. The next day, however, you can feel hung over. The more often you take them the more you need to get the same effect and, without them, you can get rebound anxiety and insomnia. Knowing all this, it's shocking that these drugs are still prescribed for anything other than short-term traumas. Yet, in the U.K., 16 million prescriptions are still written annually for these so-called minor tranquilizers to treat anxiety and insomnia.

The terrible side effects of tranquilizers were the major motivator for the development of a new class of drugs, the nonbenzodiazepines. These are a class of related but more targeted drugs, colloquially known as the Zs—zolpidem (Ambien), zalephon (Sonata), and zopiclone (Zimovane). They were introduced in the 1990s amid claims that they were a safe and non-addictive alternative to earlier drugs.

However, a review in 2005 by the U.K.'s National Institute for Clinical Excellence concluded that "there was no consistent difference" between the two types of drugs for either effectiveness or safety.[96] They too can cause tolerance and withdrawal. "Dependence can develop after as little as one week of continuous use. If you fall asleep without having taken a dose and wake some time later, do not take the missed dose. Patients who have been taking this drug for longer than 7 days should consult their doctor before withdrawing treatment," advises one drug bulletin regarding zimovane.[97] You are also not advised to take nonbenzodiazepines for more than a few weeks.

Luckily, there is an alternative.

Natural relaxants

States of anxiety are associated with the stress hormones adrenalin and cortisol. In Chapters 3, 10, and 11 we discussed how blood-sugar ups and downs and over-use of stimulants such as caffeine and nicotine can stress us out. So, the first step towards reducing anxiety is to balance your blood sugar by eating slow-releasing carbohydrates and avoid or, at least considerably reduce, your use of both stimulants and alcohol. This alone has a major effect in reducing anxiety.

> Andrew is a case in point. Managing a chain of supermarkets had left him very stressed. In the day he'd drink coffee and in the evening he'd relax with a beer or some wine, as otherwise he would experience difficulty sleeping. He was also gaining weight. He decided to go on a low-GL diet (as described in Chapter 3), quit drinking coffee and booze, and take some supplements. Three weeks later he said, 'My energy is through the roof, I don't feel stressed and I have no problem sleeping, and wake refreshed.'

Some people need a little extra help to learn how to switch out of the adrenalin state. There are breathing and meditation techniques for this, as well as psychotherapeutic avenues to explore in dealing with the perceived stresses and causes of anxiety, and many of them can be extremely helpful. Then there are natural GABA promoters that ensure you produce and release GABA when you need to. These include amino acids, minerals, and herbs, the most effective being:

- GABA
- Taurine
- Kava
- Valerian
- Hops
- Passionflower
- Magnesium.

Let's explore how these can reduce your anxiety level.

GABA: the antidote to stress

As we saw above, GABA (gamma-amino-butyric acid) is the main inhibitory or calming neurotransmitter. It not only calms down excess adrenalin, noradrenalin, and dopamine, but also effects serotonin, thereby affecting your mood. For these reasons, having enough GABA in your brain is associated with being relaxed and happy, while having too little is associated with anxiety, tension, depression, and insomnia.[98]

GABA is not only a neurotransmitter, it's also an amino acid. This means it's a nutrient and, by supplementing it, you can help to promote normal healthy levels of GABA in the brain.

There is one problem, however. In the European Union, GABA has been classified as a medicine, meaning it is no longer available over the counter in the U.K. You can buy GABA supplements in the U.S. on the Internet though.

If you can get hold of GABA, supplement 500–1,000 mg, once or twice a day as a highly effective natural relaxant. But note that while it is not addictive, that doesn't mean there are no side effects in large amounts. Up to 2g a day has no reported downside; however, if you go up to 10g a day, this can induce nausea or even vomiting, and a rise in blood pressure. So use GABA wisely, especially if you already have high blood pressure, starting with no more than 1g a day, and do not exceed 3g a day.

Taurine: GABA's best friend

Taurine is another relaxing amino acid, similar in structure and effect to GABA. Many people think taurine is a stimulant because it is used in so-called energy drinks, but it is not. It helps you relax and unwind from high levels of adrenalin, much like GABA.

Taurine has many other uses as well, including its benefits as a treatment for insomnia, depression, and even mania, the high phase manic depression, discussed in Chapter 24.

Taurine is highly concentrated in animal foods such as fish, eggs, and meat. Vegetarians are therefore more likely to be at risk of deficiency. While the body can make taurine from the amino acids L-cysteine and L-methionine (provided you've got enough vitamin B6), if you are prone to high levels of anxiety you may benefit from supplementing this relaxing amino acid. Try 500–1,000 mg of taurine, twice daily. There are no known cautions or adverse effects at reasonable doses.

Kava kava: a Pacific herb

Kava is a native Polynesian vine that has been consumed as a social and ceremonial non-alcoholic drink by Pacific islanders for over 3,000 years. The first description of this member of the pepper family came to the West from Captain Cook, on his celebrated voyages through the South Seas. The root is used both for the drink and dried to make the supplements available in some regions of the West, where it is being used increasingly to counteract stress, anxiety, and insomnia. Note, however, that kava is only available via the Internet in Europe as it has been banned from the market, although you can still buy it over the counter in the U.S. The reason is that in people who drink heavily or are on liver-toxic drugs, kava can add to the liver's burden (see page 179).

Kava is excellent at reducing anxiety. One four-week study of patients diagnosed with anxiety found that participants experienced dramatic improvements in their symptoms of anxiety after just one week, with improvement continuing through week four.[99] In the longest (six-month) study to date, by Dr. H.P. Volz in Germany, kava provided significant relief of anxiety versus a placebo, and with minimal side effects.[100] Numerous studies have compared the effectiveness of kava not just with placebos but also with the leading tranquilizer medications and found it just as effective but without the side effects common in those on the drugs.[101–103] Kava relaxes both emotions and muscles, making it useful for headaches, backaches and other symptoms caused by muscular tension. It also reduces excessive mental chatter and increases mental focus. But, most important of all, it is non-addictive.

The reason kava works is because it contains a unique resin made up of kavalactones and other compounds acting both on the limbic system, which is the emotional center of the brain (most likely through an indirect action on GABA receptors), and directly on muscles, thus promoting relaxation in two different ways, while causing no habituation, tolerance, addiction, or hangover as alcohol does.

You need 60–75 mg of kavalactones, taken two to three times daily, to get this anti-anxiety effect. As a sedative to aid sleep, take 120–200 mg before retiring. Different forms of kava have different concentrations of kavalactones, so it is always best to work out the dose from the kavalactones rather than the total amount of kava in any given powder, capsule or tincture.

Can kava be liver toxic?

Taken in the doses I've just given, kava has no known side effects except for exceedingly rare skin rashes in sensitive individuals, headache, or mild stomach upset. Recent investigations in Germany have, however, focused on the potential liver-toxic effects of excessively concentrated extracts, which may make it difficult for the liver to process the fatlike kavalactones.

When the liver processes kavalactones, it uses enzymes that are dependent on a nutrient called glutathione. The whole kava root contains both kavalactones and glutathione, but some kava extracts (especially those giving 60 percent or more kavalactones) eliminate the glutathione. Under normal circumstances this isn't a problem, but alcohol and many prescription drugs, for example paracetamol, need to be processed with the same detoxification enzymes. So if you drink a lot of alcohol and are on liver-toxic drugs such as benzopiazepine tranquilizers, kava adds to your liver's burden. There were some cases in Germany where just this happened.[104] For this reason, I don't recommend using kava extracts if you are a heavy drinker, or are on prescription medication, without your doctor's approval.

Valerian: nature's valium

Another excellent anti-anxiety herb is valerian (*Valeriana officinalis*). Derived from the dried rhizomes and roots of an attractive perennial with pretty pink flowers, it grows throughout Europe in wet soils. As a natural relaxant it is useful for several disorders such as restlessness, nervousness, insomnia, and hysteria, and it has also been used as a sedative for nervous stomach. Valerian acts on the brain's GABA receptors, enhancing their activity and thus offering a similar tranquilizing action to the Valium-type drugs but without the same side effects. As a relaxant you need 50–100 mg twice a day, and twice this amount 45 minutes before retiring for a good night's sleep. (See the next chapter for more on valerian's effect on sleep.)

Since valerian potentiates sedative drugs, including muscle relaxants and antihistamines, don't take it if you are on prescribed medication without your doctor's consent. Valerian can also interact with alcohol, as well as certain psychotropic drugs and narcotics.

Hops and passionflower: calming herbs

Hops (*Humulus lupulus*) are an ancient remedy for a good night's sleep and are probably included in beer for that reason. Hops help to calm nerves by acting directly on the central nervous system, rather than affecting GABA receptors. You need about 200 mg per day, but the effect is much less than kava or valerian and most effective when taken in combination with these and other herbs such as passionflower.

Passionflower (*Passiflora incarnata*) was a favorite of the Aztecs, who used it to make relaxing drinks. It has a mild sedative effect and promotes sleep much like hops, with no known side effects at normal doses. Passionflower can also be helpful for hyperactive kids. You need around 100–200 mg a day.

Combinations of these herbs are particularly effective for relieving anxiety and can really help break the pattern of reacting stressfully to life's challenges.

Magnesium: relaxing mind and muscle

Magnesium is another important nutrient that helps you relax. It's also commonly deficient. Magnesium not only relaxes your mind, it relaxes your muscles. Symptoms of deficiency therefore include muscle aches, cramps, and spasms, as well as anxiety and insomnia. Low levels are commonly found in anxious people and supplementation can often help. You need about 500 mg of magnesium a day. Seeds and nuts are rich in it, as are vegetables and fruit, but especially dark green leafy vegetables such as kale or spinach. I recommend eating these magnesium-rich foods every day and supplementing an additional 300 mg. But, if you are especially anxious, and can't sleep, supplement 500 mg in the evening.

Cutting out the culprits

Supplementing to alleviate anxiety is vital. But we also need to look at substances in the body which you might need to control to feel calmer.

The histamine–copper connection

While blood-sugar problems and low magnesium levels are common reasons for reacting stressfully, they are not the only biochemical imbalances that can lead to anxiety. The late Dr. Carl Pfeiffer, who founded the Brain Bio Center at Princeton, found that many of his patients who experienced extreme fears, phobias, and paranoia had very low histamine levels. Many also had high levels of copper, a toxic element in excess, which can depress histamine levels.

These low-histamine patients, Pfeiffer found, had many characteristics that were opposite to the high-histamine types described later in Chapter 23. These included more body hair, more likelihood of being overweight, rare headaches or allergies, a high pain threshold, and a suspicious nature. He found that these people also did really well on large amounts of niacin, folic acid, and B12, plus vitamin C, zinc, and manganese, which help to lower high levels of copper.

If these symptoms sound like you, it's well worth having your mineral levels checked and, if you do have high levels of copper, or any other toxic minerals, then taking the necessary steps, described in Chapter 11, to lower your levels. If you do experience extreme fears and anxiety you may also benefit from supplementing large amounts of niacin, folic acid, and vitamin B12. This should, however, only be done under the guidance of a clinical nutritionist.

Lactic acid: pushing the panic button

Some people experience panic attacks, characterized by extreme feelings of fear. These are not at all uncommon. Symptoms often experienced during a panic attack include palpitations, rapid breathing, dizziness, unsteadiness, and a feeling of impending death. Those with agoraphobia, a fear of being alone or of public places, often know that they can go out or can be alone, but are afraid of having a panic attack.

As psychological as this sounds, there is a biochemical imbalance behind many people's anxiety attacks, apart from, or as well as, any psychological factors. It's too much lactic acid. When muscles don't get enough oxygen, they make energy from glucose without it. The trouble is there's a byproduct called lactic acid. As strange as this might seem, giving those prone to anxiety attacks lactic acid can induce an anxiety attack.[105]

One way to increase lactic acid levels is to hyperventilate. Many people will do this when they're experiencing anxiety attacks. Hyperventilation changes the acid level of the blood by altering the balance of carbon dioxide. The body responds by producing more lactic acid. The solution is to breathe into a paper bag during a hyperventilation attack and concentrate on breathing deeply for a minute. This helps redress the balance. Moments of blood-sugar dips can also both bring on hyperventilation and increase lactic acid. So, keep your blood-sugar level even by eating little and often. Finally, deficiency in vitamin B1 stops the body breaking down glucose properly, again promoting lactic acid. So, make sure you are supplementing a good B complex or multivitamin. Also, check yourself out for food allergies. These are the most common biochemical imbalances that can lead to panic attacks.

Combinations of herbs and nutrients work best

The combination of relaxing amino acids and herbs is the most effective for reducing high levels of anxiety. The synergistic action of nutrients and herbs such as GABA, taurine, kava, valerian, hops, and passionflower also means the doses for each can be lower.

While the causes of high levels of anxiety are often psychological, by balancing blood sugar, reducing stimulants, ensuring optimum nutrition, plus judicially using these natural anti-anxiety herbs and nutrients, you can break the habit of reacting with fear and anxiety to life's inevitable stresses.

Here's one man's experience on a combination of these natural relaxants, which are available in combination in some supplements:

> 66 They certainly seem to take the sharp edges off daily stresses. I am conscious of the detrimental effects of relying on alcohol to wind down at the end of the day and feel I have found a good substitute. The effect is quite subtle, although still very noticeable. 99

SUMMARY

In summary, to beat stress and reduce anxiety:

- Keep your blood sugar even by eating complex carbohydrates and avoiding stimulants and sugar.

- Deal with the underlying causes of your stress and anxiety, perhaps by working with a counselor or psychotherapist.

- Supplement kava or valerian, or the amino acids GABA or taurine, depending on what's available in your country, or a combination of these relaxing herbs and amino acids, plus magnesium.

CHAPTER 18

Solving sleeping problems

None of us can live without it. We need it every day. And most of us are deficient in it. It's not a vitamin or a mineral—it's sleep. An alarming 47 percent of people have difficulty falling asleep or staying asleep throughout the night, but many more are simply not getting enough for optimal health.

Before the electric light bulb extended our days, most people slept for up to 10 hours a night. The figure now hovers around seven and continues to fall. Not only are we sleeping less in the 21st century because we've learned how to extend our daytime, but we also sleep less to get more done. Yet research clearly shows that it's a rare person who can survive on a great deal less than seven or eight hours' sleep a night.

One of the great mysteries is why we need sleep at all. Without it, even for a night, the body shows clear signs of stress—mood and concentration go, defenses drop, levels of vital nutrients such as zinc and magnesium fall, and vitamin C is used up at an alarming rate. Sleep rejuvenates both the body and the mind. During the first three hours of sleep, the body goes into rapid repair mode. This is one of the reasons why, if you are injured or sick, nothing is better than a good night's sleep.

The importance of dreaming

After a couple of hours, we enter the dream state sleep, known as rapid eye movement, or REM, Stage 1. REM sleep normally occurs 90 minutes after the onset of sleep, but if we are sleep-deprived it may occur within 30 minutes.

Dreaming occurs during REM sleep and most of us have four or more REM periods per night, even though many people have difficulty remembering the dreams that occur in them. As well as providing physical rest, sleep may provide the chance to make a back-up tape of the day's events for our large computer, the brain. While Westerners pay little heed to dreams, one African tribe believes real life is lived in dreams and daytime is the illusion. The Bolivian philosopher Oscar Ichazo describes dream reality like the stars at night: that dream thoughts are always happening, but the brightness of the Sun, daytime consciousness, blots them out. Many scientists believe that nutritional deficiency is one reason why poor or no dream recall can occur.

In a survey at the Institute for Optimum Nutrition we found that more than 40 percent of people had no or very infrequent dream recall. When researching the signs and symptoms of vitamin B6 and zinc deficiency, we found that an alarming proportion of deficient people couldn't recall their dreams. After supplementation with B6 and zinc their dream recall returned and they reported their dreams as more vivid.

So if you don't think you dream it's worth supplementing B6 and zinc, gradually increasing the dose up to 200 mg B6 and 30 mg of zinc. (It is best not to take more than this without the advice of a nutritionist.) Combinations of sleep-promoting herbs and amino acids, discussed on page 194, are also excellent for promoting good-quality sleep and dreams.

One woman told me she hadn't slept more than five hours a night for at least 10 years. After supplementing a combination of kava, hops, passionflower, GABA and taurine, she slept for 12 hours straight and woke up feeling fantastic. Another woman reported great benefits from the same combination, but not in promoting sleep. Her problem was in waking up. After supplementing these sleep-promoting nutrients she started waking up at 8am full of energy, rather than at 10am still tired. Another reported that after supplementing a combination of kava and 5-HTP she started dreaming in color for the first time in her life! Many others have reported more lucid dreams and improved dream recall, as well as deeper sleep without waking.

Given that it is an essential way of resting, recharging, and nourishing both your body and mind, sustained, unbroken sleep, and dreaming, is part of the lifestyle package that determines the quality of our lives and our health.

Are you sleep deprived?

Sleep specialists at Loughborough University have carried out a series of tests into how the brain functions when it is deprived of sleep. And the results are very clear: sleepy people have problems finding the right words, coming up with ideas, and coping with rapidly changing situations. So cutting back on sleep may make you less efficient, not more.

Even if you're not involved in any particularly brain-taxing work, a lack of sleep is likely to lower your mood and your general ability to cope with what life throws at you. How much easier is it to deal with a mistake by your bank or a late train if you're feeling alert and well rather than half awake? Sleep deprivation makes us moody and irritable, and in the long term, even depressed. Scientists have measured the body's ability to fight off infections when it is tired, and research has shown that sleep deprived individuals have a reduction in natural killer cells, a type of immune cell needed for resistance against invaders.

When you can't switch off

The problem usually begins before bedtime. You may feel unable to switch off from feelings of stress, tension, and anxiety—the buzz words of the 21st century. Sixty-three percent of people say they suffer from stress and more than half of all visits to the doctor are for stress-related conditions, including insomnia. And that is a clue to the best way of treating it.

According to a review from 2004, published in *The Lancet*,[106] the various forms of counseling and psychological help are not only more effective than pills at tackling chronic insomnia—they are also, inevitably, far safer. But in the U.K., for instance, good therapeutic help can be hard to find on the National Health Service. As a consequence, over 16 million prescriptions for what are called hypnotic (sleeping) and anxiolytic (anxiety-reducing) drugs were written out in 2004, at a cost of £37 million. (For more information on the dangers of these drugs and how to get off them, see Chapter 22.)

❓ DO YOU SUFFER FROM INSOMNIA/ANXIETY?

☐ Do you have difficulty getting to sleep?

☐ Do you wake in the night more than once?

☐ Are you a light sleeper?

☐ Do you wake up in the early hours of the morning feeling unrested?

☐ Would you describe yourself as anxious?

☐ Are you easily stressed?

☐ Do you have difficulty relaxing?

☐ Do you find yourself feeling irritable?

☐ Do you get angry easily?

☐ Do you find you are impatient with others?

☐ Are you prone to low moods?

☐ Are you easily upset or offended?

☐ Do you suffer from tense muscles?

If you answered *yes* to:

Less than 4: You are not particularly anxious or stressed although the ideal is to have no *yes* answers.

4 to 9: You have the indications of increased stress, anxiety, or insomnia, and need to take our advice in this chapter seriously. Recheck your score in one month. If your number of yeses has not fallen, go and see a nutritional therapist.

10 or more: You have a major issue with anxiety and sleep. We recommend you pursue all the options here, including seeing a psychotherapist and a nutritional therapist. If you are taking anti-anxiety medication or sleeping pills, you will need to speak to your doctor about switching to some of these safer alternatives.

Six steps to supersleep

If you are having problems getting to sleep, staying asleep, or getting enough sleep, there are six steps you can take to improve your sleep life:

- Get to the bottom of any factors interrupting your sleep.

- Manage your stress levels.

- Maintain even blood-sugar levels throughout the day.

- Balance your minerals, supplementing magnesium.

- Balance your sleep neurotransmitters—serotonin and melatonin.

- If necessary, use a natural sleep aid such as valerian.

There is always a reason why you have sleep problems—whether it's getting to sleep, waking in the night or waking too early, emotional or physical. Dealing with the cause must be the first step before you reach for the sleeping tablets—even the natural ones. So first off, look at the box below to see whether there are any triggers you can deal with right away.

Perpetuating sleeplessness—which apply to you?

- Stress
- Noise
- Heat or cold
- Irregular sleeping hours
- Shift work
- Side effects from medication (for instance, some bronchodilators for asthma, some antidepressants)
- Eating too close to bedtime
- Excessive/late caffeine intake
- Excessive/late alcohol intake
- Late cigarette smoking
- Indigestion
- Pain
- Depression
- Widely fluctuating blood-sugar levels
- Breathing problems
- Recreational drugs

- Excessive afternoon napping
- Uncomfortable or old bed
- Expecting to have problems sleeping.

Most people have at some time in their lives experienced the frustration, restlessness, and exhaustion of not being able to get enough sleep or waking up too early and not getting back to sleep. Although this is usually linked to an anxious time or to the factors listed in the box above, it is also very much affected by what you eat.

Stress, sugar, and stimulants keep you awake

Many of our bodies' daily rhythms, including those that dictate our energy and sleepiness, are finely tuned mechanisms that depend on certain hormonal patterns, body chemicals and nutrients. At nighttime, the levels of the stress hormone cortisol should dip, calming your body and preparing it for sleep. If, however, your cortisol levels are out of kilter for any reason (usually stress or a diet high in stimulants or sugar), your ability to get to sleep, to sleep through the night or to wake up refreshed is likely to be impaired. If cortisol levels are high at night, this suppresses the release of growth hormone, which is essential for daily tissue repair and growth. This effectively speeds up the rate at which your body ages. A nutritionist can run a saliva test for you to determine whether your cortisol rhythm is out of sync.

Caffeine is another well-known sleep disrupter. When you go to sleep, levels of the hormone melatonin—which is secreted by our pineal glands in response to darkness—increase. Melatonin levels start to rise two hours before sleep, then peak somewhere between 2am and 4am before starting to fall. Coffee drinkers halve the amount of melatonin produced, according to sleep expert Dr. Maurice Ohayon from Stanford University in California.[107] Research conducted at Tel Aviv University in Israel found that volunteers given regular coffee, compared to decaf, slept an average of two hours less.[108] The melatonin-depressing effects of caffeine last for up to 10 hours, making it wise to avoid caffeinated drinks from midday.

Dealing with underlying causes of stress and avoiding caffeine are clearly important. So too is keeping your blood-sugar levels balanced by eating regular meals throughout the day, including some protein-rich food at each meal (such as fish, eggs, lean meat, or a form of soy), avoiding refined foods, coffee, sugary foods, and drinks and minimizing alcohol. Many people who wake in the night and then can't get back to sleep find that keeping blood-sugar levels even during the day sets the scene for the correct patterns at night, giving more chance of a good night's sleep.

Get more GABA

If you suspect that switching off adrenalin is your problem, one obvious solution is to raise your level of GABA, the main inhibitory or calming neurotransmitter. Because GABA regulates the neurotransmitters noradrenalin, dopamine, and serotonin, it can shift both a tense, worried state towards relaxation, and a blue mood to a brighter one. When your levels of GABA are low, you feel anxious, tense, and depressed, and have trouble sleeping.[109] When your levels increase, your breathing and heart rate slow down and your muscles relax.

As we've seen, GABA is an amino acid and in many parts of the world you can buy it over the counter. However, in the U.K. it's recently been classified as a medicine, so you can't buy it this way, and will need to use the Internet.

Taking 500 mg twice daily after meals is very calming. Just don't exceed this dose because high amounts can trigger nausea. Infrequently, this is also experienced with lower amounts.

How serotonin and melatonin help you sleep

During the daytime, adrenalin levels are higher and keep you stimulated. As you start to wind down, serotonin levels rise and adrenalin levels fall. As it gets darker another neurotransmitter, melatonin, kicks in. Melatonin is an almost identical molecule to serotonin, from which it is made, and both are made from the amino acid tryptophan. Melatonin's main role in the brain is to regulate the sleep/wake cycle. Interestingly, melatonin is produced in the light-sensitive pineal gland in the center of the brain, also known as the third eye and considered by René Descartes to be the seat of the soul. Have you ever thought about where the light comes from when you dream?

As we learned earlier, many people, especially women, become serotonin deficient. Without enough serotonin you don't make enough melatonin. Without melatonin it is difficult to get to sleep and stay asleep. Waking far too early in the morning and not being able to get back to sleep is a classic symptom of deficiency of these essential brain chemicals.

Adequate amounts of B6 and tryptophan are needed for you to get sleepy. Foods that are particularly high in tryptophan are chicken, cheese, tuna, tofu, eggs, nuts, seeds, and milk. As usual, a traditional remedy—drinking a glass of milk before bed—becomes grounded in science. Other foods associated with inducing sleep are lettuce and oats. Supplementing tryptophan has also proven consistently effective in promoting sleep if taken in amounts ranging from 1–4g.[110] Smaller doses have not proven effective. You also need to take it at least 45 minutes before you want to go to sleep, again ideally with a small amount of carbohydrate such as an oatmeal cookie. The reason for this is that eating carbohydrate causes a release of insulin, and insulin carries tryptophan into the brain.

Most effective of all is supplementing 5-HTP or melatonin itself. 5-HTP (hydroxytryptophan) is the direct precursor of serotonin and by supplementing it you can increase levels of melatonin and serotonin. 5-HTP is very highly concentrated in the seeds of the African griffonia plant. Supplementing 100–200 mg of 5-HTP half an hour before sleep helps you get a good night's sleep.[111] It's also been shown to reduce sleep terrors in children when given at an amount equivalent to 1 mg per pound of body weight before bed.[112]

Melatonin, which is a neurotransmitter, not a nutrient, can also be helpful, but needs to be used much more cautiously. In controlled trials it's about a third as effective as the drugs, but has a fraction of the side effects.[113] However, supplementing too much can have undesirable effects such as diarrhea, constipation, nausea, dizziness, reduced libido, headaches, depression, and nightmares. If you do sleep badly you may want to try it in any case; take between 3–6 mg before bedtime. In Britain melatonin is classified as a medicine and is only available on prescription. Discuss this option with your doctor. It is available in other countries, such as the U.S. and South Africa, over the counter, or over the Internet.

Sometimes supplementing 5-HTP or melatonin for a month can bring you back into balance, re-establishing proper sleep patterns, after which the supplements become unnecessary to continue. This is a great way to wean yourself off more harmful sleeping pills.

Melatonin is also very useful for jetlag, when your body clock goes out of sync with the Earth. The best way to bring yourself back into balance is to supplement 1 mg of melatonin for every one-hour time difference, just before your new bedtime. So, if you fly from London to LA, which is eight hours behind, you take 8 mg on the first night, then halve it to 4 mg for the second night, 2 mg for the third, then 1 mg, then stop. Always take it just before you want to go to sleep and halve the dose each night.

Calming minerals

A lack of the minerals calcium and magnesium can trigger or exacerbate sleep difficulties because they work together to calm the body and help relax nerves and muscles. Magnesium levels may well be low if you are particularly stressed or consume too much sugar. Including some magnesium in the evening, perhaps even in a supplement, may help. Your diet is more likely to be low in magnesium than calcium—so make sure you are eating plenty of magnesium-rich foods such as seeds, nuts, green vegetables, wholegrains, and seafood. Milk products, green vegetables, nuts, seafood, and molasses are particularly good sources of calcium. Some people find it helpful to supplement 600 mg of calcium and 400 mg of magnesium at bedtime. Ensuring adequate B vitamins daily helps support the body in many ways, including its ability to deal with stress—take B-complex vitamins earlier in the day rather than in the evening, though, as they are also involved in energy production and keep some people awake.

Herbal nightcaps

It's really best to resort to sleeping aids—natural or pharmaceutical—only as a last resort. Medicinal sedatives are generally bad news in that they are usually addictive and your tolerance increases, making higher and higher doses necessary for any effect. They have a range of side effects such as daytime drowsiness, memory problems, confusion, depression, dry mouth, sluggishness, and all sorts of other unpleasant symptoms. They are also strong chemicals which need to be detoxified by the body, placing a burden on your liver.

There are many natural substances which can help you sleep, although again, they should be used when other avenues have been exhausted and then only occasionally. You'll find many of them, especially the herbs, are sold in blended formulas.

Valerian is sometimes referred to as nature's Valium. As such, it can interact with alcohol and other sedative drugs and should therefore be taken in combination with them only under careful medical supervision. It seems to work in two ways: by promoting the body's release of GABA, and by providing the amino acid glutamine, from which the brain can make GABA. Neither of these mechanisms make it addictive.[114] One double-blind study in which participants took 60 mg of valerian 30 minutes before bedtime for 28 days found it to be as effective as oxazepam, a drug used to treat anxiety.[115] Another found that the combination of valerian and lemon balm was as effective as the drug Halcion but produced no next-day drowsiness.[116] On the other hand, an expert from Loughborough University's Sleep Research Centre describes valerian as an "unreliable sleep inducer."[117] Our experience is that it works exceptionally well for many people.

Dosage: 150–300 mg about 45 minutes before bedtime.

Passionflower's mild sedative effect has been well substantiated in numerous animal and human studies. The herb encourages deep, restful, uninterrupted sleep, with no side effects.

Dosage: varies with the formula, generally 100–200 mg of a standardized extract.

Kava is a relaxant for both mind and body. If taken 20 minutes before bedtime, kava can help promote a deeper sleep with no drowsiness on waking. See the cautions and further information on page 178.

Dosage: 250 mg an hour before bed (standardized to 30 percent kavalactones).

St. John's wort, also called hypericum, has both serotonin- and melatonin-enhancing effects, making it an excellent sleep regulator.

Dosage: 300 mg (standardized to 0.3 percent hypericin).

Hops have been used for centuries as a mild sedative and sleeping aid. Their sedative action works directly on the central nervous system.

Dosage: varies, but around 200 mg per day.

Combinations of these herbs, together with 5-HTP, are the most effective natural sleep promoters of all; look for them in your health food store. Here are a couple of reports from people who found them of benefit:

> ❝❝ I was suffering from chronic insomnia for a year and a half and was not keen to take sleeping pills. I decided to try a certain combination of relaxing herbs and nutrients, seeing that they were 100-ppercent natural. I took one an hour before bed and they actually work. Over the last two weeks I have fallen straight to sleep. At long last I can feel refreshed in the morning. ❞❞

> ❝❝ My problem isn't getting to sleep—it's waking up! I have two alarm clocks and left to my own devices, I don't wake up before 11am. I'm the girlfriend from hell in the morning! Then I tried taking a combination of kava, GABA, taurine and hops before bed. The next morning I woke up at 8.30am happy and awake. I've tried this several times and it always works. ❞❞

Other solutions to insomnia

Psychotherapy

A small study published in a 2004 issue of *The Archives of Internal Medicine* found that just two hours of cognitive behavior therapy (CBT) was able to cure insomnia by encouraging patients to acknowledge the stress that was preventing them from sleeping, then helping them to develop ways of dealing with it.[118] One way CBT works is by helping the patient identify negative or unhelpful thoughts—"I just can't sleep without my pills"—and then encouraging them to challenge them—"I didn't have a problem until six months ago," "I fell asleep with no trouble after that long walk."

Such techniques are often combined with progressive muscle relaxation or a form of biofeedback to reduce the amount of active beta brainwaves before going to bed. This involves hooking a patient up to a machine that displays their brain activity on a screen so they can see how it slows down in tandem with slowed breathing and other relaxation exercises. "The challenge," declared *The Lancet* review mentioned above, "is to move these therapies out of specialized sleep clinics and into everyday applications."[119] Ask your doctor about getting psychological help.

Sleep hygiene

The essentially common-sense advice rather quaintly known as sleep hygiene forms part of most sleep regimes. The rules are simple: keep the bedroom quiet, dark, and at a temperature that is good for you, wear comfortable clothing, don't have a big meal in the evening, and avoid coffee and alcohol at least three hours before bed. Also exercise regularly, but not within three hours of bedtime. Be aware that certain prescription medications can cause insomnia, such as steroids, bronchodilators (used for asthma), and diuretics.

The idea is to create regular sleep-promoting habits. A similar but more systematic approach is known as stimulus control therapy (SCT). This involves ensuring that the bed is only associated with sleeping (and, of course, sex!). Patients are advised against having naps, and to go to bed when sleepy. They are also told to get up within 20 minutes if they haven't fallen asleep, do something relaxing until they feel drowsy, then try again—and if that fails, go through the process again until it works.

Although sleep hygiene is widely recommended, there have been very few studies of it as an individual treatment and those few have only found limited improvement. The evidence for the effectiveness of SCT is much stronger.

A study from 2005 has shown that an important element of sleep hygiene—regular exercise—does help you sleep better.[120] This may be because exercise helps burn off excess adrenalin and generally helps stabilize blood-sugar levels, but remember to try to confine your exercise times to no later than early evening to allow your body to wind down before bedtime.

Brain music

The New York psychiatrist Dr. Galina Mindlin, an assistant professor at Columbia University's College of Physicians and Surgeons, uses brain music—rhythmic patterns of sounds derived from recordings of patients' own brain waves—to help them overcome insomnia, anxiety, and depression. The recordings sound something like classical piano music and appear to have a calming effect similar to that generated by yoga or meditation. A small double-blind study from 1998, conducted at Toronto University in Canada, found that 80 percent of those undergoing this treatment reported benefits.[121]

Another study found that specially composed music induced a shift in brain wave patterns to alpha waves, associated with the deep relaxation before you go to sleep, and that this induced less anxiety in a study of patients going to the dentist.[122] This music, composed by John Levine especially to induce a relaxation response, has also been shown to calm down hyperactive children. Our favorite CD is called *Silence of Peace* (see page 458).

Sleep is not the only time that we relax and recharge. Taking regular exercise, doing relaxation exercises such as yoga, t'ai chi, meditation, or breathing exercises, enjoying a pastime such as painting or playing an instrument, spending fun time with a partner, children, or a pet—all these can help to divert attention from work and worries, leaving bedtime for sleeping, and maybe sex, if you're not too tired!

SUMMARY

In summary, if you want to ensure you get a good night's sleep, with some dreaming thrown in:

- Avoid sugar and stimulants, especially after 4pm.

- Find ways of relaxing and de-stressing in the evening.

- Make sure your supplement program includes vitamin B6 100 mg, and zinc 10 mg (up to 30 mg if no dream recall).

- Supplement 400 mg of calcium and 300 mg of magnesium in the evening and eat calcium- and magnesium-rich foods such as seeds and crunchy or dark green vegetables.

- If you suffer from insomnia, supplement either 200 mg of 5-HTP or two 2,000 mg capsules of L-tryptophan (available on prescription) before bed; or valerian; or a combination of these herbs and nutrients. Also eat tryptophan-rich meals (see the box in Chapter 15, page 151 for some ideas). If this doesn't work, ask your doctor to prescribe melatonin.

PART 4

What Is Mental Illness?

Mental illness, more than any other disease, is a stigma in modern society. Yet as with many diseases, we know a lot about what causes, prevents, and improves problems from depression to schizophrenia. Often the cause is biochemical and, with the right nutrition, many people make complete recoveries. In this part you will discover what mental illness means, how to get the right diagnosis, why long-term drug therapy is rarely the answer, and all about more effective alternatives.

CHAPTER 19

Understanding mental illness

Before discussing what to do to alleviate certain types of mental illness, it is important to understand what we mean by this term. It is often used, by layman and specialist alike, as an identity tag with no apparent clear-cut definition or understanding. In fact, the U.K. Mental Health Act of 1983 contains no definition. Instead, it states,

> 66 In practice the decision as to whether a person is mentally ill is a clinical one and the expression invariably has to be defined by reference to what the doctor says it means in a particular case rather than to any precise legal criteria. 99

In other words, it's up to your doctor or psychiatrist.

What we commonly understand by the term mental illness is a state of being that falls short of what we consider normal or acceptable. We have all experienced some degree of this. At one end of the spectrum we become unhappy for no apparent reason, or find ourselves reacting explosively to the smallest stress or insult. At the other extreme, we hear voices which just won't go away, or feel that we can't go on anymore.

In practice, what tends to happen is that a person who continuously suffers from less than normal mental states is labeled depressed, manic depressive, schizophrenic, or with some other mental disorder. He may then carry this label for life, and be tagged as a less than normal human being. Such labels do nothing of actual benefit for the individual, so in defining what we mean by mental illness it is important to avoid a label which in itself could contribute to more mental turmoil.

It might therefore be more useful to define our terms in reference to the concept of mental well-being. If a good state of mental health refers to a condition of feeling stable, happy, and satisfied that one is coping adequately with the inevitable problems of day-to-day living, then a mental-health problem would refer to a condition where one is *not* coping, where a person is unhappy a lot of the time, frequently feels distressed, and is unnaturally and frequently afraid.

With that in mind, what I call mental illness is a state of mind in which a person is unable to cope with some aspect of life, to the point where their ability to lead a fulfilling life is seriously impaired.

Mind and body: a self-organizing jungle

Every thought and feeling we have can both alter, and be altered by, the chemistry of our body. The mind and body are completely interconnected. One does not exist without the other. The Western concept that we are our minds (I think, therefore I am) and that our body is a machine has created this false idea of separation. This idea generated the notion that mental illness is a result of that part of the machine responsible for thinking and feeling, the brain, going wrong. This led to the notion of mental illness as something that must be destroyed by drugs, or surgical procedures such as lobotomies and electroconvulsive shock treatment, both of which damage the brain.

The other avenue that emerged from this concept of separation was a blind belief in psychoanalysis, and the notion that mental illness is purely the result of problems in the abstract mind, not the physical brain. This false separation continues today.

Instead of the concept of trying to fix the part that doesn't work, be it the physical brain or the abstract psyche, I prefer to conceive of us human beings as *complex adaptive systems*, more like a self-organizing jungle than a complicated computer. Rather than trying to control a person's health by playing God with hi-tech medicine, there's a new way of looking at health that considers a human being as a whole, with an interconnected mind and body that is designed to adapt to health if the circumstances are right. We have this amazing drive towards health and happiness, and an extraordinary ability to restore balance when health is lost.

Of course, this adaptive capacity is not the same for all. We all have different strengths and weaknesses. So, in this new model, our health is a result of the interaction between our inherited adaptive capacity and our circumstances. For example, on a physical/chemical level that would be between our genes and our environment (see Figure 25 opposite). If our environment is sufficiently hostile (poor diet, pollution, allergens, and so on), we exceed our ability to adapt and become unwell.

We can apply the same model on a psychological level. Our psychological environment is literally everything we see, hear, smell, touch, and taste—the total sum of all our sense inputs. Our psychological genes are your mental constructs, your mind frame, that interprets whatever comes in through the senses in order to make sense of our world. We don't see reality as it actually is, we interpret all we see based on our mental constructs, which are the result of reactions we've had to past similar experiences, which makes up the basis of our childhood conditioning. In this way we form likes and dislikes, attractions and aversions, and so on.

In this new model of health there are four aspects to mental health, and four contributors to mental illness:

Environment This includes all the nutrients and anti-nutrients we take in. As we learned in Parts 1 and 2, deficiencies in certain vitamins, minerals, essential fats, phospholipids, and amino acids can cause mental health problems, as can excesses in anti-nutrients. These can be corrected by improving your nutrition and making lifestyle changes to minimize the effects of anti-nutrients.

Genes In quite a few mental health conditions, for example schizophrenia, there is clear evidence of genetic differences, which means that a particular aspect of a person's brain chemistry is more likely to become imbalanced, especially if they are suboptimally nourished. This too can be vastly improved by specific nutritional strategies. This is also why some people need much more of a nutrient to stay well than others. We are all unique.

Sense input In many cases, mental health problems develop in times of high stress, when there is more going on than a person can cope with. Adjusting your life to minimize stress is part of the equation. The other is

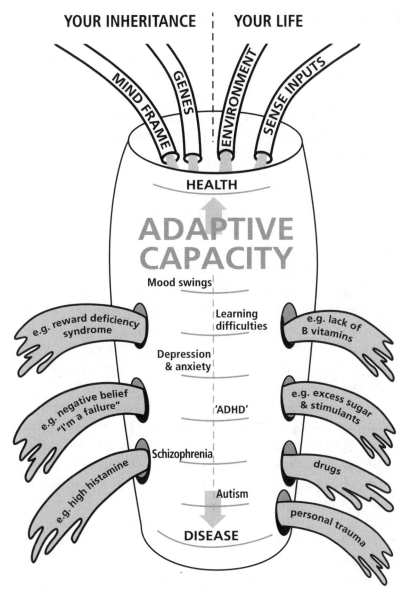

YOUR INHERITANCE ⋮ **YOUR LIFE**

MIND FRAME · GENES ⋮ ENVIRONMENT · SENSE INPUTS

HEALTH

ADAPTIVE CAPACITY

Mood swings

e.g. reward deficiency syndrome

Learning difficulties

e.g. lack of B vitamins

Depression & anxiety

e.g. negative belief "I'm a failure"

'ADHD'

e.g. excess sugar & stimulants

e.g. high histamine

Schizophrenia

drugs

Autism

personal trauma

DISEASE

Fig 25. New model of mental health

changing the way you interpret what is happening in your life. Although it is of less importance in this part of the equation, once again nutrition does make a difference to how you perceive. For example, zinc deficiency alters perceptions about body size and appetite, both of which can contribute to eating disorders (see Chapter 33).

Mind frame It's important to realize that we don't perceive reality as it actually is. We all interpret what is happening in our lives. "Don't change the world. Change the prescription of your glasses," said Swami Muktananda, a master of meditation. Most forms of psychotherapy are nothing more or less than techniques to help a person develop self-observation and become aware of negative mental patterns that lead to self-destructive behavior. Developing a more expanded and positive mind frame promotes mental well-being.

While nutrition would seem to have little to do with your mind frame, the two are related. When we cannot cope with our interpretation of reality we have to let off steam, to dissipate the fear, anxiety, or pain, which we sometimes do by eating too much, or by consuming sugar, alcohol, and cigarettes—or even more harmful drugs, such as heroin or cocaine. These compensating behaviors leave us drained of energy and nutrients, which simply makes matters worse. To cope with the fatigue we then use stimulants, which further deplete us, leading to more and more addiction, and worsening mental health. It's a vicious downward spiral.

Imagine this scenario. Peter has blood-sugar problems, is lacking B vitamins, and has reward deficiency syndrome. This is a genetic predisposition to under produce dopamine, the motivating neurotransmitter. All of these factors make him tired and unmotivated. He therefore craves stimulation and stimulants, such as sugar and caffeine, to make him feel good. Unfortunately, these make him more mentally hyperactive, with excessive thoughts. He can't switch off. So he starts drinking alcohol every day. This makes him more depressed. His doctor prescribes antidepressants. His wife leaves him and he loses his job. He feels useless, worthless, and hopelessly inadequate. He can't cope with what's happening in his life and escapes into his own world. He has a breakdown. He is prescribed major tranquilizers and, although stable, or at least not harmful to others, he is clearly suffering from mental illness.

This example shows the complex interplay between genes, environment, sense input, and mind frame. Drugs alone will not restore his health. He needs to rebalance his brain's chemistry with optimum nutrition, and rebalance his psyche with good psychological guidance and support, and, most of all, he needs the willingness to change his diet, his lifestyle, and his mind frame. This total approach is likely to be much more effective than just drugs, psychotherapy, or nutritional therapy alone.

A common and growing problem

Whatever the cause, mental health problems are incredibly common and very much on the increase. Currently, diagnosis with a mental health problem is as common as diagnosis with heart disease and three times more common than diagnosis with cancer. Official figures suggest that 6 million people in Britain, or 1 in 10, are sufferers at any one point in time.[1] In the course of a year 12 million adults attending their doctors' surgeries have symptoms of mental illness. Every five years the number of children up to the age of 14 seen by psychiatric services is doubling.[2] In fact, out of 100 people that you know, up to 20 will be affected at any point in time. The cost to the U.K. economy has been estimated as in excess of $100 billion a year.

As unwelcome as the thought may be, any one of us is a potential sufferer of a mental health problem. We are all subject to a greater or lesser degree to the stresses and strains of daily life, which for many people may be in addition to a much deeper source of stress or unhappiness coming from a particularly difficult past or present experience. The vast majority (80 percent) of disorders appear in the form of either anxiety states, depression or stress-related disorders, with the remaining 20 percent being made up of alcohol and drug dependency, dementia, and personality and psychotic disorders such as schizophrenia.

There is no question that mental health problems are more common in those who are socially deprived. Suicide rates are 11 times higher among the unemployed and 53 people per thousand are being admitted to psychiatric hospitals from deprived areas as opposed to 19 per thousand as a national average. However, this still begs the question as to why some people seem to cope reasonably well with a given situation while others will start to manifest the symptoms of mental illness.

Mental illness costs all of us a small fortune. In Britain, almost 10 percent of the National Health Service budget is spent on mental illness. This, plus sickness and disability benefits, plus the cost of informal care in the community, exceeds $20 billion, or approximately $400 per person per year.[3] We desperately need a new way of dealing with mental health problems that is both more effective and more cost-effective. The good news is that the optimum nutrition approach is both.

CHAPTER 20

Getting the right diagnosis

There's an old saying: "**Neurotics** build castles in the sky, psychotics live in them, and psychiatrists collect the rent." Some decades ago neurotic was the term for those anxious or depressed, while psychotic referred to those who had lost touch with reality.

Nowadays the diagnosis of a mental health problem is much more complex, but still based largely on a subjective judgement of a person's condition, rather than objective tests. The categories are defined in a book called the *Diagnostic and Statistical Manual of Mental Disorders*, generally referred to as *DSM-IV*, which has 17 categories for mental health problems. The main ones are shown below:

- **Disorders first diagnosed in childhood and adolescence:** retardation, learning disorders, attention deficit disorder, autism, etc.

- **Delirium, dementia, amnestic and other cognitive disorders:** delirium, dementia, Alzheimer's, etc.

- **Substance-related disorders:** alcohol, amphetamine, caffeine, cocaine, etc.

- **Schizophrenia and other psychotic disorders:** schizophrenia, various sub-types.

- **Mood disorders:** manic depression, depression.

- **Anxiety disorders:** phobias, anxiety, etc.

- **Personality disorders:** paranoid, schizotypal, histrionic, etc.

- **Eating disorders:** anorexia, bulimia, etc.

- **Sleep disorders:** insomnia, etc.

The trouble with diagnoses

The trouble with this categorization is that it completely ignores the many physical/biochemical factors that lead people into mental illness. A landmark study in 1980 found that 46 percent of people diagnosed with psychiatric disorders had a physical ailment, such as a nutritional deficiency.[4] Far too few psychiatrists test their patients for nutritional deficiencies, stimulant addictions, or hormone imbalances, all of which can bring on symptoms of mental illness.

Also, not everybody makes the same diagnosis, as this famous study by a Stanford University professor of law and psychology, Dr. David Rosenhan, clearly demonstrates.

Rosenhan and seven others, including three psychologists and a psychiatrist, gained admission to 12 hospitals on the East and West Coasts of the U.S. by faking mental illness (11 of the hospitals were totally funded by public money). The story they told to gain admission was that they heard voices. Asked what the voices said they replied that they were often unclear but as far as they could tell they said "empty," "hollow" and "thud." However, once admitted to the hospital, they acted in a normal manner. In therapy, they answered all questions truthfully, including those about their childhood and their current areas of interest. They engaged in normal activities in the hospitals and, short of revealing their true purpose, they did everything possible to gain their release. Yet, only the other patients in the hospitals were able to tell that these pseudopatients were sane. The first three pseudopatients to be hospitalized took careful notes. Their accurate accounts show that 35 of a total of 118 regular patients were suspicious of them. Referring to their continual notetaking, one regular patient remarked: "You're not crazy. You're a journalist or a professor. You're checking up on the hospital."

The hospital staff, however, were not able to detect the pseudopatients' sanity. One nurse saw the notetaking as a symptom of a sick compulsion:

"Engages in writing behavior," she put on the patient's chart. This led Rosenhan to conclude that, "once a patient is designated as abnormal, all their other behaviors and characteristics are colored by that label." Whether this generalization is true or not, the inability of the hospitals to diagnose properly, or even suspect something, shows how the thin line between sanity and insanity may be blurred. Proper use of the medical model entails careful differential diagnosis, which draws this line firmly in view for both the staff and patient.

None of the pseudopatients was discharged as cured; all bore the label "schizophrenia in remission." In other words, it would seem they were still insane. With the schizophrenia on their record they would have to bear this stigma, and even be expected to behave as schizophrenics again, concluded Rosenhan.

The uniform and simple disorder of perception, or disperception (misinterpretation of events), that the pseudopatients reported in their first interview at the hospitals was the only evidence of schizophrenia—an example of waste-basket diagnosis (if it won't fit in anywhere else, they throw it in there!). Psychiatrists assume that no one would actually want to report such a symptom unless they actually had it. The error, of course, is the lack of diagnosis based on proper tests. In one such test, the EWI (Experiential World Inventory), the patient can report disperceptions in a setting where he has no fear of recrimination, in a more or less objective fashion. There is no possibility that 200 answers can be faked.

One observation that Rosenhan made, as a result of this study, was that mental illness carries with it a connotation entirely different from that of a physical disorder. The *Diagnostic and Statistical Manual of Mental Disorders*, which as we saw above is widely regarded as the official bible of psychiatric diagnoses, might have one believe that the sane are always clearly distinguished from the insane, and that schizophrenia is always treated as objectively and straightforwardly as a broken leg. Rosenhan found that in actual practice, this was not the case. For example, sensible questions asked by the pseudopatients were frequently ignored. One patient stopped a doctor and asked: "Excuse me, Dr. X , could you tell me when I am eligible for grounds privileges?" The doctor replied: "Good morning, Dave. How are you today?" and moved on without waiting for an answer or answering the patient's question. Not only was the credibility of the patients impaired in this way (presumably because of their diagnostic labels), but they were also denied privacy even in matters of personal hygiene. They reported feeling depersonalized, even though they knew they did not belong in the mental hospital.

Not really sick?

Dr. Rosenhan further wondered whether the atrocious diagnostic performance of the hospital staff merely reflected their professional caution. Having once been informed that a patient was hearing voices, perhaps the psychiatrists felt obliged to alert all future doctors to the possibility of trouble. Thus, Rosenhan wondered if his findings resulted from a greater inclination of physicians to call a healthy person sick than a sick person healthy. To check this, he provided an esteemed psychiatric hospital, one of those involved in his first study, with yet another opportunity to redeem its reputation for adequate and proper diagnosis. The staff was informed that at some time during the next three months, one or more pseudopatients would once again attempt to be admitted into their hospital. The staff members were asked to rate each person who came for admission on the likelihood that they were a pseudopatient. Of the 193 patients admitted during the three months, 41 (or 21 percent) of them were judged, with a high degree of confidence, to be pseudopatients by at least one member of staff. The joke, again, was on the hospital staff. No pseudopatients at all had been sent to the hospital!

The study proved, basically, that insanity can easily be faked in front of professionals who do not use objective diagnostic tools such as psychometric assessments and biochemical tests. Although I hope diagnosis has improved substantially since this study, which was performed in 1973, we can conclude that psychiatric diagnoses, without objective laboratory tests and psychometric tests, are frequently erroneous; and that without an accurate diagnostic method, a label should not be applied. After all, labels tell you nothing about the underlying causes of a person's problem. We badly need a fresh approach to psychiatric diagnosis and treatment.

What divides abnormal behavior from mental illness?

A valid point for debate is whether certain abnormal behavior qualifies as mental illness. Patients who have certain mental symptoms after strokes or infections of the brain present no problem in being considered ill. In contrast, there is a group of disorders listed as personality disorders. There is nothing in this term to suggest any organic or physiological derangement, so to call them mental illness is highly debatable. Similarly, how many are inappropriately diagnosed with ADHD? The now commonplace diagnosis of attention deficit hyperactive disorder is another waste-basket diagnosis used to classify and treat children with a wide variety of symptoms and behaviors. A conference held by the National Institutes of Health in the U.S. in 1988 failed to find any substantial evidence that there is a single condition called ADHD. Some with the diagnosis are simply super-intelligent, bored, and understimulated children, whose condition is exacerbated by poor diet. Others are probably suffering from manic depression, a diagnosis that doesn't exist in children. The worst thing you can do is give these children stimulant drugs such as Ritalin. Others are dyslexic, dyspraxic, and unable to concentrate, often because they have a deficiency in essential fats.

Diagnosing manic depression and schizophrenia

Somewhere beyond the extremes of eccentric behavior are patients with two major psychoses: the schizophrenias and manic-depressive psychosis, also known as bipolar disorder. It has become popular to regard manic depression as 'better' than schizophrenia: bipolar disorder has long been felt to have a biochemical basis, and anyway, doctors claim "it is only a disorder of emotions, the patient isn't really crazy." Perhaps this is, in part, because intellectual functioning may be less impaired than in one of the severe schizophrenias.

Schizophrenia has become a dirty word, a diagnosis to be whispered, and often to be concealed from patient, family, or friends. Again, a broken leg or even blindness would be more bearable, because it is visible, explicable, and being plainly physical, something one can live with. Schizophrenia, about which some people have such strong and irrational feelings (no doubt because of their own fears or other emotional reactions), strikes everywhere in the world. This led some researchers to believe that there may be a genetic cause, creating a biochemical weakness, in many people with schizophrenia and that the genetic twist occurred very early in humanity's evolution, back in Africa. Hence the equal spread throughout all cultures, a pattern unseen in almost any other disease.

The commonly quoted figure for schizophrenia as 1 percent of all humanity is certainly far short of the actual incidence. We should add to this estimate the walking wounded who are never seen by any doctor, since only a third of those afflicted need to be hospitalized. We must also add the teenager who commits suicide before an accurate diagnosis is made. Thus the problem is one that is important from the viewpoint of numbers, as well as individual misery. Heart disease may cause more deaths, but schizophrenia causes more heartache.

There are many conflicting descriptions and explanations for the schizophrenias, but at a basic level, there is usually little difficulty in making a preliminary diagnosis; and there is usually agreement among doctors in making the diagnosis, even though they may disagree about the possible causes and the ultimate outcome for any given patient. Since the schizophrenias may vary from simple (but abnormal) feelings of disperception or persecution to complete loss of contact with reality, the doctor hesitates to apply the term schizophrenia to the mild forms of the disorder. Instead he uses the terms schizoid personality, schizophrenic reaction, or other such words. The doctor really means, "I am puzzled and will sit on the fence until I see what happens to you in the next year or so as you freewheel through life with or without medication."

At the moment, around 30 percent of people diagnosed with schizophrenia recover in the West[5] compared to 60 percent in the developing world.[6–8] The disparity between the developed and developing world rates may be based in the more tightly knit communities of poorer countries, less associated stigma, and other social factors. So, it seems clear that with appropriate help, including optimum nutrition, the right kind of psychotherapy and positive lifestyle changes, very many people who experience a psychotic episode can recover fully.

The indicators of biochemical imbalances

One way to differentiate between a psychotic condition and purely a mood disorder is to focus on disorders of perception, or disperceptions, which was the purpose of the Hoffer-Osmond Diagnostic (HOD) test. On the next page are some of the disperceptions in the HOD test that are checked if applicable:

☐ People's faces sometimes throb as I watch them.

☐ People watch me all the time.

☐ Now and then when I look in the mirror my face changes and seems different.

☐ Sometimes when I read the words begin to look funny—they move around or grow faint.

☐ Sometimes objects vibrate when I look at them.

☐ My hands or feet sometimes seem much too large for me.

☐ I sometimes feel that I have left my body.

☐ I often hear or have heard voices.

☐ I can no longer tell how much time has gone by.

☐ I often hear thoughts inside my head.

☐ I find that past, present, and future all seem muddled up.

The presence of symptoms such as these suggests that something isn't right in the way the brain is processing information, which is a good indicator that a person has a biochemical imbalance, not purely a psychological imbalance. However, some of these symptoms could also be seen as a different kind of awareness, akin to dreaming, which is brought about through stress. According to psychotherapist Ivan Tyrrell and psychologist Joe Griffin of the Human Givens Institute in the U.K., "A psychotic breakdown is almost always preceded by an overload of stress and severe depression in a person's life, which results in excessive REM sleep. We are now convinced that, when people are in psychosis, they are in fact trapped in the REM state, a separate state of consciousness with dreamlike qualities. In other words, schizophrenia is waking reality processed through the dreaming brain."[9]

A new classification of mental health problems

The modern classification of mental health problems should be made, both from symptoms, objectively measured in questionnaire tests, and from physical and biochemical tests that help determine if any of the many kinds of biochemical imbalances are causing, or contributing to, a person's problems. Here are some of the more common biochemical imbalances that can result in symptoms of mental illness.

- Stimulant and drug intoxications

- Hypoglycemia—blood-sugar problems

- Allergy—especially wheat gluten

- Under- or overactive thyroid

- Faulty methylation and B vitamin deficiencies

- Essential fat and prostaglandin deficiency or imbalance

- Heavy metal toxicity—copper, lead, cadmium, etc.

- Detoxification overload

- Pyroluria and porphyria—resulting in zinc deficiency

- Histamine imbalance—excess or deficiency

- Low serotonin

- Dopamine/adrenalin imbalance—excess or deficiency

- Acetylcholine deficiency.

The good news is that all these can now be tested and, as a result, a more accurate assessment of their contribution to a person's mental health problems can be evaluated. The modern approach to mental illness involves keeping an open mind to all the possible contributory causes, understanding that, in most cases, more than one apply. Diagnoses are made on the basis of objective biochemical tests and subjective symptom assessment. The treatment is more often specific nutritional therapy, together with psychotherapy.

Once symptoms are gone and test results are normalized, the patient can be declared better. Dr. Abram Hoffer, a psychiatrist who has pioneered this approach since the 1950s, claims a 90 percent success rate in acute schizophrenia, with thousands of cases to prove it. His definition of cure is threefold: free from symptoms, able to socialize with family and community, and paying income tax! This, of course, is a tremendous step forward in the most debilitating of all mental health problems, for which many psychiatrists still believe there is no cure.

The next chapter explains the most common biochemical causes of mental health problems, how to identify whether a person has them, and what to do if you do.

CHAPTER 21

What's your problem?

If you've got a strange set of physical symptoms, your doctor is probably going to run a basic biochemical screening blood test, just to see if anything abnormal shows up. The same is rarely done for those with mental health problems: the belief seems to be that biochemical imbalances don't manifest as psychological symptoms. Of course, the reverse is true. The brain is far more sensitive to biochemical imbalances than any other organ of the body. The very fact that most treatment of mental illness involves chemical drugs proves the direct link between a person's biochemical state and their psychological state.

So, if you do have mental health problems, it is vital to investigate whether or not you have any of the most common biochemical imbalances that can cause mental illness. Each has a clear set of symptoms. If you score high on any one of the sections in the checklist in this chapter, an objective biochemical test can be run to prove whether or not this imbalance is present. Then, a nutritional strategy can help bring you back into balance. This approach, pioneered by our Brain Bio Centre in Richmond, greater London, has helped thousands of people recover their mental health.

The easiest way to find out if there's a high probability that one or more of these imbalances is contributing to your problems is by completing the Food for the Brain Questionnaire at the website www.foodforthebrain.org. This is a free service and gives you a printout that you can copy and give to your nutritional therapist, doctor, or psychiatrist so they know what tests to run, and what to do if the results are positive. To find a treatment center or nutritional therapist with knowledge of this approach, see www.foodforthebrain.org.

Biochemical imbalances: 13 common causes of mental health problems

Blood-sugar problems

The most common underlying imbalance in many types of mental health problems is fluctuating blood-sugar levels, called hypoglycemia. If you've got this, the chances are you crave sweet foods or stimulants such as tea, coffee, and cigarettes, all of which affect your blood-sugar levels. Here are the most common symptoms:

Difficulty concentrating
Palpitations or blackouts
Fainting or dizziness or trembling
Excessive or night sweats
Excessive thirst
Chronic fatigue
Frequent mood swings
Forgetfulness or confusion
Tendency to depression
Anxiety and irritability
Feeling weak
Aggressive outbursts or crying spells
Cravings for sweets or stimulants
Drowsiness after meals.

If you've got five or more of these, the chances are you have hypoglycemia. The best way to confirm this is to have a blood test measuring glycosylated hemoglobin. Hemoglobin is a red blood cell, while glycosylated simply means sugar-coated. If your blood-sugar level goes up and down like a yo-yo along with your mood, the red blood cells get sugar-coated. In the old days we used to measure your blood-sugar level every half hour for five hours (the five-hour glucose tolerance test). Now there's this single test, and it's much more accurate than simply measuring your blood-glucose level, which can vary from moment to moment.

Meanwhile, follow the guidelines in Chapter 3 for stabilizing your blood-sugar level.

Stimulant and drug dependence

If you've read this far, the chances are you already know if you are suffering from stimulant or drug intoxication. But many people don't, because they assume that drinking lots of tea, coffee, caffeinated drinks, or alcohol, eating sugar and smoking cigarettes, while not good for their health, is hardly going to make them crazy. This is far from the truth. Intoxication with stimulants, or drugs such as amphetamines, cocaine, crack, heroin, marijuana in excess, or Ecstasy can and does bring on symptoms of mental illness. The symptoms are very similar to those for hypoglycemia, coupled with a craving for any of these substances. In addition, you can experience disperceptions, extreme anxiety, paranoia, and depression through the excessive use of some of the substances.

Complete the stimulant inventory on the next page for a week. Add up your total number of units. The ideal is five or less per week. If you are having more than 10 stimulant units a week, this is going to have an effect on your mental well-being. If you score 30 or more this could well be contributing to mental health problems. I strongly recommend you quit all these substances for at least a month (see Chapter 10) and see how that helps your mental health.

If you are currently taking prescription drugs, please read the next chapter carefully, because many of the side effects of prescription drugs get mistaken for symptoms of a person's mental health problem.

Food and chemical allergies and intolerances

If you suffer from daily mood swings, or are fine sometimes and not others, for no apparent reason, one possibility is that you are reacting to something you're eating. The most common single food that's been linked to mental health problems is wheat, which is a rich source of gluten. Wheat gluten allergy can make some people feel crazy. Other foods that can cause allergic reactions include milk products, oranges, eggs, grains

Unit	Sun	Mon	Tue	Wed	Thu	Fri	Sat
Green Tea	2 cups						
Tea	1 cup						
Coffee	1 cup						
Cola or Caffeinated Drinks	1 can						
Caffeine pills (e.g., No-Doz, Excedrin, Dexatrim)	1 pill						
Chocolate	2 oz						
Alcohol (units) Glass of wine is 1 Bottle of beer is ½ Shot of liquor is 1	1 unit						
Added sugar	1 teaspoon						
Hidden sugar (see sugar contents on ingredients lists)	1 teaspoon/5g						
Cigarettes	1 cigarette						
Marijuana	½ joint						
Amphetamines	½ pill						
Ecstasy	½ pill						
Cocaine	½ line						
Heroin	½ hit						

other than wheat, foods with yeast, shellfish, nuts, beef, pork, and onions. Food colorings such as tartrazine and other chemical additives can also cause problems. Some people also develop intolerances to tea and coffee, while alcohol, which irritates the gut wall and makes it more leaky, often increases allergic sensitivity to anything eaten. Check yourself out on the symptoms below:

Child history of colic, eczema, asthma, rashes, or ear infections
Daily mood swings
Deep depressions for no particular reason

Brain fog
Frequent, rapid colds or stuffy nose
Difficulty sleeping
Facial puffiness, circles, or discoloration around eyes
Hyperactivity
Dyslexia or learning difficulties
Aggressive outbursts or crying spells.

If you score five or more, or know you feel better off certain foods, then food or chemical allergies may be contributing to your problem. See a nutritional therapist, who can show you how to do a two-week avoidance, then challenge test with your suspect foods. Alternatively, have a quantitative IgG ELISA allergy test. This involves taking a single blood sample and testing your allergic potential to some 50 different foods and chemicals. For more details, read Chapter 12.

Under- or overactive thyroid

If your mind and body feel sluggish most of the time, you may have an underactive thyroid, referred to as hypothroidism. If your thyroid is clinically underactive your doctor may prescribe thyroid hormones to be taken directly. However, blood tests are often unable to detect sub-clinical hypothyroidism, so it may be better to go by the symptoms. You can also test your thyroid function yourself with the Broda Barnes Temperature Test. If your temperature before rising in the morning is consistently below 97.7°F, this suggests your thyroid may be underactive. Check yourself out on the symptoms below:

Physical or mental fatigue or lethargy
Depression or irritability
Dry skin and/or hair
Intolerance to cold or cold hands and feet
Constipation, gas, bloating, or indigestion
Gain weight easily
Painful periods
Muscle pain
Poor memory
Sore throat, or nasal congestion.

If you score five or more, an underactive thyroid may be contributing to your problem. Get it tested by your doctor and also see a clinical nutritionist who can show you which foods to eat and which foods to avoid to support your thyroid. Chronic stress can deplete thyroid function, as the stress hormone cortisol inhibits it. Thyroid health is also dependent on specific nutrients in the diet, most importantly iodine, which is abundant in seafood and seaweed, and tyrosine, an amino acid found in all protein-rich foods, plus zinc and selenium. (See also "How's your thyroid?" in Chapter 23, page 256, and do the home test.)

Faulty methylation and B vitamin deficiency

Niacin (B3), B6 (also known as pyroxidine), folic acid, and B12 are your brain's best friends. They oil the wheels of the brain's neurotransmitters, especially dopamine, adrenalin, noradrenalin, and serotonin. Without enough of these vital B vitamins the brain can produce chemicals that make you crazy. They help to control the process of methylation, which is how the brain keeps everything in balance, as we learned in Chapter 8. A lack of B vitamins and other nutrients or a specific genetic fault, coupled with lifestyle factors and stresses, can lead to poor methylation, usually indicated by a high homocysteine level in the blood. Because of this or other factors, some people need much larger amounts of B vitamins than others, so it's best to be guided by symptoms, rather than your dietary intake. Here are the more common ones:

Feeling unreal or disconnected
Hearing your own thoughts
Anxiety and inner tension
Inability to think straight
Suspicious of people
Good pain tolerance
Seeing or hearing things abnormally
Having delusions or illusions
Loose bowels or skin problems at onset of mental health problems
Difficult orgasm with sex
Tendency to overweight
Frequent mood swings.

If you have five or more of these symptoms, it is worth your while to increase your intake of these nutrients for two months. See Chapter 26 for more details and guidance on the amounts to take.

Essential fats—deficiencies or imbalances

Essential fats are intimately involved in brain function and imbalances in brain fats are now known to be associated with everything from dyslexia, hyperactivity, and depression, to schizophrenia and manic depression, or bipolar disorder. Changes in our intake of essential fats, especially in women during pregnancy—when the growing fetus needs these fats, particularly to build a healthy brain—could easily explain the rapid increases in mental health problems. In short, it is essential to assess your need for essential fats if you have a mental health problem. Common symptoms are the following:

Excessive thirst
Chronic fatigue
Dry or rough skin
Dry hair, loss of hair, or dandruff
PMS or breast pain
Eczema, asthma, or joint aches
Dyslexia, or learning difficulties
Hyperactivity
Diagnosis of depression, manic depression, or schizophrenia.

If you have five or more of these symptoms and you have a mental health problem, it may be worth your while to have a blood test to determine your essential fat status. Your nutritional therapist or possibly your doctor can let you know how.

Heavy metal toxicity and metallothionein deficiency

The brain and body are constantly detoxifying and getting rid of toxic elements using a removal agent called metallothionein. If this isn't working well, possibly due to a deficiency in key nutrients and/or an excess of lead; or copper (perhaps from copper plumbing in soft water areas), mercury (present until recently in vaccines), or cadmium, which is often found in smokers as tobacco is relatively rich in it, you may end up intoxicated.

Check yourself out on the symptoms below:

Anxiety, extreme fears, or paranoia
Phobias
Poor concentration or confusion
Poor memory
Angry or aggressive feelings
Hyperactivity
Emotional instability
Headaches or migraines
Joint pain
Nervousness.

If you score five or more, I'd recommend a hair-mineral analysis as a screening to test whether you've got an excess of toxic minerals. This inexpensive, non-invasive test is a good place to start. However, if you do find excesses of toxic elements, it's best to see a nutritional therapist and have a blood test.

Detoxification overload and inflammation

When your body is unable to detoxify the result is inflammation. Inflammation, externally characterized by pain, redness or swelling, is the body's alarm signal when things get out of hand. It is a natural response to too many insults and not enough nutrients. Omega-3 fats, one of the nutrients we're most deficient in, are especially important in preventing inflammation.

New evidence is now emerging that many mental health problems, as well as heart disease, cancer, and diabetes, have excessive inflammation as part of the root cause. There is evidence of inflammation in Alzheimer's, autism, depression, Parkinson's, and schizophrenia. We are beginning to learn that inflammation upsets the brain as much as the body. The most common cause of inflammation is faulty digestion, leading to an overload of substances for the liver to detoxify. We also produce toxins, such as homocysteine, in the absence of the right nutrients.

Check yourself out on the symptoms below:

Headaches or migraine
Watery, itchy eyes, red eyelids, or dark circles under the eyes
Itchy ears, frequent ear infections, or ringing in the ears

Excessive mucus, a stuffy nose, or sinus problems
Excess sweating and strong body odor
Indigestion or bloating
Constipation or diarrhea
History of eczema, asthma
Joint or muscle aches or pains, or arthritis
Mental health symptoms are often worse after eating.

If you score five or more, you may have detoxification problems and also be suffering from inflammation. Your doctor can check this by running a standard blood test that measures your ESR (standing for the erythrocyte sedimentation rate). If this is raised, you have excessive inflammation. A clinical nutritionist can also assess whether you have digestion and detox-ification problems. The antidote is more omega-3 fats, more antioxidants, and fewer oxidants (especially saturated, processed, and fried fats), and solving any underlying digestive problems.

Pyroluria and porphyria

Some people produce more of the proteinlike chemicals called hydroxy-hemopyrrolin-2-one or HPL, otherwise known as mauve factor (previ-ously thought to be kryptopyrroles) and porphyrins than is healthy. An excess of them is linked to mental illness. The madness of George III, for example, was almost certainly porphyria, which makes the urine dark red in color. This, and probably pyroluria, are genetically inherited tendencies which increase a person's need for zinc. Stress also depletes zinc. Having a high level of HPL also means there's more oxidation going on, which means an inability to detoxify, making people very sensitive to even low levels of toxins. So, if your mental health problems are strongly stress-related and the symptoms below apply to you, you may be pyroluric, or even porphyric, although the latter is much less common:

Nausea or constipation
White spots on fingernails
Pale skin that burns easily
Frequent colds and infections
Stretch marks
Irregular menstruation or impotency

Oversensitive to light, sound, smell, or stress
Poor tolerance of alcohol or drugs
Poor dream recall.

If you score five or more you may be pyroluric. You can test this by having a urine test for HPL. If high, you need more zinc and B6, among other nutrients.

Histamine excess

Histamine is an often overlooked neurotransmitter. Some people are genetically preprogramed to produce more histamine, a condition known as histadelia, and this can make a person excessively compulsive and obsessive. High-histamine types have a faster metabolism and therefore use up nutrients at a fast rate. Without good nutrition, they can easily become deficient, which can precipitate patches of deep depression. These are some of the symptoms associated with excess histamine:

Headaches or migraines
Sneeze in sunlight
Cry, salivate, or feel nauseated easily
Easy orgasm with sex
Abnormal fears, compulsions, rituals
Light sleeper
Fast metabolism
Depression or suicidal thoughts
Excessive body heat
Little body hair and lean build
Large ears or long fingers and toes
Good tolerance of alcohol
Inner tension or driven feeling
Shy or oversensitive as child
Seasonal allergies (such as hay fever)
Obsessive or compulsive tendencies.

If you have five or more of these symptoms you may be a high-histamine type. You can check this out by having a blood test for histamine. If your blood levels are high you will benefit from supplementing vitamin C, plus the amino acid methionine, together with calcium. But don't take large amounts of folic acid on its own. For more details on histadelia read Chapter 23. Histamine levels can also be determined as part of an overall neurotransmitter screening test (see page 480 or visit the Brain Bio Centre).

Serotonin deficiency

Serotonin deficiency is one of the most common findings in people with mental health problems. It is associated with sleeping problems, mood disturbance, and aggressive and compulsive behavior. Check yourself out on the symptoms below:

Depression, especially post-menopausal
Anxiety
Aggressive or suicidal thoughts
Violent or impulsive behavior
Mood swings, including PMS
Obsessive or compulsive tendencies
Alcohol or drug abuse
Sensitive to pain (low pain threshold)
Craves sweet foods
Sleeping problems.

If you score five or more you may be low in serotonin. A neurotransmitter screening test can help confirm this. Your nutritionist can arrange this blood test for you. If you're low, there are specific nutrients, including the amino acids tryptophan or 5-hydroxytryptophan (5-HTP), which can help restore normal mental health.

Adrenal imbalance

The adrenal glands and the brain produce three motivating neurotransmitters called dopamine, adrenalin, and noradrenalin. The adrenal glands also produce cortisol. Excesses of adrenalin can result in states of high stress and anxiety, while deficiency results in the opposite—low energy, no motivation, and poor concentration. There is evidence that some people may abnormally turn excessive amounts into toxins that induce disperceptions and even hallucinations. Check yourself out on the symptoms below:

Irritability
Nervousness or anxiety
Extreme fears
Raised blood pressure
Rapid or irregular heartbeat
Insomnia
Cold hands and feet
Excessive sweating
Teeth grinding
Headaches or migraine
Muscle tension
Restlessness
Seeing or hearing things.

If you score five or more you may have excessive levels of adrenalin or cortisol. If, on the other hand, you have the following symptoms, you may have adrenal insufficiency:

Depression
Difficulty concentrating
Short attention span
Lack of drive or motivation
Rarely initiates or completes tasks
Frequently tired
Can't deal with stress
Socially withdrawn.

Both excess and deficiency can be tested with either an adrenal stress index, using saliva samples, or as part of a neurotransmitter screening test. Your nutritionist can arrange these tests. For high adrenalin levels, cut back on stimulants and sugar and up your intake of vitamins B and C (also see Chapter 17). For low adrenalin levels, you may benefit from supplementing the amino acid tyrosine. Adaptogenic herbs such as Asian or Siberian ginseng or rhodiola can also help.

Acetylcholine imbalance

Acetylcholine is the brain's learning neurotransmitter. Low levels are associated with memory loss and even Alzheimer's. Levels tend to decline with age, but they don't have to if you are optimally nourished. Check yourself out on the symptoms below:

Poor dream recall
Infrequent dreaming
Difficulty visualizing
Dry mouth
Poor memory or forgetfulness
Mental exhaustion
Poor concentration
Difficulty learning new things.

If you score five or more, chances are you might be low in acetylcholine. A neurotransmitter screening test can help confirm this. Your nutritional therapist can arrange one for you. Alternatively, you can simply supplement brain-friendly nutrients, as explained in Chapter 14.

SUMMARY

In summary, these are 13 reasonably common biochemical imbalances that can lead to a whole host of mental health problems, both major and minor. Most mental health problems are down to a number of factors, however. Part 5 looks specifically at the most common mental health problems and what we know about their causes and treatment, using optimum nutrition principles.

CHAPTER 22

The dangers of drugs and how to get off them

Since the 1950s, the treatment of mental illness with drugs has become the major therapeutic tool of psychiatrists the world over. There are three main types of such drugs: antidepressants (such as Prozac), stimulants (such as Ritalin) and tranquilizers (such as Valium). Tranquilizers can be further divided into minor tranquilizers for the treatment of anxiety and sleeping problems, and major tranquilizers (such as chlorpromazine, sold as Thorazine) for the treatment of psychotic conditions, including schizophrenia.

Perilous prescriptions

Antidepressants: they work but the side effects are depressing

Antidepressant drugs may work, but they are not without considerable risk. Tricyclic antidepressants such as amitriptyline, Anafranil, and Prothiadin have over 20 side effects listed in the doctor's drug guide, the *British National Formulary*, including dry mouth, blurred vision, nausea, confusion, cardiovascular problems, sweating, tremors, and behavioral disturbance.[10] Monoamine oxidase inhibitors (MAOIs) such as Nardil and Parstelin have even worse side effects, and can be very difficult to come off: they're highly addictive. They can cause dangerously high blood pressure if taken with substances containing yeast, alcohol or caffeine. Some patients have died after taking MAOIs and failing to avoid these substances, which are found hidden in many convenience foods.

Serotonin reuptake inhibitors (SSRIs), the relatively new class of antidepressants that work by keeping levels of serotonin relatively high, are touted as having less side effects for most people. But they can create profound problems in a significant minority. Prozac, the market leader, prescribed to more than 38 million people worldwide, has 45 side effects listed in the *British National Formulary*. According to psychiatrist David Richman, between 10 and 25 percent of people experienced each of the following: nausea, nervousness, insomnia, headache, tremors, anxiety, drowsiness, dry mouth, excessive sweating, and diarrhea. These drugs also tend to flatten moods, sometimes to the point of zombielike emotionlessness, and reduce libido and sexual performance.

Prozac and another commonly prescribed antidepressant, Seroxat, show clear evidence of agitation leading to potential aggressive and suicidal behavior in as many as a quarter of patients in a number of clinical trials. However, these particular SSRI antidepressants shouldn't be singled out. Most increase suicidal tendencies. A review of 702 studies on SSRI antidepressants showed that people taking an SSRI were more than twice as likely to attempt suicide compared with those taking a dummy pill. The researchers also noted that the actual number of suicide attempts is likely to be much higher, because many of the studies did not gather information on suicide.[11]

SSRIs can also cause people to feel fuzzy, and can trigger major sexual dysfunction, resulting in an inability to climax in both men and women (in its turn leading to a loss of intimacy that, ironically, could adversely affect a person's ability to make it through depression). On top of this, research published in 2006 suggests that SSRIs might dramatically increase the risk of death in people with cardiovascular disease.[12] There have now been 90 legal actions and one recent successful litigation, with $6.4 million dollars being awarded against Eli Lilly. "I estimate that about one person a day has committed suicide as a direct result of taking Prozac since it was introduced," declares Dr. David Healy of the North Wales Department of Psychological Medicine in Bangor, who has been petitioning the government's Medicine Control Agency to warn users about these potential adverse reactions.[13] In the U.K. that means about 1,000 suicides and 10,000 attempts.[14]

While SSRI antidepressants may not be technically addictive, there is now considerable evidence that some 50 percent of those who try to quit experience alarming withdrawal symptoms. One study testing withdrawal showed that as many as 85 percent of the volunteers, people with no previous hint of depression, suffered agitation, abnormal dreams, insomnia, and other adverse effects.[15] A recent report on all treatments for depression from the U.K.'s National Institute for Clinical Excellence (NICE) says: "There is little clinically important difference between antidepressants and placebo for mild depression."[16] For mild depression, NICE does not recommend antidepressants, favoring instead exercise, guided self-help (effectively, keeping a journal) and counseling. Unfortunately, nutrition has not yet made it onto their agenda.

Antidepressants should be used only as a last resort, and even then, only for a short period of time, especially since equally effective but much safer alternatives exist (see Chapters 15 and 23).

As we saw in Chapter 15, there's now a fourth generation of antidepressants starting to replace the SSRIs as their patents run out. These are known as serotonin and noradrenalin reuptake inhibitors, or SNRIs. But these drugs come with side effects too—nausea, headaches, insomnia, sleepiness, dry mouth, dizziness, constipation, weakness, sweating, nervousness, and, as with SSRIs, serious sexual dysfunction.

If you are currently on antidepressants and would like to come off them, the best strategy is to phase out the antidepressant and phase in the nutrients and herbs that help promote a good mood, but without the side effects. You should definitely do this only with the support of your doctor, and preferably with the guidance of a nutritional therapist (see Useful Addresses, page 474).

Stimulants: 10 million children are on Ritalin

Sadly, many hyperactive children are not evaluated for chemical, nutritional and allergic factors, nor are they treated nutritionally. Instead, they're quickly put on drugs such as Ritalin (methylphenidate), which acts like an amphetamine. They might also get a slow-acting form of Ritalin, called Concerta, or a variation on that theme called dextroamphetamine, which is marketed as Adderall or Dexedrine, a habit-forming amphetamine with similar properties to cocaine.

Diagnoses of hyperactivity and ADHD have risen more than 15-fold in the last decade. Prescriptions of Ritalin, however, have risen 180-fold—from 2,000 in 1991 to 259,000 in 2004. The drug is currently given to 7 million schoolchildren in the U.S.—that's nearly 1 in 5.[17]

This is all good news for drug company sales. The bill for this class of drug now stands at over $3 billion per year in the U.S. In Britain, 359,000 prescriptions for methylphenidate (Ritalin and Concerta), costing $23 million (£12.5 million), were dispensed in 2004.[18]

According to the U.S. Drug Enforcement Administration, the harmful side effects of taking Ritalin can include increased blood pressure, heart rate, respiration and temperature, appetite suppression, stomach pains, weight loss, growth retardation, facial tics, muscle twitching, insomnia, euphoria, nervousness, irritability, agitation, psychotic episodes, violent behavior, paranoid delusions, hallucinations, bizarre behaviors, heart arrhythmias and palpitations, tolerance, psychological dependence, and even death. Some of these symptoms do not go away on stopping the drug.

Like dextroamphetamine, Ritalin is structurally and pharmacologically similar to cocaine and has a similar dependency profile. It may be even more potent. Researchers have found that it is chosen over cocaine in self-administered preference studies with non-human primates. Using brain imaging, Dr. Nora Volkow of the Brookhaven National Laboratory in Upton, New York, has shown that Ritalin occupies more of the neural transporters responsible for the high experienced by addicts than smoked or injected cocaine. The only reason Ritalin has not produced an army of addicted schoolchildren, she concludes, is that it takes about an hour for Ritalin in pill form to raise dopamine levels in the brain, while smoked or injected cocaine does this in seconds.[19] There are now growing reports of teenagers and others abusing Ritalin by snorting or injecting it to get a faster rush.

But it doesn't end there. Dr. Joan Baizer, Professor of Physiology and Biophysics at the University of Buffalo, has shown how Ritalin, which physicians considered to have only short-term effects, may initiate changes in brain structure and function that remain long after the therapeutic effects have dissipated.[20] This can in turn lead to a greater susceptibility to drug dependence in later life.

As you'll see in Chapter 28, nutritional approaches to the multitude of problems lumped together as ADHD have already proven to be more effective than these drugs. However, as with any stimulant, coming off Ritalin does result in withdrawal symptoms. These can best be minimized by keeping blood-sugar levels even. Follow the strategy given in Chapters 3 and 10.

Tranquilizers: the false calm

As I mentioned earlier, every week in Britain we take 10 million tranquilizers. And every year in Britain, around 16 million prescriptions for these drugs are written out, mainly to treat anxiety and insomnia. Major tranquilizers are also prescribed for people with schizophrenia, to calm them down.

Any way you look at it, the figures are staggering. But it's not just the numbers: the big problem is that most of these drugs are highly addictive. In fact, they are as addictive as heroin, and dependence on them can occur within two weeks of use.[21] Doctors are specifically instructed not to prescribe more than a four-week supply, yet a MORI poll in the 1980s found that 35 percent of those prescribed benzodiazepines had been on them, not for four weeks, but for over four months! The poll estimated than 1.5 million people in Britain are addicted to tranquilizers.[22]

As we saw in Chapter 17, benzodiazepine tranquilizers such as diazepam (Valium), chlordiazepoxide (Librium), clonazepam (Klonopin), and the shorter-acting alprazolam (Xanax) or temazepam (Restoril) are still prescribed, but are giving way to a new class of related but more targeted drugs, the nonbenzodiazepines. They're colloquially known as the Zs— zolpidem (Ambien), zalephon (Sonata), and zopiclone (Zimovane) —and were introduced in the 1990s amid claims that they were a safe and non-addictive alternative to earlier drugs.

However, a review in 2005 by NICE concluded that "there was no consistent difference between the two types of drug for either effectiveness of safety."[23] Nonbenzodiazepines too can cause tolerance and withdrawal. "Dependence can develop after as little as one week of continuous use. If you fall asleep without having taken a dose and wake some time later, do not take the missed dose. Patients who have been taking this drug for longer than seven days should consult their doctor before withdrawing treatment," advises one drug bulletin on zopiclone.[24] You are also not advised to take nonbenzodiazepines for more than a few weeks.

In the late 1980s, thousands of tranquilizer addicts sued the drug companies. The case was, however, abandoned in 1994 due to lack of funding.

Just how bad are the benzodiazepines? Their dangers and addictive qualities are well known, although this has not stopped the flow of prescriptions. An editorial published in a 2004 issue of the *British Medical Journal* concluded that not only was there plenty of evidence that they cause "major harm" but that there was also "little evidence of clinically meaningful benefit."[25]

A recent trial found that people on these drugs for 18 months had "negative effects on crisis reaction, intensified defense mechanisms and reduced cognitive, emotional, and conative [behavioral or active] functions, and passive coping."[26] A 2005 review of 37 trials examining whether benzodiazepines were effective for insomnia found that none of the trials was well enough designed to allow any conclusions to be drawn.[27]

Tolerance is also a major problem: after taking them for some time, a higher dose is required to get the same effect. People often experience forgetfulness, drowsiness, accident-proneness, and/or social withdrawal. Other side effects include rebound anxiety as a result of withdrawal and insomnia, and hangover (grogginess the next morning, accidents caused not only right after ingestion, but the following day). Benzodiazepines trigger serious withdrawal effects on quitting, including anxiety, insomnia, irritability, tremors, mental impairment, headaches—possibly even seizures, and death. Combining these drugs with alcohol is especially dangerous.

These symptoms can go on for months afterwards but, with the right nutritional support, can be greatly reduced (see www.foodforthebrain. org/comingofftranquillisers.) Mary's story, from the book *Natural Highs* (case generously supplied by co-author Dr. Hyla Cass at www.cassmd. com), is a case in point:

When Mary was in her thirties, she found herself stuck in an unhappy marriage, and with a young child. Seeing no escape, she was taking large doses of Valium to shut out the pain. One day, while filling yet another prescription for Mary, the pharmacist said, "In case you don't know it, you're addicted. Speak to me when you're ready to stop." This was Mary's wake-up call.

In shocked response, she simply stopped the drug cold. She was too ashamed to face the pharmacist, who would have advised a slow withdrawal program under medical supervision. Then, not knowing she was suffering from withdrawal symptoms, she simply, in her words, "went crazy" for the next two months or so. It took that long for her brain to readjust itself.

What had happened was that the Valium had caused Mary's brain to downregulate. It had adjusted to Valium's relaxing action. This led to extreme agitation (withdrawal) when she stopped it, until, in time, her brain readjusted. "When I finally got my mind back, I decided to leave my husband. I never looked back. Nor did I ever dare take another tranquilizer," declares Mary, now, at 48, a successful writer and a proud grandmother.

I'd also recommend seeing a psychotherapist to help deal with the underlying issues for your anxieties. As well as following all the advice in Parts 1 and 2, the relaxing herbs valerian and kava can be gradually substituted, but only under the guidance and support of a clinical nutritionist and your doctor. You can also get some great support and guidance from the charitable self-help group the Council for Information on Tranquillisers and Antidepressants (CITA). Their details are in Useful Addresses on page 474.

Anti-psychotic drugs: chemical straitjackets

The first anti-psychotic drug, reserpine, was introduced into psychiatric practice in 1952, shortly followed by chlorpromazine (Thorazine) in 1954. The perfecting of this type of anti-psychotic drug was achieved in the 1960s with the introduction of fluphenazine (Prolixin) and haloperidol (Haldol). Most other anti-psychotic drugs introduced since 1970 have been *me-too* drugs which have little advantage over these two standard and now cheaper drugs.

For patients who will not take these medications by mouth, oil-soluble decanoate salts are available for intramuscular injection. These weekly injections—Depixol for example—do not give as smooth a result as the daily use of the drug by mouth. Most patients can have the daily dose they need by taking the pills at bedtime with dephenhydramine (Benadryl). If they develop muscle shakes from taking the drug, a small dose of Cogentin, Artane, or Kemadrin is often given each morning (see also page 236).

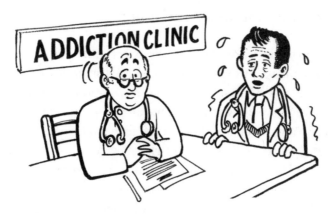

Fig 26. "Doctor, I seem to have become addicted to prescribing drugs."

Drugs such as the major tranquilizers should only be considered as temporary crutches, to be used until the biochemical imbalances are slowly corrected by nutritional therapy. According to the psychiatrist Dr. Abram Hoffer, who has been treating mental illness for over 50 years, tranquilizers never cure mental illness—they just replace one psychosis with another. No normal person can function under the influence of tranquilizers. Yet even today, one unfortunate consequence of understaffing at public mental hospitals is that excessive doses of chlorpromazine are routinely prescribed to keep a difficult patient quiet.

When a columnist with the *San Francisco Examiner*, Bill Mandel, tried 50 mg of Thorazine, he reported,

66 Simply put, it made me stupid. Because Thorazine and related drugs are called liquid lobotomy in the mental health business, I'd expected a great grey cloud to descend over my faculties. There was no grey cloud, just small, unsettling patches of fog. My mental gears slipped. I had no intellectual traction. It was difficult, for example, to remember simple words. 99

Most patients are prescribed 2–16 times the amount taken by Mandel. Tranquilizers such as these should only be used as a last resort, and even then, phased out as the patient improves on the right diet and treatment with specific nutrients, based on a proper diagnosis.

Side effects of anti-psychotic drugs

A major problem in treating mental disorders with pharmaceutical drugs, which is often played down, is the immense discomfort caused by some of the side effects. Drugs such as the now-antiquated chlorpromazine (Thorazine or Largactil) can have some annoying and sometimes serious side effects. Patients taking these drugs may find themselves unable to steady their hands. Their facial muscles may twitch involuntarily. They may try to read but find their vision is too blurred to decipher the printed lines. The eyes may turn up and refuse to come down. The patients may be restless and pace the floor until they have blistered feet. A severe skin reaction may follow even a brief exposure to the sun, so that patients on the drug are compelled to spend much of their time indoors. After long-term drug therapy, a patient may look in the mirror one morning to discover that his face has acquired a purplish-grey hue, a very slowly reversible condition. This pigment can also lodge in the heart muscle and may cause sudden death.

And imagine the agony of an intelligent young man or woman, particularly the artistic or intellectual type, who is forced to take this medication—only to find, at some point, that their imaginative facilities are simply no longer available. Is it ethical, more than half a century after the introduction of chlorpromazine, to increase the agony of the suffering schizophrenic by giving them this drug, when safer drugs and treatments are available?

If needed, a drug such as haloperidol or fluphenazine may be substituted for chlorpromazine. These produce fewer side effects, but should only be used as holding drugs until the nutrients begin to take effect. A pharmacological lobotomy is not at all necessary, nor is the frustrating disruption of patients' imaginative resources.

These anti-psychotic drugs, if given at high doses for many months, may produce tardive dyskinesia—a delayed impairment of voluntary motion causing incomplete or partial movement. The risk of getting this side effect after long-term use is around 75 percent, according to Dr. William Glazer, an expert on the condition.[28]

Since the drugs, called phenothiazines, have been found to attach to manganese, so making it less available for use in the brain, one researcher hypothesized that manganese might be useful for preventing the side effects caused by the drugs. Out of 15 people given manganese supplements, seven were cured outright of their involuntary muscle twitches, three were much improved, and four were improved. Only one person did not respond.[29] Manganese taken daily in doses of 25 mg is helpful, as is the daily use of phosphatidylcholine or DMAE, which builds up acetylcholine, the neurotransmitter involved in brain and muscle function. Vitamin E may also help, at a level of 800 IUs per day.[30]

The neuroleptic malignant syndrome is yet another, sometimes lethal, side effect of anti-schizophrenic medication. More than 20 publications have depicted the distressing effects of prolonged use of these drugs. Patients may get elevated temperature, sweating, rapid pulse, panting, soiling, rigidity, dazed mutism, stupor, and coma. If the drug is not withdrawn, death can occur within 24 hours.

Newer agents such as Zyprexa (olanzapine), which has been taken by over 15 million people around the world, are said to have fewer side effects than these older-generation drugs. However, a shocking number of health risks have recently been associated with the drug, including diabetes, pancreatitis, substantial weight gain, and again, tardive dyskinesia, and neuroleptic malignant syndrome. Evidence suggests that the manufacturer, Eli Lilly, knew of these risks long before they were forced by the U.S. Food and Drug Administration (FDA) to include them in their labeling of Zyprexa. By the end of 2004, over 125 individual lawsuits had been filed by Zyprexa users against Eli Lilly. Although sales of Zyprexa are dropping significantly, the drug is still available and is still prescribed off-label (for uses not approved by the FDA) to children and adults alike.[31]

Are any of these drugs really worth it? A 2006 analysis by Dr. David Healy of the North Wales Department of Psychological Medicine in Bangor, which compared suicide rates among schizophrenic patients before and after the introduction of psychotropic drugs, found that patients treated with the latest antipsychotic drugs had a 20-fold increased risk of suicide compared to those treated without drugs in Victorian times.[32] These findings lend support to those of the prizewinning author of *Mad in America*, Robert Whitaker, who, after analyzing U.S. government disability data, found that the outcome for schizophrenia patients in the U.S. has worsened since the introduction of psychotropic drugs.[33]

Problems with multi-drug use

Another problem is multiple drug interactions. Many psychiatric patients simultaneously take daily doses of one or more anti-psychotics, antidepressants, a minor tranquilizer, and a hypnotic to make them sleep at night. In addition, because of certain Parkinson's-like side effects of these drugs, most patients are also given drugs used to treat Parkinson's, such as Cogentin or Kemadrin. These make sleeping even more difficult. Then there are drugs for co-existing illnesses prescribed by other doctors, and self-medication with over-the-counter drugs, all of which the patient could conceivably take simultaneously. Together this adds up to a potentially dangerous constellation of pharmacological interaction and personal neglect of the patient which might prolong suffering and delay rehabilitation.

While anti-psychotic drugs can have beneficial short-term effects, the lethargic, anti-social, odd behavior of some patients, which is usually attributed to illness, is more often than not the result of medication. Every avenue of treatment, including nutrition, should be thoroughly explored before sentencing a person to the chemical straitjacket of long-term tranquilizer use.

If polypharmacy—that is, taking a cocktail of pharmaceutical drugs—in adults isn't bad enough, even more alarming is the evidence that it's on the rise in children. A survey in 2005[34] found that in the U.S. it is not uncommon to find a child on an antidepressant, a mood stabilizer, and a sleep agent all at the same time, yet there's no research to see how these drugs interact with each other. According to this study, the most frequent combination were stimulants such as methylphenidate (Ritalin) or dextroamphetamine (Dexedrine, Adderall), commonly used to treat ADHD, with another psychotropic medication. Contributing to this already dire situation is the prevalence of off-label prescriptions—the practice of prescribing a medication to children when there is not an FDA-approved indication for that disorder in children.

This study's co-author, Henrietta Leonard, M.D., a child psychiatrist with the Bradley Hasbro Children's Research Center and Brown Medical School, says that anti-psychotics like risperidone are sometimes used to symptomatically treat psychosis or aggression in children, yet most of these medications don't have FDA approval for use on psychiatric symptoms in the the young. The authors cite examples of a child on two medications for ADHD who died suddenly, and additionally describe serotonin syndrome, a serious and potentially fatal illness that can result when a person receives two medications with serotonergic properties.

SUMMARY

In summary, in almost all cases, with the right guidance, the right nutritional program and support, it is possible to get off medication. This is desirable because almost all drugs currently used for mental health problems do have unwanted side effects, especially in the long term.

However, coming off medication should never be done too quickly, or without the full support of your doctor and nutritional therapist or other health professional who can support you with less toxic nutritional approaches for keeping you in a good state of mind.

PART 5

Solving Depression, Manic Depression, and Schizophrenia

More people suffer from depression and schizophrenia than any other mental health problem. In Britain, 1 in 20, or around 3 million people, are diagnosed with depression. One in 100 are diagnosed with schizophrenia. Both conditions can be a living hell. But it needn't be this way, as both are also, for the most part, curable with the right nutrition plus psychotherapy. Yet more often than not, the only treatment given is far less effective drugs. In this part you will find out about the proven biochemical imbalances that can cause these conditions and how to solve them.

CHAPTER 23

Overcoming depression

In Chapter 15 we explored how blood-sugar imbalances, allergies, and deficiencies in vitamins, minerals, essential fats, and amino acids have all been linked to low mood. If you suffer from depression, it's best to start by correcting these. But there is much more that you can do, and that's what this chapter explores in depth.

There's no doubt that there is a need to counteract depression: the condition is 10 times more common today than it was in the 1950s. Overall in the U.K., approximately 15 percent of people are labeled clinically depressed, and half of them will consult their doctor.[1] In fact, an estimated one in three doctor consultations involve patients with mental health issues such as depression.

Depression is also the primary cause of suicide, claiming 3,000 lives a year, and is now the second most common cause of death in young people aged 15 to 24. As depressing as all this sounds, there is a lot that can be done, both with nutrition and proper counseling.

The classic symptoms of depression include:

- Feelings of worthlessness or guilt

- Poor concentration

- Loss of energy, and fatigue

- Thoughts of suicide or preoccupation with death

- Loss or increase of appetite and weight

- A disturbed sleep pattern

- Slowing down (both physically and mentally)

- Agitation (restlessness or anxiety).

If you are experiencing four or more of these, this chapter is for you. It's important to realize that there is rarely one cause for a set of symptoms that we call depression, nor a single cure.

As a general rule, however, it's a good idea to keep crucial neurotransmitters in balance. You may remember from Chapter 15 that low levels of serotonin are strongly associated with states of depression, while low levels of dopamine, adrenalin or noradrenalin are associated with a lack of motivation. Most prescription drugs aim to correct these imbalances, but have undesirable side effects. Instead, I recommend supplementing 100 mg up to 300 mg of the amino acid 5-hydroxytryptophan (5-HTP), twice a day, to boost your serotonin levels. Supplementing tyrosine at 500–1,000 mg twice a day helps boost motivation and may be helpful in those who feel a distinct lack of drive. Tyrosine is best taken on an empty stomach.

Natural ways to beat the blues

St. John's wort: the happiness herb

Another highly effective natural remedy is the herb St. John's wort (*Hypericum perforatum*). It is one of the most thoroughly researched of all natural remedies.

St. John's wort works just as well as tricyclic antidepressants, but has fewer side effects.[2] Tricyclic antidepressants such as imipramine are widely prescribed but often produce undesirable side effects. For instance, in a recent study published in the *British Medical Journal*, 324 patients were randomly assigned to treatment with either St. John's wort or imipramine. Both were equally effective in treating patients with mild to moderate depression. However, St. John's wort was better tolerated than imipramine and fewer patients withdrew as a result of adverse effects.[3]

An analysis of 23 such randomized clinical trials on St. John's wort versus placebos, involving 1,757 people in total, proves that the herb is highly effective with minimal side effects.[4] In one German study using 300 mg of St. John's wort, 66 percent of patients with mild to moderately severe depression improved, with less depression and complaints of disturbed sleep, headache, and fatigue, compared to just 26 percent of those receiving a placebo.[5] It is not, however, as effective for severe depression. The same is true for SSRI antidepressants.

A 300 mg dose of St. John's wort (containing 0.3 percent hypericin) two or three times a day helps most people with mild depression, while twice this amount may help those who suffer severely. But don't expect instant results. It often takes a couple of weeks to work.

The joy of minimal side effects

One of the consistent findings in this research, and my clinical experience, is that St. John's wort has minimal side effects. It is much gentler than antidepressant drugs. That said, there are some side effects reported. About 2 percent of people report side effects including gastrointestinal symptoms, allergic reactions, anxiety, and dizziness. These have often been exaggerated in the media, possibly because more and more people are opting to take St. John's wort instead of antidepressant drugs, and the drugs companies are fighting back with scare stories in the popular press.

Concerns about St. John's wort causing photosensitivity (increased skin sensitivity to strong sunlight) should not be alarming, having only occurred at very high doses rather than the recommended 600–900 mg a day.[6]

St. John's wort does upregulate certain liver enzymes. This means that the liver works a bit harder. The same happens with almost all drugs and substances foreign to the body, as the liver tries to detoxify them.

The prominent psychiatrist Dr. Hyla Cass is one of the world's leading experts on St. John's wort. In her excellent book *St. John's Wort: Nature's Blues Buster* (Avery Publishing, 1997), she gives 10 reasons why she prefers St. John's wort to antidepressant drugs:

1. Its side effects are not nearly as severe or frequent.

2. Mixing with alcohol doesn't lead to adverse reactions, as with the other antidepressants.

3. It is not addictive.

4. It does not produce withdrawal symptoms when you stop.

5. It does not produce habituation, or the need for increased dosages to maintain its effects.

6. It can be easily stopped and restarted without requiring a long buildup period.

7. It enhances sleep and dreaming.

8. It does not inhibit sex drive as SSRIs do in some people—and can actually enhance it in some people.

9. It does not make you sleepy in the daytime. In fact, it has shown in experiments to enhance alertness and driving reaction time.

10. According to one report, the annual rate of death by overdose on anti-depressant drugs is 30.1 per 1 million prescriptions. No one has ever died from an overdose of St. John's wort. In fact, we don't think anyone has even tried to OD with it!

Exactly how St. John's wort works is still a bit of a mystery. However, a $6 million research grant in the U.S. means we'll be hearing a lot more about this herb in the near future. Recent research indicates that hypericin, thought to be one of the major active ingredients in this herb, may act by inhibiting the reuptake of serotonin and dopamine. This may explain some of its benefits, but not all. In another study where the purported active ingredient hypericin was removed, St. John's wort still raised levels of the brain chemicals. So we have to conclude that so far, we still don't know enough about the activities and synergistic abilities of the many compounds found in this and other herbs.[7]

Chromium and atypical depression

It has long been known that supplementing the mineral chromium, usually provided in a 200 mcg tablet, helps stabilize blood sugar. This is because without chromium, insulin—the hormone that carries excess glucose out of the blood into the body and brain—can't work. But thanks to research by Professor Malcolm McLeod from the University of North Carolina

School of Medicine, chromium has proven to be not just a vital nutrient for blood-sugar stability, but a highly effective antidepressant for those with atypical depression—that is, depressed people who are gaining weight, feel tired all the time, crave carbohydrates, and could sleep forever, unlike the classic depressive who is suffering from weight loss and insomnia.[8]

McLeod's discovery happened by chance when one of his patients, George, who had been severely depressed for several years suddenly recovered completely after taking a nutritional supplement. McLeod thought it was a placebo effect and, since the supplement contained ephedra, a potentially dangerous herb, he asked George to stop taking it. What happened in the following week amazed McLeod. "It was unbelievable. I didn't believe it at first, but without the supplement his depression returned." He couldn't ignore the rapid change and concluded that it might be to do with one of six ingredients in the supplement. He then gave George an unidentified envelope containing only one ingredient to take for the next week. Six weeks later, having ruled out ephedra, guarana (which made the depression worse), kava, and two other substances, McLeod found that it was the chromium in the supplement that actually worked.

These days I am seeing more and more patients with atypical depression and often, they will get instant relief by taking 400–600 mcg of chromium a day. According to McLeod, between a quarter and half of people diagnosed with depression are dealing with this strain of it. A survey of several hundred depressed patients conducted by Andrew Nierenberg, associate director of the Depression and Clinical Research Program at Massachusetts General Hospital, backs this up. Nierenberg found that atypical depression affects anywhere from 25–42 percent of people with depression, and an even higher percentage of depressed women.[9] So given the number of people whose tendency to depression falls into this category, atypical is a bit of a misnomer.

The link between depression and blood sugar has been around for a long time. Sir Thomas Willis, the 17th-century medical pioneer who conclusively established the diagnosis of diabetes, noted that "sadness and long sorrow often precedes this disease." Two epidemiologists at the Johns Hopkins School of Medicine found that the incidence of diabetes in depressed people is 2.5 times that of the general population. Depression often precedes diabetes by two to three decades.

McLeod went on to test his theory by running a double-blind study of 15 patients with atypical depression. Five were given a placebo and 10

Do you have atypical depression?

Do you crave sweets or other carbohydrates, or tend to gain weight?

Are you tired for no obvious reason, or do your arms and legs feel heavy?

Do you tend to feel sleepy or groggy much of the time?

Are your feelings easily hurt by rejection from others?

Did your depression begin before the age of thirty?

If you answer *yes* to even one of these questions and you often feel low, the chances are chromium will help you.

were given 600 mcg of chromium picolinate, which is much better absorbed than cheaper forms of inorganic chromium, such as chromium chloride. At the end of 8 weeks, 7 out of the 10 participants taking chromium experienced a major improvement in their depression, compared to none on the placebo.[10]

A larger trial confirms McLeod's finding. Professor of Psychiatry John Docherty at Weill Medical College of Cornell University in New York gave 113 patients with depression either 600 mcg of chromium or a placebo for eight weeks and measured them on the Hamilton Rating Scale, one of the most widely used tests measuring depression. At the end of the eight weeks, in a subset of 41 patients who were overweight, 65 percent of those taking chromium saw a major improvement in their depression, compared to 33 percent on the placebo.[11]

Chromium is a remarkably safe mineral even at levels 100 times higher than this. McLeod gives 3–5 mcg per pound of body weight, and sometimes more for people with diabetes. Some people need this amount to stay free from depression. George, his original patient, has been on chromium for a decade and it has positively transformed his life. McLeod recommends taking chromium twice a day, although you should take it in the morning (at breakfast and lunch) as it can cause insomnia and vivid dreaming.

Chromium levels decline with age, so the older you are the more you need. Our diets are generally very deficient in this mineral anyway, but the more fast-releasing carbohydrates you eat, the more chromium you will lose. Stress also depletes chromium.

According to McLeod, chromium is far superior to SSRIs because it has no side effects. Even if its ability to relieve symptoms of depression is only half as powerful as an SSRI's, chromium is better for this reason. There are, however, some people who may need to take both. Chromium is also much faster acting than SSRIs, usually working in just 2–3 days while SSRIs can take 4–6 weeks to produce relief. Furthermore, chromium often reduces symptoms much more effectively than SSRIs. McLeod has found that many of his patients had complete relief in a matter of weeks just by taking chromium. The Hamilton Rating Scores of several patients dropped below 5 within 2 weeks, which means they were no longer depressed. You don't see this on SSRIs.

These results with chromium fit in well with other promising frontiers in the nutritional treatment of depression. 5-HTP, the precursor of serotonin, needs insulin to get from the blood into the brain—so chromium, which is essential for insulin to work, might be playing a leading role in this process. Omega-3s also improve serotonin reception. Given the role that stress, highly refined, and high-sugar diets, and caffeine have on blood sugar, and the lack of chromium and omega-3s in most people's diets, it isn't perhaps so difficult to comprehend why the incidence of depression would be on the increase in the 21st century.

The magnesium method

Another mineral that might help boost your mood is magnesium. The role of magnesium in depression was first discovered in 1921 by P. G. Weston, who used magnesium to help 50 of his patients relax and sleep.[12] Since then there have been many other studies demonstrating the important role played by magnesium in brain biochemistry and how it benefits mental health.

A study by George and Karen Eby in the U.S. of patients with major depression found that they recovered rapidly, in less than a week, by taking 125–300 mg of magnesium with each meal and at bedtime. The participants suffered not just from depression but from a number of related and accompanying mental illnesses, including headache, suicidal thoughts, anxiety, irritability, insomnia, short-term memory loss, and IQ loss, as well as cocaine, alcohol, and tobacco abuse, and these conditions improved too.[13]

After zinc, magnesium is generally the second most commonly deficient mineral. A major reason for this is that food contains far less magnesium than it did 100 years ago. Not only is much of the food people eat refined and stripped of all its goodness, but the raw material itself often contains far fewer vital nutrients, including magnesium, because it's grown in soil laced with chemical fertilizers. These deplete the health of the soil overall, and lower the capability of the crop to absorb nutrients. As the amount of magnesium in our diets has decreased, so the incidence of depression has increased.

But poor diet is not the only culprit. One study[14] has shown that chronic stress depletes magnesium while at the same time increasing oxidative stress in humans. So if you, like so many other people, are stressed out by the frenetic pace and complexities of 21st-century life, you need to ensure you are getting adequate amounts of magnesium.

Green, leafy vegetables are rich in magnesium because the mineral is part of the chlorophyll molecule, which makes plants green. So are nuts and seeds, particularly sesame, sunflower, and pumpkin seeds. An ideal intake is probably 500 mg a day, which is almost double what most people achieve. Eating a tablespoon of seeds a day, and at least three servings of vegetables (including a dark green, leafy one), plus 100 mg of magnesium in a multivitamin and mineral, is a good way to ensure you're getting enough. However, if you are depressed and the symptoms above sound like you, you may want to take an additional 100 mg of magnesium in the morning and at night for a few weeks and see if that helps. Don't supplement more than 300 mg in total.

Bump up your Bs

If you're depressed, you may well be low in B vitamins. You'll recall from Chapter 8 that four B vitamins in particular (B2, B6, B12, and folic acid) are vital for methylation, the process that keeps the brain's chemistry in balance; and that faulty methylation, indicated by a high level of homocysteine, is strongly associated with depression.

Low levels of folic acid, the B vitamin that's abundant in beans, nuts, seeds, and vegetables, have consistently been reported in depressed people, as have high homocysteine levels. Somewhere around a third of people with depression are found to have low folic-acid levels.[15] In a study of 213 people suffering from depression at the Depression and Clinical Research Program at Massachusetts General Hospital in Boston, people with lower folic acid levels had more melancholic depression (as opposed to atypical

—see page 243), and were less likely to improve when given SSRI antidepressant drugs.[16] In another study of 46 severely depressed patients, 24 had very high homocysteine levels and low levels of folate in their blood.[17]

Giving extra folic acid to people with this condition often helps to alleviate their depression. The first demonstration of this was back in 1990. A study at King's College Hospital in London found that giving folic acid supplements to people with depression and borderline or low folic-acid levels alongside standard treatment significantly improved recovery.[18] This study also found that a third of all patients with depression and other psychiatric disorders were deficient in folic acid. Since then other researchers have found that giving extra folic acid either on its own[19] or with antidepressant drugs[20–21] definitely helps improve a depressive state. Overall, the evidence to date is convincing.[22] But it doesn't work for everybody, and is much more likely to work for those who have raised homocysteine levels and low levels of folic acid in the blood.

Vitamin B12 is also vital for methylation and for mood, although studies giving B12 supplements on their own have not proven as effective as those giving folic acid on its own. B12, which is only present in food of animal origin, is also much more likely to be deficient in older people, as its absorption depends on stomach acid and levels of that tend to decline with age. A survey in Rotterdam, the Netherlands, of almost 4,000 elderly people found that those with low B12 levels were almost twice as likely to be depressed.

We still have much to learn about methylation and mood. My advice is not to supplement B vitamins singly, but to take a combination of B2, B6, B12, folic acid, and TMG (an amino acid that is also required to make stomach acid, which, in turn, helps you to absorb vitamin B12), all of which are required for proper methylation. These are often available in combination in homocysteine-lowering formulas. Methyl-B12 is also likely to be more effective. If your homocysteine level is high (above 10 mg/dl—see page 255 and page 480 for information on testing) I'd start with a supplement that provides 1,000 mcg of folic acid and 500 mcg of methyl-B12. Alternatively, if you can get it, you could try supplemeting SAMe at 200 mg a day (see page 157 for more on SAMe).

You might have wondered why the amounts of folic acid and other Bs I'm recommending here as homocysteine-busters are so much higher than those you'd get from a well-balanced diet. The answer is that we are biochemically unique and there is growing evidence that some people, perhaps those prone to severe depression and also schizophrenia, don't methylate properly. As a result, these people will need more of these key nutrients than others, simply to function normally—let alone optimally.

You'll remember that methylation goes on throughout the brain and body, helping to turn one neurotransmitter into another. For example, noradrenalin turns into adrenalin by having a methyl group, a kind of organic compound, added. Nutrients that can donate or receive methyl groups help the brain to function better; folic acid and SAMe, for example, help donate methyl groups. Depressed patients may not be good methylators and would therefore benefit from getting more of these nutrients.

Later on, in Chapter 26, you'll learn how megadoses of vitamin B3— which is also involved in methylation—is particularly helpful for some people diagnosed with schizophrenia. SAMe, however, while often very effective with depression, can aggravate manic symptoms, both in schizophrenia[23] and manic depression. So use it with caution.

It's all one great, big balancing act, helping your brain's chemistry to get, and stay, in sync.

The right fats to keep you happy

Talking of balancing acts, B3, B6, B12, and folic acid also have a crucial role to play in how the brain makes its essential brain fats. Throughout this book I've extolled the virtues of the essential fats from fish and seeds. However, to turn these essential fats into building materials for the brain, for example in making the receptor sites for neurotransmitters, you need these B vitamins too. That's because they drive the enzymes that turn one essential fat into another. Essential fats are also converted into hormone-like prostaglandins by these B-vitamin-dependent enzymes. Both these enzymes and the prostaglandins themselves further promote the brain's production of serotonin and other key neurotransmitters. It's one big happy family of chemical reactions. Your job is simply to make sure that your brain gets enough of all the right pieces of the equation. These are:

- Essential fats, especially omega-3 fats

- B vitamins

- Amino acids such as 5-HTP, tyrosine, and SAMe, or TMG.

In Chapter 15 we reviewed the studies to date showing the benefits of omega-3 fats, especially EPA, for people suffering from depression. What is encouraging is that some studies show omega-3 supplementation can reverse major depression. One, published in the *American Journal of Psychiatry*, has confirmed that patients already on antidepressant medication who still have pronounced symptoms of depression experience major improvements in as little as three weeks when given daily supplements of concentrated EPA.[24]

To achieve a therapeutic amount of EPA of around 1,000 mg, you will need to take something like three 1,000 mg fish oil capsules and ensure the EPA provided adds up to the 1,000 mg; or you can take a special concentrated form called ethyl EPA, which is what was used in this study. In fact, the higher your blood levels of omega-3 fats, which help build the brain's neurons, the more serotonin you are likely to make.

This also may explain why very low intakes of fat or cholesterol can lead to depression. According to a study of 121 healthy young women by Duke University psychologist Edward Suarez, low cholesterol is a potential predictor for depression and anxiety.[25] An eight-year Finnish study of 29,000 men aged 50–69, published in the *British Journal of Psychiatry*, found that those reporting depression had significantly lower average blood-cholesterol levels than those who did not, despite a similar diet.[26] The best dietary way to ensure adequate cholesterol and essential fats is to eat coldwater fish such as herring, fresh tuna (in moderation), salmon, sardines, and mackerel. It remains to be seen whether the current trend of putting millions of people on statin drugs, which are designed to lower cholesterol, will induce a tendency to depression as a side effect, especially in those whose cholesterol is already too low. It is not uncommon to be put on these drugs after a heart attack, even if the person's cholesterol level is already low.

The histamine connection

While supplementing folic acid has been seen to work in many cases of depression, it doesn't do it for everybody. The late Dr. Carl Pfeiffer, founder of Princeton's Brain Bio Center, discovered that while many depressed patients get better with massive amounts of folic acid, some get worse. He wondered why, and found that those people who got worse had high blood histamine levels. These *histadelics*, as he called them, are genetically preprogramed to overproduce histamine. High-dose folic-acid supplements further stimulate the production of histamine in these people. And this can lead to serious depression, as we'll see below.

His finding that some people get worse on massive doses of folic acid (that is, 15 mg a day) has since been confirmed by others as potentially triggering symptoms of sleep alterations, malaise, hyperactivity, and irritability.[27]

Dr. Pfeiffer's discovery is yet another example of biochemical individuality, illustrating how each of us is unique. For this very reason, to diagnose depression purely on the basis of symptoms, and then treat everyone with the same drug, or even the same nutrient ignoring the principles of synergy and biochemical individuality, is to ignore the many potential underlying reasons for depression, both biochemical and psychological.

I know about high-histamine types because I am one. I remember sitting in the waiting room of the Brain Bio Center at the age of 20, about to meet Dr. Pfeiffer, this extraordinary pioneer in nutritional medicine and mental health. He took one look at me and my white, marked nails and said, "You're high histamine. You need more zinc and B6. Do you wake up early, have a good appetite, an active mind, tend towards being compulsive and obsessive, suffer from allergies, and rarely gain weight?" Yes, that sounded like me.

And as Dr. Pfeiffer spoke, all became clear. We all make histamine, but some more than others. This is a genetic trait nicknamed histadelia. Since histamine speeds up the body's metabolism, providing more heat, and since vitamin C is an antihistamine, we think that when our ancestors lost the ability to make vitamin C—a fate they share only with other primates, guinea pigs, and bats—this put them at an advantage in colder climates during and after the Ice Age.

But histamine also makes you more prone to compulsive behavior and allergic reactions, as Dr. Pfeiffer mentioned, and gives you a tendency towards increased production of mucus and saliva, hyperactivity, and depression. Some of these traits can be an advantage, but when histamine levels become excessively high, they can lead to chronic depression and even suicide. Marilyn Monroe and Judy Garland are examples of likely high-histamine types who died a suicidal death. High-histamine types often love alcohol because it sedates an overactive mind. Many alcoholics are high histamine, and commit a kind of slow suicide through drink, as in the harrowing film *Leaving Las Vegas*.

Howard Hughes is another classic example of a histadelic, with his tremendous drive, compulsive and obsessive behavior, and tendency to depression. Dr. Pfeiffer described the high-histamine type as "built for the 21st century, complete with self-destruct." The point is that a faster metabolism means a greater need for nutrients, and insufficient nutrition leads the fast-burning high-histamine type to burn out fast. Without the right nutrients, a high-histamine person can end up severely depressed. If this all sounds familiar, you can check yourself out on the mini-questionnaire on page 222, or online at www.foodforthebrain.org.

Are you histadelic?

Histadelics have certain obvious physical signs and symptoms. Histamine promotes the production of saliva, so their teeth are frequently cavity-free. Histadelics also produce more mucus and tears, and so can cry more easily. Since Marilyn Monroe was probably histadelic we can, at this late date, understand better her remark to photographers, "You always take pictures of my body but my most perfect feature is my teeth—I have no cavities." With good salivary flow, teeth are well bathed in saliva and the histadelic may have the habit of wiping saliva from the corners of the mouth. High-histamine types are also less hairy than the norm. In men, the beard is usually light and there are few chest hairs. They have a faster metabolism, and are fast oxidizers, and the rapid oxidation of foods means a person can eat a lot and never gain weight.

Histadelics usually have relatively long fingers and toes, with the second toe longer than the big toe. When Monroe met her sister Bernice for the first time, at the age of 25, Bernice said in an interview, "the most exciting thing was discovering our toes. See how the second toe is longer than the rest. Marilyn had the same thing." Their mother, Gladys, spent many years in a mental institution, diagnosed as a schizophrenic. Abraham Lincoln is another example of a high-histamine type, with his long, skinny fingers.

Histadelics usually have an easy and well-sustained orgasm and higher than usual sex drive. They also often have the most severe insomnia. A history of allergies or periodic headache and sensitivity to pain is also common; and they're often hooked on excess sugar in coffee or tea and like alcohol and other drugs, having a high tolerance level.

Pfeiffer tested 12 hard-core drug addicts and found them all to be high in histamine. When histamine levels are too high, a person is more likely to be depressed, compulsive, and have abnormal thinking. Therefore heroin, methadone, uppers, downers, alcohol, and sugar are often craved to compensate for these feelings.

Creative or crazy?

Many great artists, writers, and pioneers are high-histamine types, passionate and compulsively driven to accomplish. And it's a fact that schizophrenia is more prevalent in families where a member has won a Nobel Prize. What's the link? During his decades at Princeton's Brain Bio Center, Dr. Pfeiffer found that histadelics comprise about 20 percent of so-called schizophrenics. However, the chances of having mental illness in the family are even higher if you're artistic or highly sexual, according to a survey published in the British scientific journal, the *Proceedings of the Royal Society B*.[28]

In the survey, British psychologists Daniel Nettle and Helen Keenoo compared the mental health, personality characteristics, and number of sexual partners in 425 people, including a proportion of artists and schizophrenics. They found that artists are much more likely to share key behavioral traits with schizophrenics and that they have, on average, twice as many sexual partners as non-artistic types.

Nettle and Keenoo carried out this research to help explain why the rate of schizophrenia, which affects about 1 percent of the population worldwide, hasn't changed over the years. From a Darwinian point of view, if schizophrenia is caused by a defective gene, why hasn't it been eradicated from the gene pool? On the other hand, if it's caused by environmental factors, then why would schizophrenia rates be relatively consistent throughout the world? Illnesses with known environmental links, such as diabetes, heart disease, cancer, and Alzheimer's, occur at different rates in countries with different diets and other environmental factors.

What the survey found was that both artists and schizophrenics had something called 'unusual cognition'– a trait that leads to a greater tendency to feel or identify with a state between reality and dreams. From Lord Byron to Dylan Thomas, the art world is littered with famous philanderers who hovered somewhere between genius and madness. While both artists and schizophrenics had a tendency to feel "overwhelmed by their own thoughts," the difference was that the artists were able to channel their ideas into creative expression and the schizophrenics became more socially withdrawn. As for sex, artists tended to be more promiscuous, but not very good in long-term relationships. As the Beat Generation novelist Jack Kerouac said, "My failure is not in the passions I have, but in my lack of control of them."

The link to depression, suicide, and schizophrenia

As we saw earlier, after seeing thousands of patients at his Brain Bio Center in Princeton over 40 years, Dr. Pfeiffer estimated that histadelics comprise about 20 percent of so-called schizophrenics and a substantial proportion of depressed patients. Here's how he described these patients:

66 The histadelic person is often the problem patient at psychiatric clinics and hospitals. Our first contact with histadelia occurred in a biochemical and psychiatric study of outpatient schizophrenics. Two out of nine chronic patients on whom we had extensive data and repeated visits showed significant positive correlations between blood histamine and the Experimental World Inventory (EWI), a psychological measure of stability. In other words, both the highly elevated EWI score and the blood histamine decreased as the patient got better.

Histadelia usually runs in families, with the onset at around 20 years of age. The easily elicited history of suicide, depression, and allergies among near and distant relatives is a strong indication of possible histadelia. This disorder has probably been termed familial psychotic depression in the past. The undiagnosed histadelic patient is treated as a schizophrenic but the patient does not respond to any of the usual drug therapies, electroshock, or insulin coma therapy. We have now treated over a thousand of these patients and our experience provides many important signs that help in making early diagnosis.

The classic symptoms are disperceptions, obsessions, compulsions, thought disorder, abnormal fears, constant suicidal depression, easy crying, confusion, and blank mind. The symptom of blank mind is elicited by asking if the patient can visualize the face of her mother or visualize why, on a highway, she might be directed to turn left though she actually wants to turn right on to a new highway (clover leaf turn). She often cannot visualize these things.

The greatest problem in the severely depressed histadelic is the constant threat of suicide. We can never meet this degree of mental over-alertness with good nutrition. We can make the patient feel normal but not stop the hyperactive mind. For some of these compulsive patients normality is just not enough. 99

Optimum nutrition for histadelics

If you suspect you are a high-histamine type and are experiencing undesirable symptoms, the best thing to do is see a nutritional therapist who can recommend a blood test to determine your histamine status. If you've had a standard blood test and your basophil count was high, this is an indicator of high-histamine status.

The ideal optimum nutrition for you depends on your histamine status. For all high-histamine types it is best to eat a diet relatively low in protein, and high in complex carbohydrates, emphasizing fruit and vegetables. Proteins like meat contain amino acids that further increase histamine levels. Vitamin C is a natural antihistamine and supplementing at least 2g a day is wise. Also important is sufficient zinc, manganese, and B6. Make sure you are supplementing 15 mg of zinc, 5 mg of manganese, and at least 50 mg of B6. Some people need double these amounts.

If you are experiencing undesirable symptoms, or have a high histamine level in your blood, go one step further and supplement 500 mg calcium and 500 mg of the amino acid methionine, morning and evening, plus a basic supplement program. Calcium supplementation releases some of the body's stores of histamine, and methionine helps to detoxify histamine by attaching methyl groups onto it—the usual mode of detoxification of histamine in the human body.

If you do have a high homocysteine level, don't take folic acid on its own. You need it in combination with the other homocysteine-lowering nutrients (B2, B6, B12, and TMG). Choose a formula using methyl-B12. It is also best to avoid doses of folic acid above 400 mcg in these formulas, as large amounts of folic acid can further raise histamine. With or without extra methionine, these nutrients will help normalize both homocysteine and histamine levels.

Phenytoin, the anti-epilepsy drug (trademarked Dilantin in the U.S.) in a dose of 100 mg, taken morning and afternoon, will usually provide some relief from severe depression or compulsion. However, the methionine plus calcium, combined with zinc and manganese, is often sufficient. The same regime of zinc, manganese, calcium, and methionine provides successful treatment in many severely allergic patients who are not depressed.

With the right nutrients, high-histamine types can lead a perfectly normal and productive life. Liz is a case in point.

> Liz started suffering from depression at the age of 14. By the time she was 17 she had become extremely anxious, fearful and depressed and was hearing voices. She was put on three drugs—Sulpiride and Depixol injections, plus Kemadrin to offset the side effects of the other drugs. The drugs somewhat sedated her but she continued to suffer from extreme depression and anxiety and continued to hear voices in her head.
>
> She consulted a nutritional therapist who identified chronic nutritional deficiencies and an excessive level of histamine. She was given the appropriate nutrients, and within six months she was no longer depressed, and rarely heard voices or became anxious. She came off all medication and continued to improve. She is now perfectly healthy and happy and recently gave birth to a baby girl. She experienced no post-natal depression.

How's your thyroid?

Another classic cause of depression is having an underactive thyroid. In the U.S., thyroid medication is the fourth most commonly prescribed drug. The thyroid gland, in the base of the throat, makes the hormone thyroxine which tells all brain and body cells to keep active. Often as a long-term consequence of stress and suboptimum nutrition, the thyroid gland can start to underproduce thyroxine. This is a classic cause of depression and lethargy, although symptoms of irritability, anxiety, and panic attacks have also been reported in those with low thyroxine levels.

The telltale signs of an underactive thyroid are lethargy, depression, poor memory or concentration, indigestion or constipation, hemorrhoids, skin problems, feeling cold and not tolerating heat well, fluid retention, and weight gain. Since thyroxine speeds up your metabolism, which produces heat, the definitive symptom is a drop in body temperature. This is something you can check yourself by taking your temperature with a thermometer. Here's how you do it.

Shake out a thermometer and keep it by your bed. When you wake in the morning, and before getting up, put the thermometer under your arm and lie there for 10 minutes. Your basal temperature should be 97.7 to 98.6°F. Do this for at least two days. (Women should do this test on day two or three of their period as body temperature fluctuates during the cycle.) If either of your temperature readings is below 97.7°F, take your temperature again over a longer period, say a week, to see if it is low on a fairly regular basis. If it's lower than 97.7°F, you probably have an underactive thyroid.

If you suspect you have a thyroid problem, your doctor can run a blood test to further investigate this possibility. However, an apparently normal thyroxine level, if at the low end of normal, backed up by lowered temperature and symptoms, may still be worth treating.

While the medical approach is to give you thyroxine, this hormone is made from tyrosine. Iodine is also needed to turn tyrosine into thyroxine. Recent research is indicating that both zinc and selenium are important too. So, try 1,000 mg of tyrosine on waking and at noon, taken on an empty stomach, together with a multimineral containing iodine, zinc, and selenium. Exercise also stimulates the thyroid. If you suspect that you have a thyroid problem you may also want to visit www.thyroiduk.org.

Building a happy lifestyle

Mood improvement doesn't stop at nutrition. Modest exercise is a good place to start. A number of studies in which people exercised for 30–60 minutes 3–5 times a week found a significant improvement in their depression when tested with their Hamilton Rating Scale, an established method of measuring mood. This was more than double the effect you would expect from antidepressants alone.[29] In an Australian study published in 2005 and involving 60 adults over the age of 60, half took up high-intensity exercise three days a week, while the other half did low-intensity exercise. Of those on the high-intensity regime, 61 percent halved their Hamilton Rating Scale score, compared to only 29 percent of those doing low-intensity exercise.[30] However, you've got to keep exercising to stay happy. An eight-year follow-up study of people prone to depression found that their depression returned if they stopped exercising.[31]

You may also consider seeing a counselor or psychotherapist. As complex as the biochemistry of mental health is, so too is the nature of the psyche. Feeling bad about yourself and lacking someone supportive to listen to you can be a major cause of depression, however good your diet might be.[32] A study by the University of Dundee that examined health behaviors in 1,289 lonely and non-lonely adults found an association between loneliness and depression.[33] Meanwhile, research by the University of Pennsylvania reported that older adults viewed loneliness as a precursor to depression.[34] A problem shared really is a problem halved. While exercise and good nutrition will give you more mental and emotional energy to solve your problems, it doesn't take away the underlying issues that fuel depression, or always give you all the tools you need to deal with it. For this reason, I recommend counseling and psychotherapy as well as nutritional approaches. See page 485 in Useful Addresses to find out how to locate the right therapist for you.

Simple lifestyle changes can help enormously too. As we saw in Chapter 15, increasing your exposure to natural daylight and using full-spectrum lights and light bulbs for indoor lighting also helps. In one study published in 2004, a third of depressed volunteers who exercised in full-spectrum lighting experienced a major improvement in their depression (a 50 percent or more decrease in their Hamilton Rating Scale).[35] Other studies from 2005 have also found a definitive improvement, even among those not specifically prone to seasonal affective disorder (SAD)—a tendency to develop the blues during winter, when natural light levels are lowest.[36] The effect could be due to the direct effect of light on raising serotonin,[37] since light affects the pineal gland, which produces serotonin's close relative melatonin. Exactly how light elevates mood isn't known, but we all know it to be true. On page 161 in Chapter 15 you'll find a simple light exercise for elevating your mood; but you might also think about taking your main holiday in the winter, choosing somewhere sunny. For indoor lighting, use full-spectrum light bulbs (see the Product and Supplement Directory, page 486).

Being outside in nature may have even more benefits than extra light and exercise. Waterfalls, mountains, beaches, and forests, places frequently associated with feelings of tranquility, are among those places where there are more health-promoting ions in the air. (It's the negative ions that are good for you, and the positive ions that are not!) After a lightning storm, most of us feel invigorated and refreshed. This is because the electrical storm has generated trillions of negative ions that ease tensions and leave us energized. Researchers now believe that SAD may be caused, at least in part, by the depletion of negative ions in the air by winter winds. Researchers at Columbia University's Department of Psychiatry measuring the antidepressant effect of negative ions in the ambient air found that 58 percent of patients treated with high-density negative ions had significant relief from their symptoms, almost identical to the number improved with drugs but with no side effects. So, consider getting yourself an ionizer.

The right music can certainly elevate your mood, as can the right essential oils. Particularly uplifting are bergamot, geranium, petitgrain, or neroli oil. The book *Natural Highs*, which I co-authored with Dr. Hyla Cass, includes many ways to give yourself a mood boost. If you've struggled with low moods or more entrenched and serious conditions for years, it's important to know that there's much you can do to banish them, and get on with building a better, happier life.

SUMMARY

In summary, if you are experiencing chronic or severe depression:

- See a nutritional therapist who can check for any biochemical imbalances, and devise a nutritional program to improve your mood. This may include supplements of St. John's wort, omega-3 fats, 5-HTP, tyrosine, B12, folic acid, B6, TMG, zinc, magnesium, and manganese, plus a diet to stabilize your blood sugar and ensure enough omega-3 fats.

- Check your homocysteine level, take homocysteine-lowering nutrients accordingly, and follow a homocysteine-lowering lifestyle (see Chapter 8).

▶

- If you have the signs of high histamine, have your histamine level checked.

- Exercise every day.

- Change your lifestyle to consciously use light, color, sound, and smell to enhance your mood.

- Consider seeing a counselor or psychotherapist.

CHAPTER 24

Mood swings and manic depression

It's not at all uncommon to have mood swings. In fact, one in two people in Britain alone say they often get mood swings, according to the 2004 ONUK survey involving 37,000 people. These swings may be generated by a huge number of factors, including too much coffee, too much stress, hormone imbalances, food allergies, and nutritional deficiencies.

Most of the people who experience mood swings can fall into depression with symptoms such as low mood, loss of appetite or weight, feeling tired, poor sleep patterns, loss of interest in hobbies and/or sex, avoiding people, irritability, poor concentration, and feeling guilty or even suicidal. Of course, there are different degrees of mood swings. About 1 in every 100 people swing between marked depression, on the one hand, and mania or hypomania on the other. Those with marked symptoms are said to have manic depression, or as psychiatrists prefer to refer it these days, bipolar disorder.

Manic depressives who have mild symptoms, in that they do not have a complete breakdown that leaves them incapable of coping outside a hospital or other supported living, can still be severely affected by the illness. They may, for instance, have exciting sex lives that get them into a broad variety of trouble and then they may suddenly become unproductive and need to take time out. On the other hand, some of them become successful politicians or millionaires. Ironically, these people may suffer the most disruption to their lives with manic depression because, by virtue of their status or less obvious swings, they may completely avoid the medical profession or other forms of help and blame other people for their irritability and other eccentricities. With no medication, their behavior may lead to divorce, loss of friends, prison, or worse.

The most severe form of manic depression carries the risk of breakdown, which can often lead to loss of job or home. Generally these sufferers spend time living on the street, in prison or in hospital. They are often known to the local police for the trouble they cause when they lose touch with reality. Fortunately, the extent of their disruptive behavior often gets them some sort of medication, though that may bring its own problems.

In practice, psychiatric diagnoses frequently change with time. Schizophrenics may frequently appear to be manic depressive at first. The two diagnoses are often swapped and changed through the course of the disease. Some psychiatrists speculate that the two diagnoses are variants of the same disease. Patients showing signs of both conditions may be labeled schizoaffective (a cross between the two diseases).

Someone showing a pure bipolar mood disorder has a high probability of being short of zinc and vitamin B6, having blood-sugar imbalances or brain allergies, or experiencing any combination of the three. However, those with mood swings and perceptual problems (such as hearing or seeing things that are not there, or experiencing strange sensations in their bodies) or having confused thought patterns (beyond simple elation or depression) may suffer from a range of chemical disorders that are often closer to the imbalances found in schizophrenia.

In this context, one of the hottest areas of research is abnormal methylation. Since methylation is vital both for building neurotransmitters, and for breaking them down, the discovery that many people diagnosed with both schizophrenia and bipolar disorder inherit a *wobble* in their methylation ability is a potential major breakthrough. This, and other factors, were fully explored in Chapter 8.

Understanding manic depression

Most people with manic depression spend the majority of their time either in a normal mood or mildly depressed. Some do remain mildly high all the time. This makes clearly assessing their mood very difficult.

Often a sufferer can be unaware of how moody they are. Their closest friends may be used to their mood swings and assume they are normal. Worse still, it is possible to be both up and down at the same time! Low mood with racing thoughts and feeling a dire need to sleep but being incapable of switching off is a common scenario.

This makes treatment options that attempt to push sufferers out of one mood swing potentially dangerous because they may push them into the other one. A number of treatment options, including some complementary therapies, can cause this, and should only be used with the guidance of knowledgeable and experienced practitioners.

Psychiatrists can be very wary about prescribing antidepressants to those with manic depression, even if they are suicidal, for fear that they will go high. Fortunately most nutritional treatments do not fall into this potential trap as they treat and prevent both types of swing simultaneously.

However, the current trend is to increasingly prescribe mood stabilizers such as olanzapine, marketed as Zyprexa by Eli Lilly. This drug is being increasingly prescribed to children as the diagnosis of bipolar disorder becomes more widely applied in the young. It is one of the top 10 blockbuster drugs, generating sales of $4.7 billion in 2005. Originally used for the treatment of epilepsy, this kind of drug is being increasingly prescribed for mania.

According to David Healy, the psychiatrist at the North Wales Department of Psychological Medicine who blew the lid on the increased risk of suicide on SSRIs, "no randomized controlled trials show that patients with bipolar disorders who receive drugs do better in the long term than those who receive no medicine."[38] One argument often given for prescribing these drugs is that the risk of suicide is high in those with bipolar disorder, yet studies tend to show that the risk is about double among those on medication. Against this background, let's take a look at the nutritional approaches.

Three ways to achieve balance

There are three safe ways of helping a person with manic depression to minimize the risk of disruptive moods. The first is to take nutrients that help to stabilize mood. These can reduce swings in either direction. The second is to take nutrients and herbs that help reduce anxiety and promote relaxation. Many mood swings coincide with a buildup of stress. Finally, there are nutrients that promote healthy sleep patterns. Insomnia is a major source of stress that only makes matters worse.

Mood, food, and allergies

Many mood swings are triggered by blood-sugar imbalances or food allergies. The brain is almost totally dependent on glucose for its supply of energy, so maintaining a stable level of glucose is important for improved mental health. People with elevated blood-sugar levels may become high, whereas low blood sugar is associated with depression. Blood-sugar balance is disrupted by too much sugar, stress, and stimulants, including cigarettes. Cigarette smoking is very harmful for manic depressives. One study conducted by Aidan Corvin and colleagues of St. James's Hospital, Dublin, studied 92 manic depressives. Fifty-three were smokers, of whom 70 percent were found to have psychotic symptoms, compared to 32 percent of non-smokers.[39]

According to the nutritional pioneer Dr. Carl Pfeiffer, daily or weekly swings in mood may be triggered by stress or regular consumption of meals containing ingredients that prompt an allergic reaction. He reported one patient who found that his blue Mondays came on because his family had chicken every Sunday. When he avoided chicken on Sunday, his Mondays were once again productive. Even sudden, large, and irregular swings in mood may be triggered by allergies. For example, sustained eating of gluten by celiacs causes nutrient malabsorption that may come to a crisis point, at which point a major mood swing occurs. (See Chapter 26, page 297, for more on how gluten affects the brain.)

Exploring the possibility of food allergies can be invaluable, as Janet's story shows:

Janet was diagnosed with manic depression at the age of 15. At times she would become completely hyperactive and manic, and at other times become completely depressed. She was put on three drugs—lithium, Tegretol and Zirtek. These helped control the severity of her manic phases, but she was still frequently depressed and anxious. Two years later she consulted a nutrition counselor who found she was deficient in many nutrients, especially zinc, and allergic to wheat. As soon as her nutrient deficiencies were corrected and she stopped eating wheat her health rapidly improved. She was able to stop all medication and, provided she stays off wheat, no longer gets depressed. She is now doing her final degree exams and continues to feel good and achieve well. However, if she has any wheat, even inadvertently in a sauce, she becomes depressed, confused, forgetful, and anxious for three to four days. Her manic phases, however, have never returned.

Allergies can also be triggered by seasonal changes. Inhalant allergies are common in the spring with trees and grass pollen, and in the autumn with weed pollens. See Chapter 12 to check this possibility.

Lithium: is it essential?

One of the most successful drugs in psychiatry is lithium, usually prescribed in the range of 300–1,200 mg a day. Though some suffer from significant side effects or simply cannot tolerate the drug, for others it has caused a dramatic improvement in their lives. Now, lithium is being prescribed more frequently to those diagnosed with schizophrenia and depressed patients as well. Compared with other psychiatric drugs, it really is a wonder drug.

Lithium may not be a drug at all. It may be an essential trace mineral. It is certainly essential for goats and some species of pig. Lithium is unusually low in British water supplies. Gerard Schrauzer and colleagues analyzed hair mineral samples from 2,648 people and found that nearly 20 percent of Americans had extremely low hair-lithium content, and the same was true for samples from Germany and Austria. Hair lithium levels are low in people with certain conditions, including heart disease, learning disabilities, and violent criminal tendencies.[40] So people may respond to lithium because they are deficient in it.

However, too much lithium does have the side effect of over-dampening emotional expression, which is a common complaint against standard lithium therapy. These high doses force mood stabilization instead of restoring healthy emotions. Nutritionally orientated psychiatrists tend to use lithium in a variety of ways. It is very effective at doses at or above 300 mg a day, and often allows reduction of other drugs. Dr. Abram Hoffer has had good results using 300 mg a day to improve patients' energy levels, eliminate depression and stabilize mood. Lithium lowers folic acid levels in the blood, and supplementing folic acid may increase lithium's ability to stabilize mood.[41] However, high-histamine types should avoid increasing folic acid levels dramatically (see Chapter 23, page 255). Depressed patients are often found to have low hair lithium levels, so low dose supplements are worth a try.

Low levels of lithium (up to 5 mg) might help us all, whether we are depressed or not. The mineral is found in kelp, dulse, and seafood, and supplements containing low doses of lithium are available (see the Product and Supplement Directory, page 486).

Omega-3 fats: miraculous for mood

Omega-3 fatty acids are now being intensively researched for their mood-stabilizing properties. The Institute of Psychiatry in London is currently running a large double-blind trial with fish oils.

The virtues of omega-3 fats for optimal mental health have been extolled throughout this book. Thanks to Dr. Andrew Stoll and colleagues at Harvard Medical School we now know that they can be extremely helpful for those with manic depression, too. They ran a double-blind, placebo-controlled trial of omega-3 fats, placing 14 adult manic depressives on the fish oils EPA (eicosapentaenoic acid) and DHA (docosahexaenoic acid) and compared them with 14 taking an olive oil placebo. Both took the supplement alongside their normal medication. Those taking the omega-3 fats had a substantially longer period in remission than the placebo group. The fish oil group also performed better than the placebo group for nearly every other symptom measured.[42]

In his book *The Omega-3 Connection*, Stoll quotes a mother of a woman with manic depression now taking fish oil,

> 66 It has been seven days with no antidepressant. I never believed this could be possible—it is definitely a record for my daughter. She has not been off antidepressants for that many days in six years, in fact, going off for one day before fish oil led to immediate suicidal ideation with her screaming for me to kill her ... For the first time in her entire life she is relaxed and her memory and cognitive abilities have returned —I cannot tell you how fortunate we feel. 99

Since his book and research were published, Dr. Stoll receives daily emails from around the world reporting miraculous responses to fish oil.

Not enough studies have been conducted to determine exactly how much is optimum, but the study used 6.2g EPA and 3.4g DHA. However, the active ingredient in the capsules is now thought to be EPA, and Dr. Stoll finds that generally 1.5–4g of EPA is adequate to improve mood in patients with mood disorders.

Fish oils have little or no side effects unless taken in enormous quantities. Gastrointestinal side effects may be a problem, but a reduction in the dose, spreading it out through the day or only taking the oil with a meal should eliminate this problem. The high doses of EPA needed to treat mood disorders make fish-liver oil supplements unsuitable for the task. Fish liver oils contain too much vitamin A, and if you take too much of this it can lead to toxicity. Vegetarians may be able to substitute a vegetarian source of alpha-linolenic acid (such as flaxseed oil) for the fish oil, as long as they take the optimum amounts of magnesium, zinc, and vitamins B3, B6, biotin, and C that are needed to convert flaxseed oil into EPA and DHA. However, you are probably better off with fish oil concentrates of EPA and DHA, since the amount the body makes from flax can be very low in some people. Antioxidants are also needed to help protect these fats.

Dr. Stoll suggests 1,000 mg vitamin E and a good general multivitamin and mineral including coenzyme Q10. For more information on essential fats, see Chapter 4.

Magnesium: finding your balance

Before the Second World War, magnesium was commonly used to stabilize mood. Since the introduction of lithium (see page 265) its use has faded, but interest in it has been increasing recently. One study of nine people with manic depression characterized by rapid mood swings found that half of them were stabilized by magnesium as least as well as would be expected with lithium.[43] Intravenous magnesium sulphate has also been used with some success for calming manic patients.[44]

Although these studies were small, magnesium does have an excellent reputation as a mild tranquilizer. Most of us are deficient in it. Diets provide around 200 mg on average, while the RDA is 300 mg. The following symptoms may indicate a deficiency: muscle tremors or spasms, muscle weakness, insomnia or nervousness, high blood pressure, irregular heartbeat, constipation, fits or convulsions, hyperactivity, depression, confusion, and lack of appetite. You can increase the levels of magnesium in your diet by increasing the amount of vegetables, fruit, nuts, and seeds.

More minerals, and vitamins too

While no specific nutrient has been proven to cause or cure manic depression, there are many that can make a difference. Dr. Carl Pfeiffer observed that many manic depressives who came to his Brain Bio Center at Princeton were short of zinc and vitamin B6 due to stress-induced pyroluria (see Chapter 21, page 221). Their mood swings often follow a weekly pattern as they tend to become workaholic and then can't relax properly on weekends. The role of B vitamins in correcting faulty methylation is also now thought to be key in a number of conditions, including manic depression. Since many of the same imbalances occur in those with schizophrenia, these are discussed in Chapter 26.

Niacin (vitamin B3) is a key nutrient in many mental health conditions, including mania, as Sonia's story shows:

Sonia was admitted to hospital with mania, having previously been mildly depressed and prescribed the antidepressant paroxetine. The physical examination failed to pick up that she had severe diarrhea, had vomited, and her hand was turning bright red. She was prescribed the anti-psychotic droperidol and the tranquilizer diazepam. She remained high and was detained under the Mental Health Act. She managed to steal some of her own B vitamins (including niacin) and swallowed 12 of them. She recovered almost completely in the next 24 hours and her detention was canceled. But she couldn't obtain any more vitamins and relapsed. She was put on a longer detention and diagnosed with manic depression. It was more than two months and numerous doses of drugs including haloperidol, depixol and lithium before she returned to normal. Today her mood is stable, and her chronic depression since childhood has cleared. She takes 3g of niacin per day, has a low sugar and gluten-free diet, and is studying to become a nutrition consultant. Her psychiatrist concedes that niacin deficiency is a credible explanation for her symptoms, and her lithium dose is being reduced.

A study of 885 psychiatric patients found that about a third of them had blood vitamin C levels that were below the threshold that has been associated with behavioral problems.[45] Another large study of psychiatric inpatients found over 10 percent showing signs of borderline scurvy.[46] Both could be explained by poor diet rather than the direct effect of the condition. However, anxiety or excitement speeds up the breakdown of vitamin C.[47] Also a double-blind trial on 40 chronic male psychiatric patients (including four with manic depression) confirms that many psychiatric patients have borderline scurvy. Supplementation with just 1g of vitamin C a day eliminates this possibility.[48]

The trace mineral vanadium is almost certainly an essential mineral. One study by Graham Naylor of the University of Dundee and colleagues showed that elevated levels of vanadium are found in the hair of manic patients and that they fall towards normal as the patient recovers.[49] Other studies confirmed that vanadium levels in various tissues are altered by mania or depression.[50] There is a credible but far from proven mechanism by which a particular form of vanadium might disrupt mood. However, it is not clear that there is enough vanadium in the human body to make such a dramatic difference to mood. Nor is it clear that vanadium changes are the cause rather than the effect of mood changes. Vitamin C disarms vanadium, turning it into a form far less likely to disrupt mood, even if it could before. However, vanadium supplementation is probably inadvisable in those with manic depression.

The best place to start is by supplementing a multivitamin and mineral because nutrients do not work on their own but in conjunction with other nutrients. One study conducted by Bonnie Kaplan of the University of Calgary, Canada, has specifically demonstrated how effective this can be for manic depression. In this study, 11 manic depressive adults were given vitamins and trace minerals in addition to their prescribed medications. Over the next six months, on average, they halved their need for the medications and every patient experienced between a 55 and 66 percent reduction in symptoms.[51]

Amino acids: use with caution

Amino acids, from which the body makes neurotransmitters, can help in manic depression, but should only be supplemented under the guidance of a health professional. Dr. Abram Hoffer gives the amino acid L-tryptophan to assist his patients when in normal phase and finds it reduces the frequency of manic phases. However, he cautions against giving it during manic phases. L-tryptophan is best absorbed with a carbohydrate snack. (Note that in some countries L-tryptophan and/or 5-HTP are restricted nutrients, and tryptophan is banned outright in some; see page 152.) The recommended amount of L-tryptophan is 1g twice a day, or 100 mg of 5-HTP twice a day. Unless under professional guidance, do not supplement these amino acids together with antidepressant medication.

The depressed phase following a period of mania may actually be burnout, and can be virtually eliminated by optimum nutrition. Dr. Abram Hoffer finds L-tyrosine, the amino acid from which we make dopamine, adrenalin, and noradrenalin, particularly effective during these depressed phases. However, it should be used with caution because high levels, in some people, can encourage mania. However, many people diagnosed with bipolar disorder do have low thyroxine levels in the depressed phase and these people can be helped by tyrosine.[52]

Taurine, which helps the body make GABA, the relaxing neurotransmitter, can help reduce mania. It has many other uses as well, in treating migraine, insomnia, agitation, restlessness, irritability, alcoholism, obsessions, and depression.

Helpful herbs

Herb-drug interactions can occur and like drug-drug interactions may not have been fully recognized yet. Also herbs can cause problems with specific conditions. St. John's wort is an example. Though it has great antidepressant effects there have been cases of it inducing mania in those with manic depression.

One herb that may well be useful, if used under guidance, is kava. It is an excellent relaxant for both muscles and emotions. It reduces mental chatter, increases mental focus and promotes good sleep. However, it should not be used with diazepam (Valium) or any of the other benzodiazepine tranquilizers, unless under expert guidance, because the two potentiate each other. This can be used to advantage in weaning people off these addictive drugs. Note that in some countries kava is not allowed to be sold; see Chapter 18 for more on this herb.

Sleep and vigilance

During manic phases sufferers tend to sleep less and less, which is a great stress on the body and mind, rapidly depleting nutrients such as magnesium, zinc, and vitamin C. During depressed phases sufferers tend to sleep too much, probably due to adrenal exhaustion and nutritional deficiency. Encouraging a regular pattern of seven hours of uninterrupted sleep can help to smooth out the curves.

The U.K.-based Manic Depression Fellowship (MDF) has pioneered a self-management training course for people diagnosed with manic depression in England and Wales. It encourages participants to detect warning signs and triggers prior to a mood swing, including loss of sleep, irritability, or changes in lifestyle, plus to take what steps they can to prevent a mood swing happening. Daily recording of mood, sleep, and medication are encouraged. This can give an early indication of a mood swing. These records can also assist when negotiating with medical professionals for a change in treatment. Mood monitoring can also easily be combined with a food diary to assist in detecting allergies. Feedback from the MDF training course has been encouraging. One participant said:

> 66 The self-management program turned my life around. Now I'm better equipped to cope with [self-manage] most of my mood swings. 99

Other therapies that encourage self-observation and help to undo negative behavior patterns can be most helpful for those with manic depression. Cognitive behavioral therapy (CBT) aims to improve mood and behavior by investigating and challenging unhelpful thought patterns. It aims to set up a virtuous circle where beneficial beliefs applied to real-life situations produce good thoughts and positive behavior that reinforces the beliefs. Having proven successful with depression, CBT is currently being researched for its efficacy with manic depression. A good book on the subject is *Think Your Way to Happiness* by Dr. Windy Dryden and Jack Gordon (see Recommended Reading, page 471).

SUMMARY

In summary, here's what you can do to stabilze your mood swings:

- Avoid sugar, stimulants, cigarettes, and excess stress.

- Check yourself out for food allergies (see Chapter 12).

- Increase your magnesium intake by eating plenty of vegetables, fruit, nuts, and seeds and consider supplementing 300–500 mg a day, found in good multivitamin/mineral formulas.

- Take fish oil supplements providing between 1.5 and 4g EPA.

- Check your homocysteine level and supplement the right amount of homocysteine-lowering nutrients (see Chapter 8).

- Supplement a good multivitamin and mineral every day, plus 1,000 mg of vitamin C.

- Become more aware of what triggers your mood swings and how to control your thoughts to improve your stability.

- Consult a clinical nutritionist who can advise you about nutrients and herbs that can help keep you in balance, as well as explore potential food allergies or intolerances.

CHAPTER 25

Demystifying schizophrenia

Schizophrenia is a loaded word, feared by patient and public alike. It conjures up images of dangerous and crazy people. In truth, most members of the public have no real idea what is meant by this word, often believing that sufferers have split personalities, like Jekyll and Hyde.

The diagnosis of schizophrenia is in fact a kind of *waste-basket* diagnosis for a collection of symptoms, most of which we've already covered. These include:

- Depression

- Anxiety

- Fears, phobias, and paranoia

- Disperceptions and thought disorders

- Illusions and delusions

- Auditory and visual hallucinations

- Anti-social behavior

A person labeled schizophrenic may have any or all of these, but at a level of severity that makes either them unable to cope or others unable to cope with them. The lack of firm, objective signs is perhaps the crux of the continuing argument as to whether schizophrenia has any physiological or biochemical basis or is just in the mind. However, more and more evidence is emerging to suggest that most people with this label do have biochemical imbalances, or predispositions, sometimes also triggered by traumatic life events.

Most of us have, at some time or other, experienced some level of psychosis, temporarily losing touch with reality as we collectively know it. The experiences of schizophrenics are reproduced in certain toxic or feverish states. The normal person recovering from the delusions brought on by a high fever can breathe a great sigh of relief at the thought that his experience was only temporary. The person under the influence of the hallucinogenic drug LSD can at least rely on the clock, since the drug-induced schizophrenia will wear off with time. Some people's experience of so-called schizophrenia can be likened to a nightmare state from which they may awaken intermittently. For some, schizophrenia is like living in a non-stop nightmare.

Whose problem is it?

The symptoms that characterize people with schizophrenia can be separated into two classes: those that bother them, and those that bother the people around them. The two may not be the same, and there is often considerable friction between the patient and those around them.

Consider the case of the man who says he has visions and hears the voice of Jesus. Hallucinations are considered by doctors to be evidence of psychosis. But what if this man is a lay preacher to one of the churches teaching that if you only have enough faith, Christ will appear in person? To him, people who say he is mentally ill are simply non-believers. Many of the stresses and frustrations of everyday life could be relieved if one had a firm belief in being a chosen child or disciple of God. (Many people have this without being delusional about it, of course.)

This kind of discord creates certain practical difficulties. Take a young woman. We'll call her Kate. Kate keeps insisting to her family that she is carrying the new Christ-child in her abdomen because she hasn't had a menstrual period for three months. This failure to menstruate is actually owing to a lack of zinc in her body because of stress, and eating a zinc-deficient diet high in refined sugar. Her family is upset and annoyed by her continued delusion as well as by her untidiness, lack of co-operation, and general unpleasantness around the house. A complaint is then made to the family doctor—by the family, not by Kate. Kate refuses flatly to even talk to the doctor, insisting that she is in good health: "It's just that my family don't understand me and my new role in society." This kind of situation can create a dilemma for the doctor.

Although the diagnosis is reasonably clear, should the doctor insist on treating a patient who has not asked for help? Of course, if the patient asks for treatment there is no problem. If the patient presents some clear evidence that he or she may harm someone, intervention is clearly justified. However, aside from the unethical taint of unsolicited treatment, a major goal should be to keep patients out of hospital whenever possible. Sometimes that alone is a victory, because with some of today's mental hospitals, there is the probability that the patient may be better off at home. One situation that creates great difficulty occurs when the doctor suspects that the patient may be suicidal or homicidal. Since the conservation of human life has high priority, the doctor must try to treat the patient. Being only human and acting on the basis of insufficient tests, the doctor is sometimes wrong, no matter how great their ability. Patients, after such a false alarm, are often bitter and unforgiving. Indeed, they frequently incorporate the memory of such a forced hospitalization into their delusional systems.

Spiritual crisis or awakening?

Some so-called schizophrenic breakdowns are spiritual awakenings. These can and do take the form of visions, inner voices, electricity shooting up the spine, clairvoyance, elation, and so on. For whatever reason, some people have such experiences, which are described in mystical traditions the world over. But often they lack an understanding or support to ground these experiences, and end up in a mental hospital. To the unprepared, these experiences can shatter their beliefs about the nature of reality, and be very scary indeed.

Whether real schizophrenia or something else, many people end up being given major tranquilizers, whether voluntarily or involuntarily. These drugs do not cure schizophrenia, although they can make extreme symptoms bearable. Most psychotropic drugs, as they are often classified, leave the patient drowsy and drugged and have nasty side effects (for which other drugs have to be given), as well as carrying the long-term risk of brain damage.

Route to a cure

With 1 in 100 people diagnosed as suffering from schizophrenia, generally speaking, and many more suffering from depression, anxiety, extreme fears, and phobias, help is badly needed. But what treatment is available? For the seriously mentally ill, this means psychiatric help. Some psychiatrists still view mental illness as a psychologically based disease, a perplexing nightmare often intertwined with suspicious family interactions. The treatment may be endless psychoanalysis, and an enormous drain on financial resources with little more than a slim chance of help. (As one patient said after years of psychoanalysis, "I may know myself a lot better but I'm still mentally ill!").

Other psychiatrists lean more heavily on drug treatments, but these too have only a small chance of really helping. At best, they can give partial relief, but virtually no one taking these major tranquilizers gets well enough to hold down a job. Fortunately, by understanding the biochemical imbalances that can lead to these symptoms, and correcting them with specific nutrients rather than drugs, there is every reason to hope that people suffering from these extreme symptoms of mental illness can recover and lead productive lives.

The starting point is the recognition that schizophrenia, as a specific disease, does not exist. Each person must be considered as an individual, with their own spread of symptoms and biochemical imbalances, determined by objective tests. These symptoms are not incurable. The nutritional approach to the so-called schizophrenias, especially if started before long-term drug therapy, gives sufferers an 80 percent chance of achieving a major recovery. As Dr. Abram Hoffer says, having successfully treated over 5,000 sufferers since the 1950s with optimum nutrition, this means freedom from symptoms, ability to socialize with family and friends, and paying income tax! Let's take a look at the approach Hoffer used in the following chapter.

CHAPTER 26

Schizophrenia can be cured

There is no such single disease as schizophrenia, nor is there likely to be any single cure. It is more accurate to talk about *the schizophrenias*, because there are many ways to end up with the symptoms and behaviors that will get you this label.

As we've seen, about 1 in 100 people develops so-called schizophrenia, which affects men and women equally. Remarkably, this is relatively true the world over. Since most diseases vary from place to place, one theory is that schizophrenia has a genetic origin that began before humanity migrated out of Africa. It also occurs far more commonly in genius families. There's an old saying that goes "What's the difference between genius and madness? Genius has limits." One theory for the leap in intelligence that occurred only in us humans is that, at some point in the evolution of our species, there was a biological shift in how our brains used fats—almost like a new microchip, so to speak. Indeed, one of the big differences in our brains, compared to less intelligent mammals, is the quantity of special essential fats. Those well placed to adapt to this evolution become super-intelligent while those with a slight variation in their brain chemistry flip over into schizophrenia. This fascinating theory is explained fully in David Horrobin's *The Madness of Adam and Eve* (see Recommended Reading, page 471).

Although, I'm sure that there are cases where people go crazy for purely psychological reasons, there is now overwhelming evidence that in most people so diagnosed, something isn't right in the brain. Researchers from the London Institute of Psychiatry have confirmed that the frontal cortex of the brain is involved in schizophrenia. Using functional magnetic resonance imaging (fMRI), they have also been able to show that the deterioration in brain function in schizophrenia is not irreversible.[53]

The best results I've seen in helping those with so-called schizophrenia are achieved by investigating a number of possible avenues, most of which we've already touched on in other chapters. These include:

- Blood-sugar problems

- Essential fat imbalances

- Too many oxidants and not enough antioxidants

- Abnormal methylation and high homocysteine

- Niacin deficiency

- Pyroluria and the need for zinc

- Wheat and other allergies.

I am not saying that so-called schizophrenia is purely a result of nutritional deficiency, although we know that certain nutrients, if lacking, do cause these symptoms in anybody. I'm rather saying that the collection of biochemical imbalances that lead an individual to have a distorted experience of life can be minimized and, in many cases, completely corrected by providing the right intake of nutrients for that particular person. These nutrients tune up different aspects of our brain, and it is likely that the drugs currently used employ similar mechanisms, but with much more undesirable side effects. They are like sledgehammers compared to nutrients, and although useful in the short term are best avoided in the long term.

I say this because the best, and most consistent, positive results in the treatment of this debilitating condition have been reported by ourselves at the Brain Bio Centre in Richmond; by Dr. Bill Walsh at the Pfeiffer Treatment Center, which is run according to the ideas and practices of the late Dr. Carl Pfeiffer; and by Dr. Abram Hoffer, former director of psychiatric research for Saskatchewan and now retired as a practicing psychiatrist. The method we all use is to assess a number of potential biochemical abnormalities, then devise a personalized regime of diet and supplements.

Pfeiffer reported that over 95 percent of the schizophrenic patients at his center had at least one biochemical disorder, and that 90 percent of the patients whose biotype had been identified showed great improvement, even complete recovery, when they followed an appropriate nutrition-based program. Hoffer also claims a 90 percent cure of acute schizophrenia, meaning recently diagnosed patients who have lived with the condition for no more than two years, while those who had been on long-term prescribed medication generally experienced less dramatic improvements. Both treated thousands of schizophrenic patients. And at the Brain Bio Centre, we have also seen extraordinary recoveries, often complete ones. We have certainly come to expect spectacular improvements in those who stick to the program.

Now let's take a look at the various biochemical imbalances that can be the true culprits in a diagnosis of schizophrenia.

Problems with essential fats

One of the big areas of research in schizophrenia is brain fats. As we've seen, we build our brain from specialized essential fats. Of course, this isn't a static process. We are always building membranes in the brain, then breaking them down, and building new ones—a process partly controlled by methylation (see Chapter 8, page 70). The balance of essential fats in these brain membranes makes a difference. The breaking down, or stripping of essential fats from brain membranes, is done by an enzyme called phospholipase A2 (PLA2). This is often overactive in people diagnosed with schizophrenia, and this leads to a greater need for these fats, which are quickly lost from the brain. The effect explains earlier findings that schizophrenic patients have much lower levels of fatty acids in the frontal cortex of the brain.[54–55]

Having an overactive PLA2 also explains another anomaly. If a person swallows niacin, or vitamin B3, they get a blushing reaction and go bright red for a few minutes. The same thing happens if you paint a patch of niacin on the skin. But not so in many schizophrenic patients.[56–57] Craig Hudson and colleagues at Stratford General Hospital in Ontario, Canada, have discovered that the blushing reaction is caused by the very same fats that the PLA2 enzyme strips out.[58] They've developed a niacin skin test to determine which patients will respond best to treatment with essential fats.

Essential fats are also communication chemicals, especially the prostaglandins, which are the most complex end-products of the body's transformation of the essential fats we consume. In this respect the omega-3 fat EPA, as well as the omega-6 fat AA or arachidonic acid, derived from GLA (such as evening primrose oil) or obtained directly from meat, are the most interesting. These fats can also influence gene expression—that is, the process by which the information in a gene is used to make proteins that determine the characteristics of that organism.

So, what's the evidence that increasing a person's intakes of these essential fats makes a difference?

The World Health Organization conducted a survey of the incidence and outcome of schizophrenia in eight countries in Africa, Asia, Europe and the Americas. They found that while the incidence was surprisingly similar in all countries, the outcomes were very different. In some countries, schizophrenia seemed to be a relatively mild and self-limiting disease, whereas in others it was a severe and life-long condition. Of all the factors considered which might explain this, by far the strongest correlation was with the fat content of the diet. Those countries with a high intake of essential fats from fish and vegetables, as opposed to meat, had much less severe outcomes.[59]

Dr. Iain Glen at the mental health department of Aberdeen University found that 80 percent of schizophrenics are deficient in essential fatty acids or EFAs. He gave 50 patients EFA supplements and reported a dramatic response.[60] A larger placebo-controlled, crossover, 10-month study of the effects of EFA supplementation in schizophrenics, including supplements of zinc, B6, B3 and vitamin C with omega-6 fats, also produced significant improvements in schizophrenic symptoms.[61] A trial by Dr. Malcolm Peet, a psychiatrist with the U.K. National Health Service in Sheffield who uses an approach that integrates nutrition, and the late Dr. David Horrobin, who wrote *The Madness of Adam and Eve* (see page 277), gave 2 or 4g of the omega-3 EPA in a highly concentrated form to patients diagnosed with schizophrenia. Compared to those taking the schizophrenia drug cloazapine, there was improvement.[62]

But not all results are positive. A trial using only omega-3 fats versus a placebo found no significant improvement in mental health.[63]

To date, the evidence strongly suggests that some people diagnosed with schizophrenia do need, and respond well to, increased amounts of both omega-6 fats, such as evening primrose oil or borage oil, and omega-3, fats, together with the co-factor nutrients (zinc, B6, folic acid, B3, and vitamin C) that help convert them into vital brain fats. The question is, who is likely to respond?

First, from the few studies that have been done in this area, it does seem that people in the early stages of developing psychotic symptoms respond better to this nutritional approach than those who have suffered for a long time. There are also three promising tests: one is a blood test testing essential fat levels in red blood cells. The other is the niacin skin flush test, and the third is an ingenious breath test which measures the release of the gas ethane, a breakdown product of the enzyme PLA2 which, if you remember, strips out the brain's essential fats. The more ethane released in the breath, the more essential fats you need. These tests can be used to determine if a person is more likely to respond to essential fat therapy.

Too many oxidants, not enough antioxidants

There's another part to the essential fat story. These fats are also prone to destruction in the brain, and in the diet, by oxidants (see Chapter 9). Indeed, there is evidence of more oxidation in the frontal cortex of those with schizophrenia. Therefore, as well as increasing the intake of essential fats, it makes sense to give a person a diet (and lifestyle) that minimizes oxidants from fried or burned food and maximizes intake of antioxidant nutrients such as vitamins A, C, and E. These alone have been shown to help. Vitamin C is also an anti-stress vitamin and may counter too much adrenalin, which is often found in those diagnosed with schizophrenia.

Vitamin-C deficiency is also far more common than realized in mentally ill people, often because they don't look after themselves properly and eat poorly. Pronounced vitamin-C deficiency can make you crazy, as reported by Professor Derri Shtasel from the department of psychiatry at the University of Pennsylvania School of Medicine in Philadelphia. She describes a case of a woman who was confused and hearing voices, as well as having physical symptoms. She was tested for vitamin-C status and found to be very deficient. After being given vitamin C she had fewer hallucinations, her speech improved and she became more motivated and sociable.[64] Vitamin C has been shown to reduce the symptoms of schizophrenia in research trials,[65] and a number of studies have shown that people diagnosed with mental illness may have much greater requirements for this vitamin—often 10 times higher than those without mental illness—and are frequently deficient.[66]

Increased levels of oxidation are a common finding in schizophrenia and also other types of mental illness from autism to Alzheimer's disease. Oxidation in turn stresses the brain's ability to control normal methylation, which is not only vital for balancing neurotransmitters, but also repairs DNA damaged by oxidation. Later on we'll also see that high levels of mauve factor, which is one of the best indicators of excessive oxidation in the brain, are frequently found in schizophrenia and manic depression or bipolar disorder, with vitamin B6 and zinc playing a role in its reversal.

Abnormal methylation and high homocysteine

You are unique. That uniqueness is expressed biochemically in your genes—the instructions within every single cell in the brain and body that tell the stuff you are made out of how to assemble itself to build proteins, enzymes, neurotransmitters, hormones, and more.

Consider the diagrams on the following pages.

Figure 27 describes the chemical reactions that occur between eating the amino acid methionine and initiating methylation, which as we've seen is the process that is vital for keeping the brain's chemical balance in check. Each of the boxed initials stands for an enzyme that drives a step in the process. These enzymes can be upregulated, meaning they work harder than they should, or downregulated, meaning they are sluggish, or just right.

Whether they're set just right depends on many factors, including your genes. We all inherit different settings for the enzymes pictured, as well as others. These different settings are called polymorphisms, and each one has a particular code name. For example, a polymorphism of the MTHFR gene, which makes the MTHFR enzyme, is called C677TT. Roughly 1 in 10 people have C677TT, which ultimately lessens their ability to create SAMe, the amino acid that's the most important methyl donor in the body.

In Figure 28 the nutrients needed to drive enzymes such as MTHFR

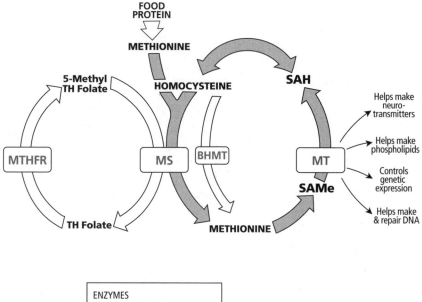

Fig 27. The methylation cycle. The amino acid methione, from dietary protein, becomes homocysteine, and is then turned, step by step, into SAMe by a process that involves a number of enzymes shown in white boxes.

are listed. As a result, these people with the MTHFR gene variation need more folic acid, B2, and B12, required by the adjoining enzymes.

This particular polymorphism is much more common in people diagnosed with schizophrenia. In fact, having this variation doubles your risk for schizophrenia and triples the risk for manic depression, according to research in Japan,[67] while a further six studies have found that inheriting this variation significantly raises the risk of developing schizophrenia.[68] For these people, lacking enough folic acid would compound the problem, resulting in an inability to produce the right levels of neurotransmitters such as serotonin, important for mood, and dopamine, which is key for motivation.

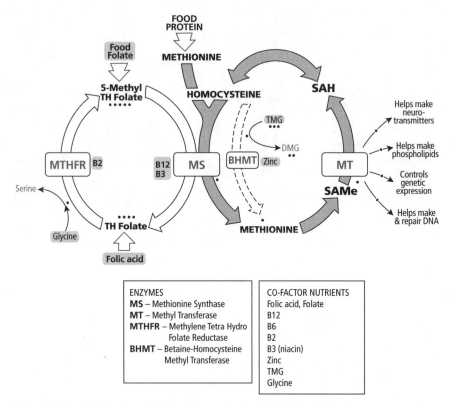

Fig 28. Nutrients needed in the methylation cycle. These enzymes are dependent on nutrients shown in grey boxes. Provided you have enough of these nutrients the enzymes help to liberate methyl groups, shown as dots. The cycle on the left liberates a methyl group from folate to turn homocysteine into SAMe. Another way of doing this is by taking in TMG (plus zinc) via the BHMT enzyme system. SAMe donates these [.] methyl groups to keep your brain and body chemistry in balance. It then needs to be reloaded by the folate cycle. See www.patrickholford.com/methylation to view an animated version of this cycle.

But let's look at other critical enzymes. As you'll see, methionine synthase or MS is dependent on vitamin B12, and a lack of B12 is another risk factor for both schizophrenia and depression. Another critical nutrient in this pathway is niacin (vitamin B3). As you'll see later, niacin deficiency induces schizophrenia-like symptoms and large amounts often reverse these symptoms. Without enough B3, once again you don't get to make enough SAMe and without SAMe methylation doesn't work properly and a person's balance of brain chemicals can go out of whack.

You might think that you could sort everything out by just giving SAMe. For many people that does work, but for some, SAMe actually induces mania and some of the symptoms of schizophrenia. So SAMe is fine for depression but often unwise for those with more manic, *hyper* symptoms—people we often find are called overmethylators. When we test them, their levels of neurotransmitters are often too high. It's as if their whole metabolism is working overtime, leaving them in a state of overstimulation.

Moving on round the methylation pathway, we come to another enzyme called methyltransferase (MT). This one marks the most critical part of the entire methylation cycle because it's where the work, so to speak, is done. Actually, there are many different kinds of MT enzymes with a variety of jobs to perform. These include:

- Making dopamine, noradrenalin, and adrenalin—needed for motivation

- Making serotonin and melatonin—needed for mood and for sleep

- Making myelin—the insulating layer around brain cells

- Building and breaking down and building phospholipids from essential fats.

For example, giving people with schizophrenia omega-3 fats often lowers homocysteine.[69] Everything in the brain in interconnected and it is providing the right balance of the brain's critical nutrients that holds out the most hope for those with schizophrenia.

There's another kind of MT called catechol-O-methyltransferase or COMT, which inactivates neurotransmitters such as adrenalin and noradrenalin, as well as histamine. (In Chapter 23 we learned that high-histamine types benefit from being given more of the amino acid methionine; methionine actually helps the COMT enzyme to break down excess histamine.)

The last player in this dance is the byproduct of SAMe, once it has donated its methyl group to the MT enzymes to do their work. This is called s-adenosyl homocysteine or SAH. Normally SAH is then turned into homocysteine, then rapidly converted again to SAMe, provided you have enough B12, folic acid, B6, and B2; then round it goes again. But if you don't have enough of these nutrients, homocysteine can accumulate and end up in high levels in the blood. As you'll see in the figure, homocysteine can convert back into SAH. If there's too much homocysteine or too much SAH, the SAH—which looks chemically similar to SAMe—starts to mess up the ability of the MT enzymes to do their job. It's a kind of negative feedback loop.

Although it's not yet commercially available, a test that measures the ratio between a person's SAMe and SAH levels would be a very good indicator of whether or not their methylation was working properly. This area desperately needs to be reasearched, but funds are hard to find for research that doesn't have a patented drug at the end of it. (If you'd like to help go to www.foodforthebrain.org/schizophreniaresearch.) In the meantime, the best indicator of a methylation problem is a raised homocysteine level.

The H factor

Not only is homocysteine often high in those with schizophrenia, even when there is no evidence of B vitamin deficiency,[70] but also the higher the homocysteine level, the worse the symptoms.[71] Dr. Joseph Levine of the Ben Gurion University in Beersheva, Israel, found that the average level of homocysteine in a group of 193 patients with schizophrenia was way above the average level. Levine found that the reason for the high average in the group was largely down to especially high levels in the young male patients in it.[72] Other psychiatric studies have reported similar findings.[73]

The consistent findings of raised homocysteine levels in people with schizophrenia strongly suggest that the right combination of homocysteine-lowering nutrients might improve methylation and thereby lessen the symptoms of schizophrenia.

Earlier studies have shown that folic acid on its own can help. Researchers at King's College Hospital psychiatry department in London have found high doses of folic acid to be highly effective in schizophrenic patients.[74] They used 15 mg a day, which is 75 times the RDA!

Vitamin B12, which like folic acid is involved in methylation, has also been shown to help schizophrenic patients.[75] B12 is difficult to absorb, especially in large amounts, and some doctors have reported good results giving weekly, or twice-weekly, injections of 1 mg of vitamin B12. Some supplements provide sublingual vitamin B12, which is absorbed in the mouth. It's hard to absorb much this way, but does sidestep the most common reason for B12 deficiency—a lack of *intrinsic factor* in the gut needed for absorption of this vitamin. So, sublingual liquid B12 supplements providing 50 mcg daily may be able to help normalize a B12 deficiency. Weekly B12 shots, at least to start with, tend to produce a much more rapid improvement.

I prefer giving large oral doses of 100 mcg of B12 or more, which is 100 times the RDA. This is not toxic and even though a relatively small percentage is absorbed, it will be enough, given the size of the dose, to raise cellular levels of B12.

However, since nutrients work in combination, the best results are likely to be achieved by combined supplementation.To date two research groups have put this theory to the test. The first, a study at Ben Gurion University in Israel headed by Dr. O. Shumeiko, gave 18 schizophrenic patients with an average homocysteine level of 15μM a combination of 2 mg folic acid, 25 mg pyridoxine (vitamin B6), and 400 mg B12 once a day for three months. The results were excellent, with the majority of patients showing a big reduction in symptoms.[76] Last year, a research group headed by Dr. Joseph Levine in Israel conducted a similar double-blind controlled trial giving 43 schizophrenic patients with homocysteine levels in the blood above 15μM either B6, B12, and folic acid or a placebo for three months. As would be expected, homocysteine levels declined with this vitamin therapy compared with the placebo in all participants, except for one who refused to follow the regime. The clinical symptoms of schizophrenia also improved significantly in the patients taking the vitamins.[77]

At the Brain Bio Centre in Richmond, we always check homocysteine levels and supplement not only B2, B6, B12, and folic acid, but also TMG and zinc. The reason for this can be found in Figure 28. There's another pathway for clearing homocysteine from the blood that is zinc dependent, and uses the nutrient TMG (found abundantly in root vegetables) to add a methyl group onto homocysteine and turn it into methionine.

The niacin connection

One of the classic vitamin-deficiency diseases is pellagra. At the turn of this century there were said to be 25,000 cases annually in the U.S., focused in the southern states where corn, lacking in tryptophan, was a staple food. The amino acid tryptophan can be converted into niacin. A lack of dietary tryptophan and a lack of niacin can trigger pellagra. The classic symptoms of this condition are the 3 Ds—dermatitis, diarrhea, and dementia. A more extensive list of symptoms might include headaches, sleep disturbance, hallucinations, thought disorder, anxiety, and depression.

Officially it doesn't really exist any more in the Western world, due to improved nutrition and the fortification of foods with niacin. Yet I come across people that fit this description every year. For instance, a girl diagnosed with schizophrenia came to see me. I always ask what other symptoms a person remembers at the time they started to feel mentally unwell, She remembered loose bowels and eczema—classic symptoms of pellagra. At the time, her doctors and psychiatrists obviously didn't make the connection. I doubt that many doctors or specialists even hold the possibility of nutrient deficiency on their checklist of causes of so-called schizophrenia. She proved B3-deficient after blood tests and made great improvement when she began taking niacin, plus other nutrients.

Two other cases illustrate another important point. In this case, two male teenagers, both diagnosed as schizophrenic and hospitalized, didn't have the associated symptoms of diarrhea and dermatitis. Both responded so well to 1,000–2,000 mg of niacin (100 times the RDA) that within days they both became lucid, were discharged and have continued to improve, requiring less or no medication. From their diets one wouldn't suspect they had been chronically deficient in vitamin B3, yet their body chemistry responded to 100 times the amount needed by most. Some practitioners call this *vitamin dependency*, but we are all vitamin dependent. It's just that some people need more, perhaps for genetic reasons, than others.

The use of megadoses of niacin was first tried by Drs. Humphrey Osmond and Abram Hoffer in 1951. So impressed were they with the results in acute schizophrenics that, in 1953, they ran the first double-blind therapeutic trials in the history of psychiatry. Their first two trials showed significant improvement giving at least 3g (3,000 mg) a day, compared to placebos. They also found that chronic schizophrenics, not first-time sufferers but long-term inpatients, showed little improvement. The results of six double-blind controlled trials showed that the natural recovery rate was doubled. Later they found that even chronic patients, treated for several years with niacin in combination with other nutrients, showed a 60 percent recovery rate.

Why niacin therapy fell out of favor

Over the next 20 years over a dozen trials tested the effects of niacin therapy, often with negative results, so niacin therapy fell out of favor. The main reason other researchers have often failed to corroborate Hoffer's claims for megavitamin treatment is that the regime he had proven successful wasn't properly followed in subsequent trials—for example, they used the wrong substances or a dosage that was much too low, or used it for too brief a period, or they discontinued tranquilizer medications too quickly.[78]

In 1973, an American Psychiatric Association task force report examined Hoffer's theory by reviewing a number of studies including Hoffer and Osmond's, the subsequent trials, and also some that failed to differentiate between acute and chronic patients. For example, Dr. Richard Wittenborn, consultant to the American Psychiatric Association, said this in a study of 86 schizophrenic patients: "Despite the reassuring clinical observations of Hoffer and others, the present findings challenge claims of general efficacy for a two-year regimen of niacin supplementation in the treatment of schizophrenia."[79]

However, Wittenborn had included both acute (recently diagnosed) and chronic (long-term) patients in his study. When he separated these subgroups, as Hoffer suggested, and looked at his findings again, his results did indeed support Hoffer and Osmond's claims for the benefits of niacin therapy. In a second paper he concluded that acute patients "may respond well with high dosage niacin as supplementary to other medication and treatment," observing that "persons whose premorbid history suggests a participatory lifestyle tend to return to a participatory pattern of living after a year or more of high niacin supplementation. No such trend was indicated for the control patients." While five out of nine acute patients undergoing conventional treatment experienced a reduction in schizophrenic symptoms after two years, this positive outcome was seen in eight of the nine patients who also received niacin supplementation. While this may seem only a moderate improvement, the overall score for important social markers (happiness, friends, a job, hobbies, etc.) worsened in the group who received conventional treatment only and improved significantly in the niacin group.[80]

Wittenborn sent a copy of this second paper to Dr. Hoffer with an apology for his previous publication. Hoffer reports that "when Wittenborn's first report came out it was treated as gospel by our critics. The second report was totally ignored."

Since then, Dr. Hoffer has published 10-year follow-ups on schizophrenics treated with niacin, compared to those not treated with niacin. In the niacin patients there were substantially fewer admissions, days in the hospital, and suicides. He continues to treat acute schizophrenics with niacin, plus other nutrients, including vitamin C, folic acid, and essential fats, and reports a 90 percent cure rate in acute schizophrenics who follow his nutritional program.

Here's a typical case from Dr. Hoffer.

In October 1990 a 24-year-old woman arrived in my office. Six months earlier she had begun to hallucinate and become paranoid. During three weeks in the hospital she began taking a tranquilizer. For several months after a premature discharge, she almost starved until a retired physician took her into her home to feed her. When I saw her she still suffered visual hallucinations, but no longer heard voices. I started her on 3g of niacin and 3g of vitamin C, daily. Three days later she was much better. By February 1991 she was well. By February 1995 she no longer needed drugs. She is still well and lives with her sister.

Now in his nineties and still actively working in Canada helping people recover from schizophrenia, Dr. Hoffer has recorded 4,000 cases and published double-blind trials. He is convinced that his approach is a major breakthrough in the treatment of mental illness. His autobiography, *Adventures in Psychiatry* (Kos Publishing, 2005), makes fascinating reading for anyone with an interest in medical science or schizophrenia. We owe an enormous debt to this man, a true pioneer who helped bring psychiatry into the 21st century, and whose discoveries have yet to be fully acknowledged. At the time of writing a controlled trial testing large-dose niacin in under way at the Beersheva Mental Health Center in Israel.

Five reasons why niacin works

Just how niacin works is still a bit of a mystery. Knowing that people with schizophrenia had hallucinations, Dr. Hoffer's explanation is that niacin stops the brain from producing adrenochrome from adrenalin, a chemical known to induce hallucinations. Niacin also protects vitamin B12 from oxidation, helping to normalize methylation, which as we've seen is a vital process for keeping adrenalin and noradrenalin levels in balance; this in turn will prevent the abnormal production of adrenochrome in the brain. These nutrients are methyl donors and acceptors, and act intelligently in the brain to keep everything in check (see Figure 29 below). Once again, some people may simply need more to stay healthy.

Niacin, together with vitamin B12 and folic acid, also helps to raise abnormally low histamine levels, an imbalance of which is also associated with hallucinations, but niacin may also help to lower high histamine levels by improving methylation.

Niacin improves dilation in the blood vessels, and so helps to flush out copper and other toxic elements which are associated with mental illness, and improves oxygen supply to the brain. Niacin is also needed for the brain to make use of essential fats. The happy neurotransmitter serotonin also needs niacin. Serotonin is made from the amino acid tryptophan, but only in the presence of enough niacin. So there are many possible ways this vitamin could affect brain function.

Hoffer has also found that patients who test positive for pyroluria (see page 292) are more likely to respond well to increased intakes of niacin. Again, this might be due to its antioxidant properties. So large doses of niacin are most likely to be most effective for acute, not chronic, schizophrenics who are pyroluric, with symptoms of hallucinations, anxiety, and thought disorder, and possibly high homocysteine levels.

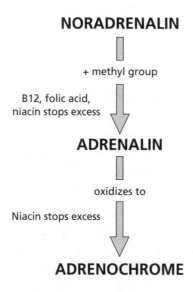

NORADRENALIN

+ methyl group

B12, folic acid,
niacin stops excess

ADRENALIN

oxidizes to

Niacin stops excess

ADRENOCHROME

Fig 29. How niacin, B12, and folic acid help keep your brain healthy

A safe and effective dose

The amount of niacin that's needed is around 1–6g a day. A minimum therapeutic level is 1g a day. These levels are in the order of 100 times the RDA. Levels of niacin much higher than these, particularly in sustained-release tablets, can be liver toxic. Out of perhaps 100,000 people taking megadoses of niacin at levels of several grams over the past 40 years, there have been two deaths due to liver failure. In a third case, jaundice resulted from a slow-release preparation. When the same patient was placed back on standard niacin, he no longer got jaundice. In any event, anything over 1g is best taken under the supervision of a qualified practitioner. If you become nauseated, that is an indication to stop supplementation and resume three days later, with a lower amount.

Niacin comes in different forms. Niacin (formerly known as nicotinic acid) causes a harmless blushing sensation, accompanied by an increase in skin temperature and slight itching. This effect can be quite severe, and lasts for up to 30 minutes. However, if 500 mg or 1,000 mg of niacin are taken twice a day at regular intervals, the blushing stops.

Some supplement companies produce a no-flush niacin by binding niacin with inositol. This works, so it's probably the best form, but it is more expensive. Niacin also comes in the form of niacinamide, which doesn't cause flushing either. It has to be said, however, that both of these forms appear to be slightly less effective than niacin. This may be because the flushing effect of niacin improves blood flow, and hence nutrient supply to the brain.

Are you pyroluric? The zinc link

Possibly one of the most significant *undiscovered* discoveries in the nutritional treatment of mental illness is that many mentally ill people are deficient in vitamin B6 and zinc. But this deficiency is no ordinary deficiency: you can't correct it by simply eating more foods that are rich in zinc and B6. It is connected with the abnormal production of a group of chemicals called 'pyrroles'. A person with a high level of pyrroles in the urine needs more B6 and zinc than usual, since they rob the body of these essential nutrients, increasing a person's requirements to stay healthy. More than 50 percent of people diagnosed with schizophrenia have pyroluria, also known as mauve factor.

The test for pyroluria is remarkably simple and very inexpensive. When you add a chemical known as Erhlich's reagant to urine, it will turn the color mauve if you have the condition. In the 1960s, pyroluria was found in 11 percent of normal people, 24 percent of disturbed children, 42 percent of psychiatric patients and 52 percent of schizophrenics.[81] Dr. Carl Pfeiffer and Dr. Arthur Sohler at Princeton's Brain Bio Center worked out that these abnormal chemicals would bind to B6 and zinc, inducing deficiency. With this knowledge, effective therapy was at hand. Since 1971, thanks to Dr. Pfeiffer's pioneering work, thousands of pyroluric patients have been successfully treated with B6 and zinc, both at Dr. Pfeiffer's Brain Bio Center and in other treatment centers around the world.

Here's a case in point from Dr. Pfeiffer.

Since she was 11, Sara's life had been a nightmare of mental and physical suffering. Her history included chronic insomnia, episodic loss of reality, attempted suicide by hanging, amnesia, partial seizures, nausea, vomiting, and loss of periods. Her knees were so painful (X-rays showed poor cartilage) and her mind so dispercep- tive that she walked slowly with her feet wide apart, like a peasant following a hand plough drawn by tired oxen. Psychiatrists at three different hospitals gave her various labels—schizophrenia, para- noid schizophrenia, and schizophrenia with convulsive disorder. At times her left side went into spasms with foot clawed and fist dou- bled up. Both arm and leg had a wild flaying motion. Restraints were needed at these times. Psychotherapy was ineffective and most tranquilizers accentuated the muscle symptoms.

Then Sara tested positive for pyroluria and was given B6 and zinc. Her urinary pyrrole level was at times as high as 1,000 mg%, the normal range being less than 15. She was diagnosed as B6- and zinc-deficient and treatment was started. Over three months her knees became normal, the depression subsided along with the seizures, her periods returned, the nausea vanished, and so did the abdominal pain. She has had no recurrence of her grave illness, has finished college, and now works in New York. She takes zinc and B6 daily. When under stress of any kind, she increases her intake of vitamin B6.

The signs and symptoms of pyroluria

Thanks to the thorough investigative work of Woody McGinnis, a medical doctor in Phoenix, Arizona, we now know what causes mauve factor in the urine and how it works.[82] (His excellent paper on this subject, "Discerning the mauve factor," is available in the Reports section of the website www.foodforthebrain.org. This lists every known reference on this subject, substantiating points in this section.)

Mauve factor, a substance excreted in the urine, is—as Dr. McGinnis has found—a type of pyrrole called 3-ethyl-5-hydroxy-4,5-dimethyl-delta-3-pyrroline-2-one, or HPL for short. Mauve factor was previously thought to be kryptopyrrole and, to this date, some laboratories still refer to kryptopyrrole levels in their tests, when in truth it is HPL that is being measured. An excess of HPL is called pyroluria. High HPL is also found in those with porphyria, a related condition (responsible, as we saw earlier, for the madness of George III). It is likely that having a high level of HPL is a consequence of either a genetic predisposition and/or a set of environmental circumstances, including suboptimal nutrition and excessive stress.

Pyroluria is common in people with mental health problems. Levels tend to fall when a person gets better and increase when they get worse. Emotional stress raises HPL and HPL itself can be seen as a powerful promoter of harmful oxidation, lowering the brain's levels of all sorts of key antioxidants, including glutathione.

Symptoms of pyroluria usually beginning in the teenage years after a stressful event such as exams or the split-up of a relationship. People with the condition often become reclusive and socially withdrawn, depending on the family and avoiding any stressful situations. Pyroluria is very common, for example, in autistic children.

Pyrolurics often have weak immune systems and may suffer from frequent ear infections as children, colds, fevers, and chills. Other symptoms include fatigue, nervous exhaustion, insomnia, poor memory, hyperactivity, seizures, poor learning ability, confusion, an inability to think clearly, depression, and mood swings. In girls there can be irregular periods and in boys relative impotence. The pyroluric patient can have bad breath and a strange body odor, have a poor tolerance of alcohol or drugs, wake up with nausea, and have cold hands and feet, and abdominal pain.

A lack of dream recall is very common. It is normal to remember dreams, and many people, whether or not they have mental health problems, report better dream recall once they start supplementing optimal amounts of vitamin B6 and zinc. Other telltale signs include pale skin, white marks on the nails and, in extreme cases, poor hair growth, and loss of hair color. White flecks on the nails are found in two-thirds of those with pyroluria, while many also have skin problems such as acne or eczema.

Not all these symptoms are present in all pyrolurics, but if you are experiencing a number of them, it is well worth testing for. As we've seen, a simple urine test measures the level of HPL in the urine (remember, these are sometimes still called kryptopyrroles), which should not be above 15 mg% (or 0.8 units). You can also check the probability of pyroluria, based on symptoms, using the online Food for the Brain questionnaire at www.foodforthebrain.org.

David is another case in point.

David was diagnosed as having schizophrenia at 20, having suffered from acute depression, paranoia, and extreme mental confusion. He was also seeing and hearing things. He was put on the drug Stelazine which calmed him down, but he felt disoriented and couldn't go back to college or relate with friends and family in a normal way. He was living a reclusive life, with his family. He came to see me at the Institute for Optimum Nutrition. He tested positive for pyroluria, and zinc deficiency, as well as having blood-sugar problems. Within days of adding B6 and zinc supplements, changing his diet, and avoiding sugar, coffee, and alcohol, he became symptom-free. He was able to stop taking Stelazine and, within months, was accepted at a university to continue his education.

Mark Vonnegut, the son of American novelist Kurt Vonnegut, is another example of someone who had a rapid recovery after been diagnosed with pyroluria at the Brain Bio Center at Princeton. At the time Mark was stricken with insomnia, which led to *crazes* while in college, and had no dream recall. He showed the usual rapid improvement when given daily zinc and enough B6, and started dreaming again. After recovering from pyroluria, Mark wrote *Eden Express* about his time in a mental hospital. It's a book that must be read for an understanding of the difficulties patients encounter in these institutions.

The key deficiency

Many of these symptoms are now recognized as classic signs of zinc deficiency, but this possibility is rarely tested for or corrected with zinc supplements. Most people with pyroluria are zinc deficient and giving extra zinc both corrects the symptoms and lowers HPL scores to normal. The failure to check for pyroluria and zinc deficiency is a tremendous oversight within psychiatry: zinc is, after all, probably the most commonly deficient mineral. The average intake in Britain is between 7 and 9 mg a day, while the European RDA is 15 mg, so almost half the population gets less than half the RDA of zinc. Seeds, nuts, meat, fish, and whole foods are all rich in it.

There's more to the story, however. People with pyroluria often come from families with a history of mental health problems. Dr. Pfeiffer also noted that it was more common in all-girl families. Although nothing is proven at this stage, it is likely that pyroluria is a genetic predisposition that makes an individual need more vitamin B6 and zinc to feel well. Like so many imbalances discussed in this book, it illustrates how we are all biochemically unique and need to discover our own optimum nutrition to stay healthy and mentally well.

Pfeiffer's observations about the importance of B6 have since been borne out.[83] Those with pyroluria are usually B6 deficient and, with supplementation, their symptoms improve and HPL levels normalize. Two of the frequently reported symptoms—poor dream recall, and mild morning nausea leading to poor appetite at breakfast—are thought to relate directly to functional vitamin B6 deficiency in people with pyroluria.

I believe that any person with a mental health problem should be routinely tested for pyroluria, using a urinary HPL test. To sum up, if you test high for HPL, this indicates increased oxidative stress, a factor that is linked to both schizophrenia and autism, but also to brain damage if left unchecked, as well as a relative deficiency in vitamin B6 and zinc in particular, although boosting your intake of other antioxidants may be wise.

Since oxidation raises homocysteine, puts further stress on methylation potential, and destroys essential fats, if you find you're pyroluric you will need to increase the amount of homocysteine-lowering B vitamins you take, such as B12 and folic acid, as well as essential fats. Supplementing relatively large amounts of zinc, starting with 25 mg and going up to 50 mg a day, and vitamin B6, starting at 100 mg and going up to 500 mg a day, is also advisable if you've been diagnosed.

As for the rest, you will need to eat a healthy diet that provides good levels of all these nutrients. Pyrolurics seem to do better on diets relatively low in protein, or at least not high-protein diets. Some people with the condition react badly to high-protein foods such as meat. This may be because they lack adequate amounts of B6 and zinc to digest, absorb, and use protein.

Allergic to wheat or milk?

Many people with mental health problems are sensitive to gluten, especially wheat gluten, which can bring on all sorts of symptoms of mental illness. This has been known since the 1950s, when Dr. Lauretta Bender noted that schizophrenic children were extraordinarily subject to celiac disease (severe gluten allergy).[84] By 1966 she had recorded 20 such cases from among around 2,000 schizophrenic children. In 1961 Drs. Graff and Handford published data showing that four out of 37 adult male schizophrenics admitted to the University of Pennsylvania Hospital in Philadelphia had a history of celiac disease in childhood.[85]

These early observations greatly interested Dr. Curtis Dohan at the University of Pennsylvania. He suspected that the two were linked and decided to test his theory by randomly placing all men admitted to a locked psychiatric ward in a Veterans Administration Hospital in Coatsville, Pennsylvania, either on a diet containing no milk or cereals, or on one that was relatively high in cereals. (Milk was eliminated from the diet because some people do not benefit when only glutens are removed.) All other treatment continued as normal. Midway through the experiment, 62 percent of the group on no milk and cereals were released to a full privileges ward. Only 36 percent of those patients receiving a diet including cereal were able to leave the locked ward. When the wheat gluten was secretly placed back into the diet, the improved patients once again relapsed.[86]

These results have since been confirmed by other double-blind, placebo-controlled trials. In one, published in the *Journal of Biological Psychiatry*, 30 patients suffering from anxiety, depression, confusion, or difficulty in concentration were tested, using a placebo-controlled trial, as to whether individual food allergies could really produce mental symptoms in these individuals. The results showed that allergies alone, not placebos, were able to produce the following symptoms: severe depression, nervousness, feeling of anger without a particular object, loss of motivation, and severe mental blankness. The foods/chemicals that produced the most severe mental reactions were wheat, milk, cane sugar, tobacco smoke, and eggs.[87]

In the 1980s, when more accurate methods of allergy testing became available, the American allergy expert Dr. William Philpott followed up Dr. Dohan's theory by testing 53 patients diagnosed with schizophrenia. Sixty-four percent reacted adversely to wheat, 50 percent to cow's milk, 75 percent to tobacco, and 30 percent to petrochemical hydrocarbons. The emotional symptoms caused by allergic intolerance ranged from dizziness, blurred vision, anxiety, depression, tension, hyperactivity, and speech difficulties to gross psychotic symptoms. At the same time, the individuals also experienced various adverse physical symptoms such as headaches, feeling of unsteadiness, weakness, palpitations, and muscle pains.[88]

Celiac disease remains vastly underdiagnosed. In recent screening surveys, it has been shown to occur in as many as 1 in 100 people,[89] although it is more common in those with mental health problems. For example, the incidence in children with mental health problems is 1 in 44.[90] Many people with celiac disease will have symptoms of irritable bowel syndrome (IBS) and/or depression. A third of patients who have panic attacks will also have symptoms of IBS. People with celiac disease are three times more likely to develop schizophrenia than those without the disease, according to researchers in Denmark and the Johns Hopkins School of Public Health in the U.S.[91] So if you have mental health problems and any of these symptoms, it is vital to check for possible celiac disease, which is now easy to do with a home test kit (see Useful Addresses, page 474).

Historical and cultural correlations would support the view that gluten has some kind of pathological effect on certain individuals with schizophrenia. Schizophrenia was extremely rare in southern Pacific nations prior to the introduction of cereal grains, though levels are now similar to those in Europe.

Why some can't stomach it

A class of peptides made in the body called endorphins and enkephalins are extremely potent painkilling substances. They perform this task by locking onto receptors in the brain to abolish the perception of pain. These receptors are heavily clustered in the frontal lobes and the lower limbic regions of the brain, where abnormalities have been found in those with schizophrenia. The wheat protein gluten, especially a kind of gluten called gliadin which is not present in oats, mimics endorphins and enkephalins, and is capable of reacting with the brain's endorphin receptors in either a stimulatory or suppressive way, very similar to certain drugs which have been known to produce psychosislike symptoms in patients. Casein proteins in dairy products are also thought to have amino acid sequences similar to those in enkephalins, so may also be capable of interacting with brain receptors. The term exorphins (a contraction of external endorphins) has been coined to describe these substances in relation to their pharmacological effects.[92]

At the Brain Bio Centre in Richmond, we routinely test for the presence of these exorphins in the urine. According to the pioneering research of Robert Cade, professor of medicine and physiology at the University of Florida, the gliadin byproduct gliadorphin was found in very large amounts in 48 percent of schizophrenics, indicating sensitivity to gliadin, while 86 percent had high IgG antibodies (see page 113) to gluten and 93 percent to casein, indicating allergy.[93]

There is now more than enough evidence to investigate the possibility of food and chemical sensitivities in people diagnosed with schizophrenia, especially to wheat and milk. At the very least, a trial period of two weeks without wheat or milk products is well worth exploring.

To find out more about the best tests for allergies see Chapter 12.

And what else?

Histamine imbalances are another biochemical twist in the tale of schizophrenia. In Chapter 23 we explored histadelia—how very high histamine levels can lead to compulsive and obsessive behavior, and significant depression. And in Chapter 17 we explored how very low levels of histamine are associated with feelings of anxiety, paranoia, and hallucinations.

Beyond histamine, where do we go? In this chapter we explored only seven of many promising avenues that can induce severe symptoms of mental illness, associated with a diagnosis of schizophrenia. As in the case of so many complex diseases, from chronic fatigue syndrome to autism, there is also evidence of immune system weaknesses, of links with viral infections,[94] of gut-related problems, liver detoxification problems,[95] and even links with difficult births and Caesareans.[96] A newcomer to this field of science will be understandably confused and wonder where to begin.

I have two answers. The first is at the beginning of this book. By working through Parts 1 and 2, and making the changes to your diet and lifestyle, this gives you the best possible chance to give your brain and body a tune-up. My second answer is to see a nutritional therapist, preferably one trained at the Institute for Optimum Nutrition, who is qualified to help you unravel the many strands that can lead to mental illness. Ideally, come to our Brain Bio Centre in Richmond.

In my view, people diagnosed with schizophrenia are like canaries in a coal mine (if you recall, the hapless birds were lowered into mines to check if the air was safe to breath). More sensitive than the rest of us to the insults of modern living and eating, to the suboptimal nutrition we almost all are victims of, those diagnosed with schizophrenia need all the help they can get through a personalized program of optimum nutrition. With this, and the right level of personal and social support, many can be released from the hellish symptoms of schizophrenia and the chemical straitjacket of the major tranquillizers to lead happy and productive lives.

SUMMARY

The starting point to tackling a diagnosis of schizophrenia is to:

- Balance your blood sugar.

- Check for, and correct, essential fat imbalances.

- Up your intake of antioxidants and especially vitamin C to 3g a day.

- Check your homocysteine level and change diet and lifestyle, and supplement homocysteine-lowering nutrients accordingly.

- Consider high-dose niacin, B12, and folic acid supplements.

- Get checked for HPL to see whether you have pyroluria and, if so, supplement extra zinc and B6.

- Check yourself for wheat, milk, and other allergies.

PART 6

Mental Health in the Young

Are children today having a *kid life crisis*? Mental health problems are very much on the increase in children—from autism to learning difficulties, hyperactivity, and depression. A major reason for these increases is often suboptimum nutrition. Here you'll find out how to maximize your child's potential and help them be and stay mentally and emotionally healthy.

CHAPTER 27

Learning difficulties, dyslexia, and dyspraxia

Nowadays children with learning and behavioral problems tend to get put into one of a number of boxes. Are they dyslexic, having problems with words and writing? Are they dyspraxic, having problems with coordination? Do they have attention deficit hyperactive disorder (ADHD), the official term for what used to be known as hyperactivity, with poor attention span, poor concentration, and hyperactive behavior?

Rightly or wrongly, the treatment depends on the box. If your child is diagnosed as having ADHD, the drug Ritalin will most likely be offered, but not if the diagnosis is dyslexia. But does ADHD actually exist? A top group of child psychiatrists and psychologists, convened by the National Institutes of Health in the U.S. in 1988, failed to find any substantial evidence that there is a disease called ADHD.[1] ADHD is purely a descriptive label given to children with a variety of behavioral and learning difficulties, and the diagnosis tells us nothing about the cause or treatment. In other words, almost every child is different, showing their own unique pattern of difficulties in learning, coordination and behavior and, as you will see, with optimum nutrition many of these difficulties often go away without recourse to drugs.

In truth, there are substantial clinical overlaps between learning difficulties, dyslexia, dyspraxia, and ADHD. While a minority of children are purely dyslexic, more often the same individual will show features of two, three, or all of these conditions in differing degrees of severity. Around half the dyslexic population is likely to be dyspraxic, and vice versa, and the mutual overlap between ADHD and dyslexia/dyspraxia is also around 50 percent.[2]

Unfortunately, there is usually no such overlap in diagnosis or treatment. ADHD lies in the realm of psychiatry, with stimulant medication the most likely course of action (see Chapter 28). Current evidence suggests that up to 20 percent of the population may be affected to some degree by one or more of these conditions, and the associated difficulties usually persist into adulthood, causing serious problems not only for those affected but for society as a whole.

Dyslexia is characterized by specific problems in learning to read and write due to sutble probelms in visual percetpion (just testing you!) Problems with arithmetic and reading musical notes are also common, as are poor working memory, difficulties with the sounds of words, and a poor sense of direction. Dyslexia affects around 5 percent of the population in a severe form, though many more when milder forms are also included. If you suspect your child might be dyslexic, many schools have special needs teachers who can test them for dyslexia. If your child's

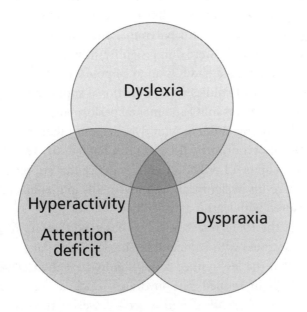

Fig 30. Dyslexia, dyspraxia, and ADHD overlap

school doesn't, contact International Dyslexia Association (see Useful Addresses, page 474), who can put you in touch with an educational psychologist who can carry out this test. This can help your child in a number of ways: by being aware they have a difficulty, by working with a special needs teacher to help minimize that difficulty, by the special privileges in time for exams, and by using computers at school that are routinely offered to those with dyslexia.

Dyspraxia is less well known but its prevalence is similar to that of dyslexia. It is characterized by clumsiness and difficulties in carrying out complex, sequenced actions. Poor coordination results in difficulties with acts such as catching a ball, tying up shoelaces, or doing up buttons, but more seriously results in extremely poor handwriting and difficulties with organization, attention, and concentration.

Where nutrition comes into learning

The link between optimum nutrition and later intelligence starts very early—during pregnancy and then in the very early stages of life. Dr. Alan Lucas's 16-year study at the Medical Research Council shows just how critical optimum nutrition is in the early years. In this study, more than 400 premature babies were fed either a standard or an enriched milk formula containing extra protein, vitamins, and minerals. At 18 months, those fed standard milk "were doing significantly less well" than the others, and at eight years old had IQs up to 14 points lower![3]

A large number of studies using nutritional supplements have shown dramatic improvements in IQ and mental performance later in childhood too, especially among children with dyslexia and other learning difficulties, even Down's syndrome (discussed in Chapter 30). The many studies discussed in Chapter 13 provide ample evidence that supplementation of nutrients can result in significant improvements in mental abilities, especially in children with learning difficulties.

As early as the 1960s researchers had observed that improved vitamin status was associated with increased intelligence.[4] Similarly, researchers at MIT found that the less refined foods children eat the cleverer they are, with diets high in refined carbohydrates—such as sugar, commercial breakfast cereals, white bread, and sweets—lowering their IQ by up to 25 points.[5] Stephen Schoenthaler, professor of criminology and sociology at the California State University, Stanislaus, later confirmed that the main effect of diets high in sugar and refined carbohydrates is that they lower the levels of nutrients in the diet.[6]

To further investigate the effects of poor nutrient intake on intelligence and learning abilities, Schoenthaler and his colleagues gave 245 school-children aged 6–12 years a daily multivitamin/mineral containing just 50 percent of the RDAs or a placebo for three months. The supplements were designed to raise nutrient intakes just to the equivalent of a "well-balanced diet," and confirmed that vitamin-mineral supplementation can significantly raise the non-verbal intelligence of some schoolchildren by up to 16 points if they are too poorly nourished before supplementation for optimal brain function.[7]

Investigating what this means for children with learning difficulties, Dr. Richard Carlton and colleagues at the Stony Brook University Medical School, New York, provided nutritional supplements on an individualized basis to 19 learning-disabled children. All of them showed significant academic and behavioral improvements within a few weeks or months, and some children gained three to five years in reading comprehension in the first year of treatment. Most importantly, all the children in special education classes became able to attend mainstream schooling, and their grades rose significantly.[8]

In another study, this time with 32 children with learning and behavioral difficulties, Dr. Michael Colgan supplemented half of the children according to their individual nutritional needs and reduced sugars and refined foods in their diet. The other children were given a standard multivitamin/mineral supplement daily, though no dietary changes were made. All the children attended a remedial reading course designed to improve reading age by one year, and over 22 weeks teachers carefully monitored the reading age, IQ, and behavior of the children. Those taking the multivitamin/mineral showed an average increase in IQ of 8.4 points and in reading age of 1.1 years. However, the group on individually tailored supplements and less sugar and refined carbohydrates had an improvement in IQ of 17.9 points and their reading age went up by 1.8 years, suggesting that subtle nutritional variables exert a substantial influence on learning and behavior.[9]

If your child is having problems with schoolwork, it's well worth seeing a nutritional therapist who can tune up their nutrition to maximize intellectual performance.

One theory as to how certain nutrients help improve intelligence is their antioxidant activity in the protection of essential fats needed for optimal brain function (see Chapter 9), though another is that they aid in the metabolism of energy, not just to the body but also to the brain. A key nutrient used as fuel for the brain, the amino acid L-glutamine, has been shown to significantly improve the IQ of intellectually impaired children, compared to controls.[10] Glutamine is also important for the health and integrity of the digestive system, an important consideration in autism, a related condition discussed in Chapter 29.

Fats are essential for brain development

We discussed the importance of essential fats for proper brain function in Chapter 4. Children with dyslexia, dyspraxia, and learning difficulties are very often deficient in these essential fats and/or the nutrients needed to properly utilize them, and the benefits of increasing the intake of these fats have been clearly documented in many studies.[11–12]

A study of 97 dyslexic children by Dr. Alex Richardson and colleagues at Hammersmith Hospital, London, revealed that fatty acid deficiency clearly contributes to the severity of dyslexic problems. Those children with the worst fatty acid deficiencies showed significantly poorer reading and lower general ability than the non-deficient children.[13] In a follow-up trial, at a school in Durham, working with educational psychologist Dr. Marlene Portwood,117 children with learning, behavioral, and psychosocial difficulties were given either a supplement of omega-3 and omega-6 or a placebo for three months. Then, without their knowing, the two groups were swapped. In both periods the group given the omegas showed significant improvement in reading, spelling, and behavior. After the swap, the improvement in those children, who were now getting the placebo, was maintained, but no longer improved.[14] Most significantly, 7 out of 16 children on essential fats were no longer classified as having ADHD, compared to 1 out of 16 on the placebo, by the end of the three months.

How do you know if your child is deficient in essential fatty acids? You could start with the checklist in Chapter 4. A key indicator is dry skin or eczema, and in a study of 60 children at the Royal London Hospital, Dr. Christine Absolon and colleagues found twice the rate of psychological disturbance in children with eczema compared with those without.[15]

So the many visible symptoms of essential fatty-acid deficiency—rough dry patches on the skin, cracked lips, dull or dry hair, soft or brittle nails, and excessive thirst—can be important indicators as to an underlying cause of learning difficulties, concentration problems, visual difficulties, mood swings, disturbed sleep patterns, and in some cases behavioral problems. This is because the related conditions of dyslexia, dyspraxia, learning difficulties, and ADHD all involve poor nerve-cell communications in the brain, and fatty acids crucially influence how your brain cells talk to each other.[16]

To test the value of supplementing essential fatty acids in dyspraxia, Dr. Jacqueline Stordy of the University of Surrey gave essential fat supplements (containing DHA, EPA, AA, and DGLA) to 15 children whose performance on standardized measures of motor and coordination skills placed them in the bottom 1 percent of the population. After 12 weeks of supplementation they all showed significant improvements in manual dexterity, ball skills, balance, and in parental ratings of their dyspraxic symptoms.[17]

Stordy also assessed the benefit of essential fat supplementation in dyslexia, and found that after just four weeks of supplementation with the omega-3 fatty acids EPA and DHA, night vision and dark adaptation (usually very poor in dyslexics) had completely normalized.[18]

More and more studies are now being published that show a clear benefit in supplementing essential fats. One recent study at Greenfield School in Durham in the U.K. gave a combination of EPA, DHA, and GLA for three months to a group of children with persistent behavior difficulties, and at high risk of exclusion. The study found a massive reduction in inattention, impulsivity, and hyperactivity in the group overall with two-thirds of the children showing major improvements in behavior.[19] Another, called the Sure Start project, gave 47 young children aged 2–3 years an essential fat supplement; this too showed considerable improvement in behavior. At the start parents rated their children's behavior as very poor, poor, moderate, good, or very good. Some 47 percent of the children were rated as poor or very poor and 17 percent as good or very good. After five months, 67 percent of children were rated as good or very good and only 4 percent as poor or very poor.[20]

Brain pollution

Another possible explanation for improvements in intelligence resulting from improved nutrient intake is that they help detoxify toxic metals like lead, which are known to have detrimental effects on intelligence.[21]

A number of studies have proved the connection between high lead levels and low intelligence. One researcher, Dr. Herbert Needleman, who has tested thousands of children, has not yet found a single child with high lead who has an IQ above 125.[22] Normally 5 percent of the population falls above this measurement. In Britain, lead levels in an estimated 50 percent of all children were high enough in the 1980s to actually impair intelligence. Since the advent of lead-free gasoline, blood-lead levels are fortunately dropping.

Copper is another toxic element that has been reported to be high in dyslexic children.[23] Since zinc and vitamin C are both antagonists of copper, this is another possible explanation for their reported benefits.

SUMMARY

In summary, I recommend the following for anyone who is dealing with learning difficulties, dyslexia, or dyspraxia:

- Ensure an optimal intake of nutrients from your diet as well as a good-quality multivitamin/mineral supplement.

- Minimize your intake of sugar and refined or processed foods that provide ample calories but few nutrients and prevent you from eating more nutrient-rich foods.

- Ensure an optimal intake of essential fats from seeds, their cold-pressed oils, and oily fish, plus sufficient antioxidants, especially vitamin E, to protect them from damage.

- Minimize your intake of fried food, processed food, and saturated fat from meat and dairy.

- Consider having a hair-mineral analysis to check for any heavy metal toxicities (see Useful Addresses on page 474).

These are a good start. But also check out the additional factors outlined in the next two chapters, and the guidelines at the end of each.

CHAPTER 28

The attention deficit disaster

Some children just can't sit still. With a short attention span and volatile moods, they get into fights and disrupt the class at school. These are classic signs of an ever-increasing pattern of attention, learning, and behavior problems labeled attention deficit hyperactivity disorder, sometimes abbreviated to ADHD or hyperactivity. These children have a hard time at school and at home, performing badly and getting into trouble, and are often shunted from school to school. Untreated, the hyperactive six-year-old might grow up to be come a delinquent teenager, often going off the rails with drugs and alcohol. Now affecting an estimated 1 in 10 boys and 1 in 30 girls in the U.K. and, according to a recent estimate in *The Lancet*, as many as 8–10 percent of children worldwide,[24] ADHD is often blamed on poor parenting or schooling. But there is a variety of other possible causes: heredity, smoking, alcohol or drug use during pregnancy, oxygen deprivation at birth, prenatal trauma, environmental pollution, allergy, and inadequate nutrition.

The good news is that more often than not, children with ADHD have one or more nutritional imbalances that, once identified and corrected, can dramatically improve their energy, focus, concentration, and behavior.

The rise of Ritalin

Sadly, many hyperactive children are not evaluated for chemical, nutritional, and allergic factors, nor are they treated nutritionally. Instead, they are quickly put on drugs such as Ritalin, which as we saw in Chapter 22, is a habit-forming amphetamine with many properties similar to those of cocaine. If you remember, Dr. Nora Volkow of the Brookhaven National Laboratory in Upton, New York, has shown that Ritalin is actually more potent than cocaine. She has concluded that the only reason Ritalin has not produced an army of addicted schoolchildren is that it takes about an hour for it in pill form to affect the brain, while smoked or injected cocaine works in seconds.[25] Despite these facts, prescriptions of Ritalin have risen 180-fold—from 2,000 in 1991 to 259,000 in 2004. The drug is currently given to 7 million schoolchildren in the U.S., or nearly 1 in 5.[26]

It's thought that the calming effect of stimulants like Ritalin on hyperactive children comes about because there is not enough of the neurotransmitters dopamine and noradrenalin in the part of the brain that is supposed to filter out unimportant stimuli. Dr. Joan Baizer at the University of Buffalo has shown that Ritalin, previously thought to have only short-term effects, initiates changes in brain structure and function that remain long after the therapeutic effects have dissipated.[27]

This is not good news when you consider the U.S. Drug Enforcement Administration's list of Ritalin's side effects. On top of increased blood pressure, heart rate, respiration, and temperature, people taking Ritalin can experience appetite suppression, stomach pains, weight loss, growth retardation, facial tics, muscle twitching, euphoria, nervousness, irritability, agitation, insomnia, psychotic episodes, violent behavior, paranoid delusions, hallucinations, bizarre behaviors, heart arrhythmias and palpitations, and psychological dependence—and can even die from it.[28]

There's another problem: Ritalin doesn't work. The U.S. National Institutes of Health concluded that there is no evidence of any long-term improvement in scholastic performance on Ritalin.[29] In September 2005 a massive review of 2,287 studies on ADHD drugs was published by the Oregon Evidence-based Practice Center at the Oregon Health and Science University in the U.S. It concluded that although 27 different drugs are prescribed for ADHD, "the evidence is not compelling that the drugs improve the thinking or quality of life of adults or help with adult anxiety or depression." Children often take these drugs for a long time but, the report said, there was "no evidence on long-term safety… in young children or adolescents." Finally, it found that the available evidence was of little use to clinicians trying to decide which of the 27 drugs might be useful for particular patients because very few comparisons between the drugs had been done in the light of how they affected academic perform-ance, quality of life, or social skills.[30]

Is your child hyperactive?

It can be difficult to draw the line between the behavior of a child that is within the normal limits of high energy and abnormally active behavior. Do these characteristics apply?

Overactive	Doesn't finish projects
Fidgets	Wears out toys, furniture, etc.
Can't sit still at meals	Doesn't stay with games
Talks too much	Doesn't follow directions
Clumsy	Fights with other children
Unpredictable	Teases
Doesn't respond to discipline	Gets into things
Speech problem	Temper tantrums
Doesn't listen to whole story	Defiant
Hard to get to bed	Irritable
Reckless	Unpopular with peers
Impatient	Lies
Accident prone	Bed wetter
Destructive	

Score 2 if a symptom is severe, 1 if moderate and 0 if not present. A score below 12 is normal. Higher scores indicate your child may benefit from the following nutritional strategies.

Another major review by the Agency for Healthcare Research and Quality, part of the U.S. Department of Health and Human Services, found that studies of ADHD drugs were of such poor quality that they could find "no evidence to support the claims made about [them]." What's more, a child given Ritalin or other stimulant drugs is more likely to become addicted to smoking and abuse other stimulant substances later in life, such as cocaine. The long and short of it is, don't let your child be prescribed these drugs.[31]

The use of stimulant drugs to control children's behavior has risen dramatically in the last decade. Ritalin is now given to up to 20 percent of children in some American schools, and researchers looking at its effectiveness have found that it can worsen the behavior of more children than it helps.

In contrast, nutritional treatment has proven very helpful for many hyperactive children and has few, if any, side effects. Given the substantial overlap between learning difficulties, dyslexia, dyspraxia, and ADHD, I will begin by reiterating the vital importance of optimal nutrient and essential fatty acid intakes and checking for brain pollutants, as discussed in the last chapter, before considering other potential factors in this distressing condition for children, parents, and teachers alike.

Eat to calm down

As we've now seen abundantly, studies have shown that academic performance improves and behavioral problems diminish significantly when children are given nutritional supplements. Although it is unlikely, on the basis of the studies to date, that ADHD is purely a nutrient deficiency disease, some children are deficient and do respond very well.

In one study by Dr. Abram Hoffer, a pioneer in orthomolecular medicine, large amounts of vitamin C (3g) and B3 (niacinamide 1.5g or more) significantly improved the behavior of 32 out of 33 children with ADHD.[32] Some children may be zinc or magnesium deficient, both of which can produce symptoms associated with ADHD. The symptoms of magnesium deficiency, for example, are excessive fidgeting, anxious restlessness, coordination problems, and learning difficulties despite having a normal IQ. (See below for more on magnesium vis-à-vis ADHD.)

Given that a possible effect of Ritalin is to correct a noradrenalin deficiency in the part of the brain that is supposed to filter out unimportant stimuli, it is interesting to note that magnesium plays a key role in promoting production of noradrenalin. Dr. Lendon Smith reports that around 80 percent of children are able to stop taking Ritalin after as little as three weeks once they start supplementing 500 mg of magnesium daily. Other nutrients also involved in the production of noradrenalin include manganese, iron, copper, zinc, vitamin C, and vitamin B6,[33] and many of these nutrients are also involved in the proper metabolism of essential fats (see page 315).

B6 and magnesium

Despite the tremendous results reported for nutritional approaches, Ritalin is far more commonly prescribed than nutritional supplements. The late Dr. Bernard Rimland assessed the relative effectiveness of different nutrient strategies compared to drugs such as Ritalin, and found that supplementing B6 and magnesium was 10 times more effective than Ritalin!

In fact, the best drug was Mellaril, not Ritalin. However, neither of these drugs was as effective as vitamin B6 and magnesium or the brain nutrient DMAE, prescribed as Deanol in the U.S., which was also twice as effective as Ritalin (see page 322).

Dr. Neil Ward of the University of Surrey has found one way that children become deficient in these important nutrients. In a study of 530 hyperactive children, he found that a significantly higher percentage of children with ADHD had taken several courses of antibiotics in early childhood than the children without ADHD.[34] Further investigations revealed that children who had had three or more antibiotic courses before the age of three tested for significantly lower levels of zinc, calcium, chromium, and selenium.[35]

A Polish study from 1997 that examined the magnesium status of 116 children with ADHD found that magnesium deficiency occurred far more frequently in them than in healthy children (95 percent of the children with ADHD were deficient), and also noted a correlation between levels of magnesium in the body and severity of symptoms. The children were divided into two groups, one supplemented with 200 mg of magnesium a day for six months, the other receiving no supplements. The magnesium status of the group receiving supplements improved and their hyperactivity was significantly reduced, while hyperactive behavior worsened in the control group.[36]

Vitamins vs drugs—which work best?

Dr. Bernard Rimland studied the effect of the nutrient approach to ADHD on 191 children. Dr. Humphrey Osmond decided to compare this to the reported results with drugs. He reported the total number taking each drug, the number helped, the number worsened and the relative efficacy ratio. This is the number helped divided by the number worsened. So if twice as many are helped as worsened, the ratio is 2. If the same numbers of people are helped as worsened then the ratio is 1. The results showed that as many ADHD sufferers are worsened by medication as are helped. In stark contrast 18 times as many sufferers are helped as harmed with a nutritional approach, with 66 percent responding positively.

Medication	Total	No. helped	No. worsened	Relative efficacy ratio
Dexedrine	172	44	80	0.55
Ritalin	66	22	27	0.81
Mysoline	10	4	4	1.00
Valium	106	31	31	1.00
Dilantin	204	57	43	1.33
Benadril	151	34	25	1.36
Stelazine	120	40	28	1.43
Deanol	73	17	10	1.70
Mellaril	277	101	55	1.84
All drugs	1591	440	425	1.04
Vitamins	191	127	7	18.14

Andrew's story is a classic example of how effective magnesium can be in helping restless, hyperactive children. When he was three years old, his sleep-deprived parents brought him to the Brain Bio Centre in Richmond. Andrew was hyperactive and seemed never to sleep. Not surprisingly, he was grumpy most of the time. We recommended that his parents give him 65 mg of magnesium daily in a pleasant-tasting powder added to a drink before bed. Two weeks later, Andrew's mum phoned to say that he was sleeping right through every night and had been transformed into a delightful child during the day too.

A similar story can be told for zinc. Even without supplements, significant improvements in behavior can result from dietary changes that increase nutrient intakes. As we saw in Chapter 27, Professor Stephen Schoenthaler of the department of social and criminal justice at California State University, has conducted extensive investigations into the relationship between poor diet, nutrient status, and bad behavior. In his many placebo-controlled studies conducted over 18 months in Alabama, Florida, and Virginia, involving over a thousand long-term young offenders, improving their diets improved their behavior by between 40 and 60 percent. Blood tests for vitamins and minerals showed that around a third of the young people involved had low levels of one or more vitamins and minerals before the trial, and those whose levels had become normal by the end of the study demonstrated a massive improvement in behavior of between 70 and 90 percent.[37]

Essential fatty acids

Many children with ADHD have known symptoms of essential fatty acid deficiency such as excessive thirst, dry skin, eczema, and asthma. It is also interesting that males, who have a much higher requirement for essential fatty acids than females, are more commonly affected: four out of five ADHD sufferers are boys. Researchers have theorized that ADHD children may be deficient in essential fatty acids not just because they have inadequate dietary intake (though this is not uncommon), but rather because their need is higher, they absorb them poorly, or they don't convert them well into prostaglandins that help the brain communicate.[38]

It is of interest then that EFA conversion to prostaglandins can be inhibited by most of the foods that cause symptoms in children with ADHD such as wheat, dairy products, and foods containing salicylates. Conversion is also hindered by deficiencies of the various vitamins and minerals needed for the enzymes that power the conversions, including vitamin B3 (niacin), B6, C, biotin, zinc, and magnesium. Zinc deficiency is common in ADHD sufferers.

Research carried out at Purdue University in the U.S. confirmed that children with ADHD had an inadequate dietary intake of the nutrients required for EFA conversion to prostaglandins, and subsequently had lower levels of the fatty acids EPA, DHA, and AA (all produced in the body from EFAs) than children without ADHD.[39] Supplementation with all these pre-converted fatty acids and with GLA reduced ADHD symptoms such as anxiety, attention difficulties, and general behavior problems.[40–42]

Research at Oxford University has proven the value of these essential fats in a double-blind trial involving 41 children aged 8–12 years who had ADHD symptoms and specific learning difficulties. Those children receiving extra essential fats in supplements were both behaving and learning better within 12 weeks.[43] There are more studies confirming this finding (see page 306): the evidence for the benefits of supplementing essential fats in children with ADHD symptoms is now substantial. But it's not only omega-3s that they need.

Stephen's story, courtesy of the Hyperactive Children's Support Group, is a case in point.

Stephen, aged six, had a history of hyperactivity, with severely disturbed sleep and disruptive behavior at home and at school. Threatened with expulsion from school because of his impossible behavior, his parents were given two weeks to improve matters. They contacted the Hyperactive Children's Support Group and evening primrose oil, a source of the omega-6 fat GLA, was suggested. A dose of 1.5g was rubbed into his skin morning and evening. The school was unaware of this, but after five days the teacher telephoned the mother to say that never in 30 years of teaching had she seen such a dramatic change in a child's behavior. After three weeks the evening primrose oil was stopped, and one week later the school again complained. The oil was then reintroduced with good effect.

Many children do not eat rich sources of omega-3 and omega-6 EFAs and could benefit from eating more oily fish (such as wild or organic salmon, sardines, herring, and mackerel), seeds such as flax, hemp, sunflower, and pumpkin or their cold-pressed oils, and walnuts or walnut oil. (See Chapter 4, page 39, for a detailed discussion of the best way to boost your child's intake of EFAs.) It is also important to replace foods that are known to hinder the conversion of EFAs to prostaglandins while supplementing the nutrients needed for the conversion, discussed above.

Other culprits behind ADHD

Toxic nasties

Looking beyond low levels of essential nutrients, excess anti-nutrients can also induce ADHD symptoms. Just as in learning difficulties (discussed above), top of the list is lead, which produces symptoms of aggression, poor impulse control and short attention span. Another is excess copper, which is found in some children with ADHD. Studies have also revealed a link between high aluminum and hyperactivity. Many toxic elements deplete the body of essential nutrients, for example zinc, and may contribute to nutritional deficiencies. A hair-mineral analysis to rule out heavy metal intoxication is therefore an important component of an overall nutritional approach.

Just an allergy?

Of all the avenues so far researched, though, the link between hyperactivity and allergy is the most established and worthy of pursuit in any child showing signs of this syndrome.

Manufacturers now use an extraordinary number of artificial additives in food, and we can each end up eating as much as 5 kg of additives every year. Some children clearly aren't coping well with this chemical onslaught. A preliminary study by Dr. Joseph Bellanti of Georgetown University in Washington, DC, found that children with ADHD are seven times more likely to have food allergies than other children. According to his research, 56 percent of ADHD children aged 7–10 tested positive for food allergies, compared to less than 8 percent of controls. A separate investigation by the Hyperactive Children's Support Group found that 89 percent of children with ADHD reacted to food colorings, 72 percent to flavorings, 60 percent to MSG, 45 percent to all synthetic additives, 50 percent to cow's milk, 60 percent to chocolate, and 40 percent to oranges.[44]

The yellow food coloring tartrazine (E102) is the best known of many chemical additives linked to allergic reactions and ADHD. In a double-blind, placebo-controlled study, Dr. Neil Ward at the University of Surrey found emotional and behavioral changes in every child who consumed tartrazine, observing that the additive decreased blood levels of zinc by increasing the amount of zinc excreted in the urine.[45] Four out of the 10 children in the study had severe reactions, three developing eczema or asthma within 45 minutes of ingestion.

Other substances often found to induce behavioral changes are wheat, dairy, corn, yeast, soy, citrus, chocolate, peanuts, and eggs.[46] Associated symptoms that are strongly linked to allergy include nasal problems and excessive mucus, ear infections, facial swelling and discoloration around the eyes, tonsillitis, digestive problems, bad breath, eczema, asthma, headaches, and bedwetting. It's relatively simple to identify foods that may be causing or aggravating symptoms by excluding them for two weeks before a carefully observed reintroduction. Testing in this way is not always conclusive, so it may be worth considering a proper allergy test using the IgG ELISA method. Such a test can identify foods that an individual reacts to from a single blood sample, though they do cost $250–$500, depending on the number of foods tested and the chosen laboratory (see Useful Addresses, page 474, and Chapter 12). While most intolerances are IgG mediated, some are IgE mediated so, ideally, it's best to have both an IgE and an IgG test.

Up to 90 percent of hyperactive children benefit from eliminating foods that contain artificial colors, flavors, and preservatives, processed and manufactured foods, and culprit foods identified by either an exclusion diet or blood test.[47] Child psychiatrist Eric Taylor from the London-based Institute of Child Health was skeptical of the reports from parents that their children responded to chemical-free diets designed to eliminate their allergens, so in the early 1990s he and his colleagues designed a study to rigorously test this proposition. They placed 78 hyperactive children on a *few-foods* diet, eliminating both chemical additives and common food allergens. During this open trial, the behavior of 59 of the children (76 percent) improved. To check for a reverse placebo effect, the researchers secretly reintroduced the foods and additives that had provoked reactions in 19 of the children. The children's behavior rapidly became worse and so did their performance in psychological testing.[48]

Combining vitamins, minerals, and essential fats while eliminating allergens can be remarkably effective at relieving the symptoms of ADHD.

Eight-year-old Richard is a case in point. Diagnosed with ADHD, he was out of control and his parents were at their wits' end. Richard had also been constipated his entire life. Through biochemical testing at the Brain Bio Centre in Richmond, they found that he was allergic to dairy products and eggs and was very deficient in magnesium. By looking at his diet they saw that he was eating far too much sugar on a daily basis.

He was given a low-sugar, low-GL diet (with a focus on whole foods and complex carbohydrates) free of dairy and eggs, and was also given magnesium and omega-3 supplements. Within three months, his parents reported that Richard had calmed down considerably and had become much more manageable. His constipation had also cleared completely.

Some have also reported success with the Feingold diet, removing not only all artificial additives but also foods that naturally contain compounds called salicylates. Although there have been few double-blind studies on the Feingold diet, researchers at the Univesity of Sydney, Australia, found that of 86 children with ADHD, 75 percent of them reacted adversely to a double-blind challenge with salicylates.[49] Foods rich in salicylates include prunes, raisins, raspberries, almonds, apricots, canned cherries, blackcurrants, oranges, strawberries, grapes, tomato sauce, plums, cucumbers, and Granny Smith apples. As the list is very long and contains many otherwise nutritious foods this should be considered only as a secondary course of action, and must be carefully planned and monitored by a nutritional therapist to ensure adequate nutritional intake.

Understanding how a low-salicylate diet helps children with ADHD offers us an alternative. Salicylates inhibit the conversion and utilization of essential fatty acids, which we know from the discussion above are essential for proper brain function and are also often low in children with ADHD. So instead of avoiding the inhibitor (salicylates), it may be sufficient to increase the supply of EFAs, which has indeed been shown to help.

Sugar problems

A diet high in refined carbohydrates is not good for anyone, and many parents believe than eating sweets promotes hyperactivity and aggression in their children. In contrast, some recent research has suggested that sugar itself is not to blame for hyperactivity, and can even have a calming effect on certain individuals. Yet dietary studies do consistently reveal that hyperactive children eat more sugar than other children,[50] and reducing dietary sugar has been found to halve disciplinary actions in young offenders.[51] It seems then that reactions to sugar are not due to allergy as such, but a craving brought on by low blood-sugar levels.

Other research has confirmed that the problem is not sugar itself but the forms it comes in, the absence of a well-balanced diet overall, and abnormal glucose metabolism. A study of 265 hyperactive children found that more than three-quarters displayed abnormal glucose tolerance.[52] As the main fuel for the brain and body, when blood-glucose levels fluctuate wildly all day on a roller-coaster ride of refined carbohydrates, stimulants, sweets, chocolate, fizzy drinks, juices, and little or no fiber to slow the glucose absorption, it is not surprising that levels of activity, concentration, focus, and behavior will also fluctuate wildly, as is seen in children with ADHD. The calming effect sometimes observed after sugar consumption may well be the initial normalization of blood sugar from a hypoglycemic state during which the brain and cognitive functions controlling behavior were starved of fuel.

The advice then is to remove from the diet all forms of refined sugar and any foods that contain it, and replace them with whole foods and complex carbohydrates (brown rice and other whole grains, oats, lentils, beans, quinoa, and vegetables), which should be eaten throughout the day. Carbohydrates should always be balanced with protein (half as much protein as carbohydrates at every meal and snack) to improve glucose tolerance. Two easy examples are eating nuts with fruit, or fish with rice. Supplementing 200 mcg of chromium also helps stabilize blood sugar.

Bipolar children

Some children diagnosed with ADHD have bipolar disorder, or manic depression. They may oscillate from states of mania and hyperactivity to crying spells and depression. The trouble is that bipolar disorder simply isn't diagnosed in childhood. In fact, it used to be thought that the condition didn't start before the age of 20, but this is a myth. Bipolar disorder can and does occur in infancy, but the majority of these children get wrongly classified as having ADHD. Drs. Janet Wozniak and Joseph

Biederman from Harvard Medical School found that 94 percent of children with mania met the criteria for a diagnosis of ADHD.

This is bad news, because the last thing a bipolar child needs is stimulant drugs such as Ritalin. Dr. Demitri Papalos, associate professor of psychiatry at Albert Einstein College of Medicine in New York City, studied the effects of stimulant drugs on 73 children diagnosed as bipolar and found that 47 of these children were thrown into states of mania or psychosis by stimulant medication.[53] His excellent book, *The Bipolar Child*, co-authored with his wife Janice Papalos, helps to differentiate between those suffering from bipolar disorder (see Chapter 24) and ADHD. These are the differences they've observed:

- Children with bipolar disorder essentially have a mood disorder and go from the extreme highs of mania, tantrums, and anger into extreme lows. Some may go through four cycles in the year, while for others these cycles can happen in a week. This rapid cycling is rarely seen in adults.

- Bipolar children also have different kinds of angry outbursts. While most children will calm down in 20–30 minutes, bipolar children can rage on for hours, often with destructive, even sadistic, aggressiveness. They can also display disorganized thinking, language, and body positions during an angry outburst.

- Bipolar children have bouts of depression, which is not a usual pattern of ADHD. They may show giftedness, perhaps in verbal or artistic skills, often early in life. Their misbehavior is often more intentional, while the classic ADHD child can misbehave through their own inattention. A bipolar child can, for example, be the bully in the playground.

The nutritional approach outlined at the end of this chapter is much more likely to be helpful, together with those outlined in Chapter 24. Ritalin, and other stimulant drugs, can be an absolute disaster.

Reward deficiency syndrome

Some children with ADHD disturbances suffer from reward deficiency syndrome,[54] characterized by a constant need for stimulation. This is thought to occur because they either don't produce enough of the motivating neurotransmitter dopamine (from which adrenalin and noradrenalin are made), or don't respond strongly enough to their own dopamine. Drugs like cocaine and Ritalin both increase dopamine production and dopamine sensitivity, at least in the short term. For these children, Ritalin can seem a miraculous cure. But in the long term, they cause downregulation so you need even more stimulation. This is probably why children given Ritalin are more likely to abuse other dopamine-promoting drugs and are more likely to become dependent on such drugs later in life.[55]

For these children, the stimulating brain nutrient DMAE is highly effective. Researcher and psychiatrist Dr. Charles Grant discovered that in addition to increasing acetylcholine, in higher doses DMAE can actually block the acetylcholine receptor. This allows more dopamine to be released, thereby stimulating the brain. This action could explain DMAE's proven success with reward deficiency syndrome and ADHD. Unlike Ritalin, DMAE doesn't increase the need for external stimulation and doesn't have all the undesirable side effects.

The optimum nutrition approach to ADHD involves a combination of all the above factors and practitioners have reported significant improvements in at least two-thirds of children. This is substantially better than any drugs currently prescribed for ADHD. Ritalin, the most frequently prescribed, helps about a third of children and makes a third worse.

SUMMARY

In summary, I recommend that anyone with ADHD:

- Follow the guidelines at the end of Chapter 27 regarding nutrients, sugar, essential fats, and heavy metals.

- Eliminate chemical food additives and check other potential allergens such as wheat, dairy, chocolate, oranges, and eggs.

- Supplement DMAE.

One last note. ADHD is a complex condition requiring supervision and treatment by a qualified practitioner who can devise the

▶

correct nutritional strategy for your child. Individual assessment of supplement requirements is essential and should always be accompanied by a healthy diet. A minimum of three to six months is required before you see any substantial results, but a general slowing of the hyperactivity and increased concentration can happen within weeks. As the children start to feel better and behave better, the positive feedback they receive from their parents and teachers can encourage them to commit to the program and considerable improvements can quickly follow. Gut problems, allergies, and poor liver detoxification are also worthy of consideration in ADHD cases, and are discussed in the next, related chapter on autism.

CHAPTER 29

Answers for autism

Few **conditions are as mysterious** as autism. All of the overlapping conditions in the previous two chapters—dyslexia, dyspraxia and ADHD—are often present in autism, but there are other symptoms that lead to a diagnosis of autism. These include difficulties with speech, abnormalities of posture or gesture, impaired understanding of the feelings of others, sensory and visual disperceptions, fears and anxieties, and behavioral abnormalities such as compulsive/obsessive behavior and ritualistic movements.

The U.S. State Department of Developmental Services has found that the incidence of autism more than tripled between 1987 and 1999.[56] The figures for the U.K. range from 3–10 times more cases in the last decade. While autism used to occur primarily from birth, or at least was detected within the first six months, over the past 10 years there has been a dramatic increase in late-onset autism, most frequently diagnosed in the second year of life, in both the U.S. and U.K. According to the National Autistic Society, the incidence may now be higher than 1 in every 100 children. However, even this may be an underestimate. One survey of children 9–10-years-old in northeast London found that 116 in 10,000 had autistic spectrum disorders.[57] This equates to 1 in 86 children and at least 1 in 50 boys, and strongly suggests that something new is triggering this epidemic. Possible culprits include diet, vaccinations, and gut problems, which are also very much on the increase in children.

Six-year-old Ethan is a case in point. He had been diagnosed with autism at the age of two and a half. He had frequent ear infections and was a very picky eater, often restricting his diet to two foods—chicken nuggets and chips. Tests revealed that he had a number of food allergies and was low in magnesium. An analysis of his diet showed that he was taking in enormous amounts of sugar. Reducing sugar, supplementing magnesium, and excluding the foods he was allergic to brought about some significant changes. Within a few weeks, his parents noticed and others began commenting that he seemed much brighter, more smiley and affectionate, and had better eye contact. He ceased having ear infections and the range of foods that he would eat broadened considerably.

Unraveling autism

As in all conditions like this, there is the question of whether it is inherited or caused by something in the diet or environment. Autism is four times as common in boys as girls. Parents and siblings of autistic children are far

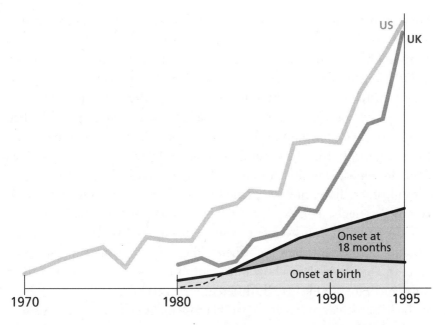

Fig 31. Rise in autism in the U.S. and U.K., and shift in relation to onset

more likely to suffer from milk or gluten allergy, have digestive disorders such as irritable bowel syndrome, and have high cholesterol, night blindness or light sensitivity, thyroid problems, and cancer. Being breast-fed also increases the risk. At first glance, one might suspect that autistic children may inherit certain imbalances. However, an alternative explanation might be that other family members eat the same food and may be lacking the same nutrients.

Given the overlaps with dyslexia, dyspraxia and ADHD, all of the factors discussed in the previous two chapters are equally relevant when considering the causes of autism. Specifically, you'll need to consider balancing blood sugar, checking for brain-polluting heavy metals, excluding food additives, correcting possible nutrient deficiencies, and ensuring an optimal intake of essential fatty acids. There is growing evidence that these approaches can really make a big difference to the autistic child. In fact, it is probably better to consider all these conditions as part of the autistic spectrum of diseases, with dyslexia and mild hyperactivity at one extreme and autism at the other.

Nutrient deficiencies

We've known since the 1970s that nutrients can make a big difference to autistic children, thanks to the pioneering research by the late Dr. Bernard Rimland of the Institute for Child Behavior Research in San Diego, California. He showed that vitamin B6, C, and magnesium supplements significantly improved symptoms in autistic children. In one of his early studies back in 1978, 12 out of 16 autistic children improved, then regressed when the vitamins were swapped for placebos.[58] In the decades following Dr. Rimland's groundbreaking study, many other researchers have also reported positive results with this approach.[59]

Still others have, however, failed to confirm positive outcomes with certain nutrients. For example, a French study of 60 autistic children found significant improvements resulted from a combination of vitamin B6 and magnesium, but not when either nutrient was supplemented alone.[60] This study shows how important it is to get the balance of these nutrients right. It's likely to be different for each child.

B6 in particular may help in part because many children with autism or learning difficulties have a condition known as pyroluria (see Chapter 26, page 292), a condition in which, for genetic reasons, high levels of a compound called HPL are excreted in the urine and cause a deficiency of zinc and vitamin B6. In children who have facial swelling, and a history of frequent colds and middle ear infections, pyroluria should be suspected, and can be tested with a simple urine test (see Useful Addresses, page 474).

A lack of the right fats

We've already discussed how essential fatty acids are essential for brain function, and deficiencies are common in autism sufferers.[61] Research by Dr. Gordon Bell at Stirling University has shown that some autistic children have an enzymatic defect that removes essential fatty acids from brain cell membranes more quickly than it should. Consequently, supplmenting the omega-3 fatty acid EPA, which can slow the activity of this enzyme, has clinically improved behavior, mood, imagination, spontaneous speech, sleep patterns, and focus of autistic children.[62-63]

Visual problems and vitamin A deficiency

Dr. Mary Megson, a pediatrician in Richmond, Virginia, believes that many autistic children are lacking in vitamin A. Otherwise known as retinol, vitamin A is essential for vision. It is also vital for building healthy cells in the gut and in the brain. There is no real doubt that something funny is going on in the digestive tracts of autistic children. Could this be related to vitamin-A deficiency, she wondered?

The best sources of vitamin A are breast milk, organ meats, milk fat, fish, and cod liver oil, none of which are prevalent in our diets. Instead, we have formula milk, fortified food, and multivitamins, many of which contain altered forms of retinol such as retinyl palmitate which doesn't work as well as the fish- or animal-derived retinol. What would happen, wondered Dr. Megson, if these children weren't getting enough natural vitamin A?[64] Not only would this affect the integrity of the digestive tract, potentially leading to allergies, but it would also affect the development of their brains, and disturb their vision. Both brain differences and visual defects have been detected in autistic children. The visual defects, she deduced, were an important clue because lack of vitamin A would mean poor black and white vision, a symptom often seen in the relatives of autistic kids.

If you can't see black and white, what you lose is shadow. Without shadow you'd lose the ability to perceive three-dimensionality and, as a consequence, you couldn't make sense of people's expressions so well. This might explain why autistic children tend not to look straight at you. They look to the side. Long thought to be a sign of poor socialization, it may in fact be the best way they can see people's expressions because there are more black and white light receptors at the edge of the visual field than in the middle. Your whole visual world would become fragmented snapshots.

Of course, the proof is in the pudding. Dr. Megson has reported rapid and dramatic improvements in autism simply by giving cod liver oil containing natural, unadulterated vitamin A. Often she has seen results within a week of starting cod liver oil.[65] Here are some of the comments her patients have made after cod liver supplementation. "Now I know where my fingers are." "Now I can see my arms at the same time I see my fingers!" "My box is getting bigger every day. Now I can see emotion on the faces on TV."

The allergy link

In addition to these likely deficiencies, the most significant contributing factor in autism appears to be undesirable foods and chemicals that often reach the brain via the bloodstream because of faulty digestion and absorption. Much of the impetus for recognizing the importance of dietary intervention has come from parents who've noticed vast improvements in their children when changing their diets. Certain offending foods and substances appear to adversely influence a large number of children, including:

- Wheat and other gluten-containing grains

- Milk and other dairy products containing casein

- Citrus fruits

- Chocolate

- Artificial food colorings

- Paracetamol

- Salicylates (see Chapter 28, page 319)

- Nightshade family foods (potatoes, tomatoes, aubergines).

The strongest direct evidence of foods linked to autism involves wheat and dairy, and the specific proteins they contain—namely gluten and casein. These are difficult to digest and, especially if introduced too early in life, may result in an allergy. Fragments of these proteins, called peptides, can mimic chemicals in the brain called endorphins, so they're often referred to as exorphins. These exporphin peptides have damaging opioid-like effects in the brain, leading to the many symptoms we describe as autism. Researchers at the Autism Research Unit at Sunderland University have found increased levels of these peptides in the blood and urine of children with autism.[66] See www.foodforthebrain.org for a report on all the research linking wheat and milk sensitivity to autism.

What's going on in the gut

To understand how these common foods can be so harmful to sensitive individuals, we need to look at how they get into the body via the gut. Opioid peptides are derived from the incomplete digestion of proteins, particularly food containing gluten and casein. One such peptide, IAG, derived from gluten in wheat, is detected in 80 percent of autistic patients,[67] while another, gliadorphin-7, has been found in very large amounts in 54 percent of autistic children, but only in very small amounts in just 32 percent of non-autistic children.[68] So the first problem is the poor digestion of proteins. Earlier in this chapter we learned how zinc and vitamin B6 can help autistic children, and here it is worth noting that these two nutrients are essential for proper stomach acid production and therefore protein digestion. But even then, these partially digested protein fragments shouldn't enter the bloodstream. So how do they? Vitamin A deficiency is certainly one culprit, but there may be more.

A large proportion of parents with autistic children report that their child received repeated or prolonged courses of antibiotic drugs for ear or other respiratory infections during the first year of life, prior to the diagnosis of autism. Broad spectrum antibiotics kill good as well as bad bacteria in the gut, weakening the intestinal membranes. This can lead to what is known as leaky gut syndrome, in which large molecules that shouldn't be absorbed through the gut membrane do get through.[69] Dr. Andrew Wakefield, in a now controversial study, published in *The Lancet* in February 1998, of 60 autistic children with gastrointestinal symptoms, found much greater incidences of intestinal lesions than in non-autistic children with similar digestive problems. Over 90 percent of autistic children showed clinical evidence of chronic inflammation of the small and large intestine as a result of infection, at levels greater than six times those found in non-autistic children with inflammatory bowel disease.[70]

Despite a concerted effort to discredit Wakefield's research, recent studies are confirming the link between autism, digestive problems, immune system abnormalities, and the MMR vaccine. Wakefield's own research has shown that, in a group of 15 autistic children versus healthy children, there is clear evidence of immune dysfunction.[71] Three studies have shown measles antibodies in the central nervous system, with the potential to damage both brain and gut.[72–74]

So restoring a healthy gut in autistic children is very important. Supplementing digestive enzymes and probiotics is known to produce positive clinical results in autistic children, as these nutrients help heal the digestive tract and restore normal absorption.[75] Improving the healthy balance of bacteria in the digestive tract, which can be helped by taking probiotic supplements, may also help by digesting exorphins in the gut before they can be inappropriately absorbed.[76] The amino acid L-glutamine is especially important in restoring the integrity of the digestive tract. Drinking 5g dissolved in water just before bedtime can help heal the gut.

Cutting out wheat and dairy

Clearly though, removing suspect foods from the diet is key, and there are many anecdotal reports of dramatic improvements from parents who remove casein and gluten from their autistic children's diet.[77] It can take some time for the harmful peptides to be removed from the blood and brain, so results can be slow to emerge. Dr. Robert Cade, professor of medicine and physiology at the University of Florida, has observed that as the levels of peptides in the blood decrease, the symptoms of autism decrease. "If they can be reduced to normal range," he says, "most patients either improve dramatically or become completely normal." (See Figure 32.) But you need to rigidly adhere to a gluten/casein-free diet to accomplish this.[78]

The Autism Research Unit at Sunderland University recommends a gradual withdrawal of foods, waiting three weeks after the removal of casein (dairy) before removing gluten (wheat, oats, barley, rye) from the diet. Keep a food diary and note behaviors and symptoms alongside. This

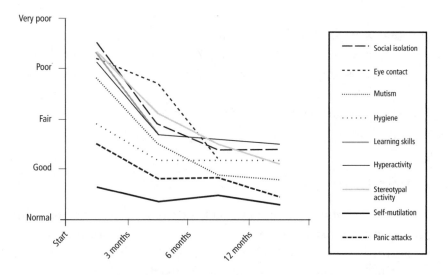

Fig 32. Symptom improvement in 70 autistic children on a gluten/casein-free diet over 12 months

can help to identify other problematic foods, which commonly include citrus fruits, chocolate, artificial food colorings, salicylates, eggs, tomatoes, avocados, aubergine, red peppers, soy, and corn.[79] Because you need to ensure that these foods are replaced rather than just removed, as well as be fully aware of all those foods that contain gluten and/or casein (see below), this is best done under the guidance of a nutritional therapist (see Useful Addresses, page 474).

Grains containing gluten include wheat, oats, barley, and rye. This makes unsuitable most bread, cookies, cakes, pasta, breakfast cereals, bulghur, couscous, pizza, pita bread, wraps, chapattis, naans, egg noodles, pastry, bagels, croissants, noodles, pies, sausages, prepared meals, and processed foods. Check ingredients lists carefully and avoid flour, malted flakes, and wheat starch. Most alternatives are based on rice or corn, and gluten-free breads, pasta, cereals, cookies, crackers, cakes, and bars are now readily available in health food shops and some supermarkets.

> **Casein is in all dairy products**, including cow's milk, butter, cheese, yogurt, ice cream, and milk chocolate. Sometimes goat's or sheep's milk are better tolerated, though a better alternative is to make use of the many soy alternatives now available, including milk, cheese, yogurt and ice cream. If soy is suspected, alternatives made from rice are also now available.

A need to detox

Another way peptides can harm the autistic child involves the liver. This organ's job is to detoxify harmful chemicals and break down hormones and neurotransmitters to avoid excesses, keeping the brain's chemistry in check. Through a process called sulphation, the liver inactivates excessive amounts of many neurotransmitters in the brain that modulate mood and behavior, thereby keeping the brain in balance. Thus any reduction in sulphation can upset the brain. Ninety-five percent of autistic children have low sulphate levels, compared to 15 percent of controls, which can result in the inadequate inactivation of these neurotransmitters. Not only that: reduced sulphation also affects the mucin proteins that line the gastrointestinal tract, increasing gut permeability and inflammatory bowel disease. And this is where peptides, known to be high in autistic children, come in, in their turn reducing sulphate production. It's a vicious circle.

Sulphate production is also dependent on the enzyme sulphite oxidase, levels of which are often low in autistic children, as indicated by high levels of sulphite in their urine. Sulphite oxidase is dependent on adequate levels of the mineral molybdenum, so supplementing this can be helpful. About 20 percent of autistic children respond well to such supplements.[80] Also potentially helpful is a highly usable form of sulphur called MSM (short for methylsulfonylmethane).

Autistic children often have dysbiosis—that is, the presence of undesirable microorganisms in the gut, whether bacteria, yeasts, fungi, or parasites. Treatment with anti-fungal drugs such as Nystatin can produce remarkable improvements, but children often get worse before they get better. This is because fungi such as candida produce all sorts of toxins as they die off. Other less aggressive anti-fungal agents—including caprylic acid from coconut, charcoal, and the yeast *Saccharomyces boulardii*—can be equally effective, causing less severe reactions.

The metallothionein connection

The idea that autistic children have a problem detoxifying led Dr. William Walsh at the Pfeiffer Treatment Center in Naperville, Illinois, to look for differences in trace and toxic elements in autistic versus non-autistic children. He found that autistic children, almost invariably, have a high blood copper/zinc ratio and high levels of copper.[81] This discovery led to the theory that a type of protein called metallothionein could be defective in autistic children, leading to an inability to rid the body of toxic metals such as copper, mercury, cadmium, and so on (see Chapter 11).

Metallothionein is not just needed by the brain and body to filter out such harmful heavy metals; it's also needed for the development of brain cells and the working of synapses, the junctions across which messages move from one neuron to the next. And it acts as a major antiooxidant in both body and brain.

Autistic children may have a genetic defect that leads to less metallothionein, or they could have been exposed to high levels of toxic metals when young. As metallothionein contains zinc, which it releases to latch on to an undesirable element such as copper or mercury, autistic children may also have a zinc deficiency that prevents it from doing its job. In any event, the child ends up overloaded with toxic metals, which are well known to induce many of the symptoms associated with autism.

Of course, as eloquent as this theory sounds, does it work? The answer is a resounding *yes*. By giving autistic children specific nutrients that help detoxify the body and get the metallothionein working properly, the Pfeiffer Treatment Center has reported consistent remarkable recoveries. Some of these cases are reported on www.hriptc.org.

Oxidation in the brain?

Evidence is increasing that children with autism have excessively high oxidation in the brain that may be the root cause of many associated problems.[82] Researchers in the U.S. compared indicators of methylation capacity (levels of methionine, and the ratio of S-adenosylmethionine (SAMe) and S-adenosylhomocysteine (SAH) in 80 autistic and 73 control children. They found that methylation capacity was severely decreased in autistic children compared to controls. The researchers also found that the autistic children had increased vulnerability to oxidative stress.[83] A further two studies show similar results: that autistic children tend to have reduced methylation capacity and higher levels of homocysteine alongside increased oxidative stress.[84–85] A good review of this evidence is available in the reports section of the www.foodforthebrain.org website. We've already discussed many imbalances that would increase the amount of oxidative stress on the brain and nervous system, including pyroluria (see page 292), metallothionein deficiency, a leaky gut, or a simple lack of antioxidant nutrients. All of these need to be considered in a child with autism.

The MMR vaccine debate

The official line is that there's no good evidence of a danger of the MMR vaccine causing autism in children. There's some truth to this, in that Dr. Andrew Wakefield's research at the Royal Free Hospital,[86] while important, is the first hint of a problem and it may be too early to jump to conclusions. Of course, the last thing the medical profession wants is a whole lot of children not being vaccinated, since that increases the risk of epidemics. Here's what Wakefield says: "Although MMR cannot by any means be described as a cause of autism, a child genetically predisposed to asthma, eczema, food allergy or intolerance, perhaps with possible disruption of the gut flora or with a fungal overgrowth, deficient in vitamins, minerals, and essential fatty acids, may be at risk from MMR. For them MMR could be described as the straw that broke the camel's back, tipping the balance of normal childhood development into a retrogressive state."[87] However, despite many attempts to discredit Wakefield, a recent review of all the available evidence on autism and vaccination concludes "there has not been a single credible study that can robustly refute the claims of the parents that their children's acquired autism has been caused by MMR or related measles-containing vaccines, or thimerosal-containing vaccines."[88] A recent study found that in 55 out of 824 children with autism, the parents reported clear signs of regression associated with the MMR vaccine. If correct, this means that 6.7 percent of autistic children, or 1 in 15, are attributed to the MMR vaccine, according to parents.[89]

For most children, the MMR vaccine is unlikely to be a problem, but having said this, no one really knows the full consequences of giving a child three immune attacks—mumps, measles, and rubella—all at the same time. Getting all three illnesses at once simply doesn't occur in nature, so there's a logical argument for single vaccines if a parent so chooses, especially for children with weakened immune systems. Perhaps for these children, with nutrient deficiencies, lacking essential fatty acids, susceptible to food allergies, infections, and/or gut problems, these triple vaccines are the last straw.

So just what is the evidence against MMR? First, studies have shown a high incidence of autism in children whose mothers had received live virus vaccines (particularly the MMR or rubella vaccine) immediately prior to conception, during pregnancy, or immediately following birth.[90] Secondly, there are two classifications of autism: the first where autistic traits are noted from birth and the second where symptoms are noted at 18 months plus. Autism onset at 18 months was uncommon until the mid-1980s, when the MMR vaccine came into wide use. After that the incidence shot up.[91] Thirdly, there is now evidence that measles antibodies can lie in the central nervous system, potentially damaging brain and gut. In fact, many autistic children are found to have measles antibodies in the gut. It's a bit like having a chronic infection. It seems that this triple vaccine makes measles persist. The antidote for measles is vitamin A. This is one of the most important infection fighters for this virus.

Some have proposed that the problem may not be the vaccine itself, but a preservative used in multidose vials of many childhood vaccines until very recently. Thimerosal, a preservative containing high levels of mercury, was used in many vaccines up until 2001. Before this, each vaccine injection exposed the child to levels of toxic mercury in excess of the U.S. federal government's own safety guidelines, and a child receiving all their jabs could have received a total of 187.5 mcg of mercury—enough to give them heavy metal poisoning.[92] Mercury is known to inhibit the enzyme that digests gluten and casein, possibly increasing a child's susceptibility to wheat and milk allergy.

Although it is too early to conclude, it is entirely possible that late-onset autism may be triggered by multiple vaccinations, allergies, toxic overload, or nutritional deficiencies, and especially combinations of any of these that send a child's gut and brain into distress.

Tackling autism naturally

The optimum nutrition approach to autism involves healing the digestive tract, avoiding sources of casein and gluten plus any other identified allergens, eating healthy foods and supplementing nutrients that help support digestion, absorption, liver detoxification, the immune system, and the brain.

This approach, although hard work, is much more effective than conventional drugs. One survey of 8,700 parents, asked to rate the effectiveness of drugs and other interventions, reported that Ritalin was the most commonly prescribed. Only 26 percent of the parents reported an improvement, while 46 percent said their child got worse on Ritalin. The most efficient drug in this survey, Nystatin, which is an anti-fungal drug, still only helped 49 percent of children taking it, according to their parents.[93] Worth considering is secretin. This is a human digestive enzyme, patented as a drug, that seems to trigger improvements in brain function in many autistic children. See www.autism.com/ari for details on this approach.

With this optimum nutrition approach tremendous improvements can result, as the case of Habbo illustrates:

Habbo was diagnosed as autistic at the age of four. He had serious speech and language problems, was severely behind in social and emotional development, and attended special education for children with developmental delay. He had shown some improvement with the use of special multivitamins, minerals, and DMG (dimethyl glycine) prior to visiting the clinic, attached to the European Laboratory of Nutrients. He was then given comprehensive biochemical testing for deficiencies and imbalances. The clinic found low levels of five vitamins (A, beta carotene, B3, B5, and biotin) and three minerals (magnesium, zinc, and selenium). He also had low levels of omega-3 fats and GLA, an omega-6 fat, and the amino acids taurine and carnitine. His digestion was poor, he had abnormal gut flora and indications of a yeast infection. Food allergy testing showed clear sensitivity to milk products and some other foods.

He was given a special diet free from milk and casein, a personalized supplement program, and later some Nystatin, which is an anti-fungal drug. He also started a program of Applied Behavior Analysis, working with a therapist.

He improved steadily and was able to attend his local primary school from the age of six.

According to the Autism Research Institute's evaluation list, his improvements were:

Speech/language	from 36–89%
Sociability	from 13–68%
Sensory/cognitive awareness	from 22–97%
Health/physical behavior	from 64–96%

(Where 100% means non-autistic behavior)

At the time of his fifth birthday, Habbo had absolutely no interest in presents or visitors. One year after the evaluation, just before his eighth birthday, he made a list of eight presents he would like to have, including a computer. His parents told him the evening before to wake them at 7.30am on his birthday, and that's exactly what he did. During the day he couldn't wait for his friends to arrive and celebrate the special day.

(Case kindly supplied by Emar Vogelaar from the European Laboratory of Nutrients in the Netherlands.)

SUMMARY

Given the promising research on the many factors discussed in this part of the book so far, the following nutritional strategy, in addition to the recommendations at the ends of Chapters 27 and 28, is a very real alternative to drug-based approaches:

- Eliminate wheat and dairy from the diet completely, replacing with now readily available alternatives, while also checking the possibility of other food sensitivities under the guidance of a nutritional practitioner.

- Supplement cod liver oil, vitamin B6, magnesium, zinc, vitamin C, molybdenum, L-glutamine (before bed), and high-strength probiotics (minimum 4 billion microorganisms) daily.

- Check for pyroluria and if present, ensure the supplement regime includes zinc and vitamin B6.

- When considering the MMR vaccination, if your child has a weak immune system or you suspect nutrient deficiencies, low essential fatty acids, susceptibility to food allergies, infections, and/or gut problems, consider giving them single vaccines if they are available. Alternatively, address all of these issues with a nutritional therapist prior to their receiving the triple vaccine.

As the recommended amounts of the supplements listed above depend on the age of your child, it is certainly best to see a nutritional therapist who can work out your child's ideal nutritional strategy.

CHAPTER 30

The way up from Down's syndrome

Many of the prenatal tests offered to pregnant women are investigating whether the baby has Down's syndrome. The condition causes so much concern in prospective parents that, in the U.K., at least 90 percent of pregnancies with a Down's baby are terminated.

The typical description of the syndrome makes bleak reading. Though many people born with Down's live for 40–60 years, that is still at least 15 years short of the U.K. average of about 75. About 4 in 10 will have heart problems, and half of them will require surgery. Thyroid problems are also common. They have developmental delays in walking, saying their first words, and so forth, and they have learning disabilities. On top of that they have an increased risk of Alzheimer's disease, starting as early as the age of 30. They often have difficulties in seeing and hearing. They also have a number of minor problems including dry skin, and more coughs and colds.

A person with Down's syndrome is born with 47 chromosomes instead of the normal 46. Chromosomes carry the genetic information that makes us who we are. In most people, 23 of them come from each parent. People with Down's have an extra 21st chromosome (or part of it) from either parent. Each chromosome contains the information to make a particular set of proteins. The extra chromosome leads to the overproduction of the proteins coded for on chromosome 21. The syndrome is clearly genetic. But just because a condition has its roots in genetics does not mean the condition cannot be treated by changing the chemical environment in which the genes bathe. In the vast majority of cases, something can be done to prevent, stop, or even reverse a genetic disorder by changing the environment in which the gene operates. This means finding out what is optimum nutrition for the condition: there is a way up from Down's.

Megavitamin therapy

Treating Down's through nutrition all began with Dr. Henry Turkel's pioneering work in Michigan in the 1930s, using treatments including large amounts of antioxidants (to protect against damage caused by highly reactive oxidants—see Chapter 9), enzymes, and other nutrients. By the 1960s he was getting remarkable results with severely retarded children, as the case of Wendy testifies.

> Wendy was four years old but her mental age was 21 months. She achieved an IQ of 44 and was classified as retarded. When she began megavitamin therapy her attention span went from 10 seconds to 15 seconds to 10 minutes. Within three months she began speaking in complete sentences. After six months of treatment her IQ score had jumped to 72. By the age of 8 her IQ score was 85, classifying her as no longer retarded, with low-average ability—a 40-point shift in 4 years.[94]

Wendy's remarkable transformation, which led to her no longer being classified as educationally subnormal, was verified by an independent psychologist. When researcher Dr. Ruth Harrell heard of Turkel's amazing results, she decided to explore the ideas that many learning-disabled children might have been born with increased needs for certain vitamins and minerals. In her first study she took 22 children with learning disabilities and divided them into two groups. One received vitamin and mineral supplements, while the other received placebos. After four months, the IQ in the group taking the supplements had increased by between 5 and 9.6 points, while those on placebos showed no change. For the next four months, both groups of children were given the supplements and the average improvement rose to 10.2 points. Of those children with Down's taking the supplements, three of the four gained between 10 and 25 units in IQ and also underwent positive facial and skeletal changes![95]

The results seemed too good to be true. After all, Down's syndrome is a genetic disease, so how could vitamin supplements increase the intelligence of six of the children so dramatically? This sort of improvement in intelligence would put most of our educationally subnormal children back in mainstream education! These findings have since been confirmed by three researchers—and contradicted by three more.[96]

Why the apparent contradiction? Researcher Dr. Alex Schauss believes he may have found the confounding variable: it appears that only those children taking thyroid treatment, commonly needed by those with Down's, plus the supplements, improved. Neither supplements nor thyroid treatment on their own are expected to help improve intelligence in children with Down's syndrome. Also, you need the right kind of supplements, and this is likely to vary from child to child.

Pinning down the right nutrients

The Trisomy 21 Research Foundation was founded to do just that— research and identify what optimum nutrition was for Down's. (Trisomy 21 is another name for Down's syndrome.) Their approach does not involve large quantities of individual nutrients but rather targets nutrients to deal with the particular biochemical difficulties that people with Down's have.

A popular misconception is that Down's babies are born with abnormal brains. However, at birth their brain appears to be normal. Within the first four–six months most of the damage that might be done to the brain is done. Nutritional therapy can help prevent the damage. Much is now known about what the effect of the extra chromosome is. One of the biggest problems is that it leads to the overproduction of a key enzyme known as superoxide dismutase (SOD).

SOD is a critical part of a chain of enzyme reactions that protects us from oxidants, so extra SOD may seem an advantage. But it isn't, because it's only part of the oxidant hit squad. Its role is to produce hydrogen peroxide (H_2O_2), a dangerous substance that is usually then disarmed by the next two enzymes in the pathway. However, these two enzymes are not found on chromosome 21. So only part of the hydrogen peroxide produced in Down's people is disarmed. The rest begins to damage the brain and body.

It now appears that the extent of that damage can be reduced by an optimal intake of nutrients that help to disarm the hydrogen peroxide and boost the body's antioxidant defenses. There are a number of nutrients that will assist, including the protective antioxidants of vitamins C and E, lipoic acid, selenium, and bioflavanoids. Essential fats are also important since these are destroyed by oxidation.

Problems with SAMe and tryptophan

Another problem caused by Down's is the disruption of a key brain chemical pathway involving the amino acid s-adenosyl methionine (SAMe). This causes a number of biochemical problems, including the conversion of folic acid, which is vital to brain and nerve function, into an unusable form. This difficulty can be minimized by providing extra folic acid and vitamins B6 and B12. One investigation showed that it is possible to correct SAMe-related problems in Down's cells in a test tube by using chemical variants of folic acid and vitamin B12.[97] Many parents have reported improvements after supplementation with methyl donors (DMAE, choline, DMG, and TMG) and methylation catalysts (folic acid, B6, and B12). SAMe itself has also been used to treat children with attention-deficit disorders, as has MSM, a highly absorbable form of sulphur, which is an essential mineral the body uses to make SAMe. These are explained in Chapter 7.

Down's people also suffer from the overproduction of collagen, disruptions of their hormones, deficiency in key growth factors, accumulation of toxic ammonia, and deficiency in the amino acid tryptophan (needed for the production of the key neurotransmitter serotonin). These problems are addressed by a large variety of nutrients in the NuTriVene formula recommended by the Trisomy 21 Research Foundation, which contains not only vitamins and minerals but also specific amino acids and some other nutrients.

Dr. Lawrence Leichtman, a geneticist and pediatrician, is a founder member of the American College of Medical Genetics and a member of the Scientific Advisory Committee of the Trisomy 21 Research Foundation. To date, he has treated over 700 patients at his Genetics and Disabilities Diagnostic Care Center in Virginia Beach, Virginia. In a trial observing Down's children for 3 years, 113 of whom (aged 1 month to 12 years) were using the NuTriVene-D formula, and 32 of whom (aged 4 months to 12 years) were on multivitamins, both groups showed benefit, but those on NuTriVene-D had the best improvements. Their growth rate went up. They had fewer infections and their white blood cell counts and levels of immunogloblin A, which are an indication of immune strength, improved. There were also clear improvements in speech, coordination, and learning abilities.[98] Madison, daughter of Dixie Lawrence, who directs an adoption agency in Louisiana, is a case in point.

> Madison was given the TNI formula [a specific supplement program] and, at around 33 months old, was started on piracetam with choline and vitamin B5. Five days later she potty-trained herself. On the fifth or sixth day she started saying the odd word and this soon developed into brief sentences. She developed an imagination, unheard of in Down's children of that age. She plays ball with a strong and accurate arm.

To date, the results are promising, but proper double-blind trials testing this formula have yet to be carried out. One such trial, giving 19 children large amounts of vitamins and minerals over three months, did not find any benefit.[99]

Piracetam and choline

Piracetam is not part of the NuTriVene-D formula, but many parents give their Down's children both, sometimes together with choline. Piracetam is an intelligence booster and general stimulant (see Chapter 38). Its effects and safety are so impressive that it prompted the creation of a new category of pharmaceuticals called nootropics, designed to boost intelligence.

There has been considerable media interest, not all positive, in the use of piracetam in Down's children in the U.S. One double-blind study giving Down's children piracetam or a placebo, carried out by Nancy Lobaugh and colleagues of Sunnybook and Women's College Health Center of the University of Toronto, claimed that piracetam therapy did not enhance cognition or behavior but was associated with adverse effects.[100]

The study has, however, been criticized, not for its design but for the interpretation of the results. Dr. Stephen Black of Bishop's University, Quebec, states that a number of positive effects were overlooked. Of 72 outcomes measured, including attention, memory perceptual abilities, executive function, and fine motor skills, 46 produced results that were better in those on piracetam compared with those on the placebo. Eleven out of 18 parents reported that they had noticed cognitive improvement in children taking piracetam, compared to 2 out of 18 parents of children taking the placebo, despite being unaware whether their child had been on piracetam when they made their comment. Teachers also reported that children had significantly "fewer total problems" when taking piracetam. The well-publicized negative effects were apparently spontaneous comments by the parents rather than questionnaire responses. Black suggests that there has been bias in the reporting of the study, and concluded, "A more justifiable conclusion would have been that while dramatic effects were not observed, and there were adverse effects with certain children, small gains in cognition and behavior were also evident."[101]

Getting help with optimum nutrition

There are currently two multinutrient supplements specifically designed for those with Down's on the market: NuTriVene-D (see Product and Supplement Directory, page 486) and MSB Plus Version 4. Both products are very similar, differing mainly in dosage size. They include a daily supplement, a daily enzyme, and a nighttime formula. The daily supplement consists of vitamins, minerals, amino acids and other essential nutrients. The digestive enzyme compensates for deficiencies in Down's children and their associated malabsorption problems. The nighttime formula is designed to provide essential nutrients for increased growth (nighttime is the main period of growth for a child) and to ease common sleep disorders found in Down's children. It is also possible to have a custom-made version based on blood and urine analysis of the patient.

Any supplement program for the treatment of Down's must be undertaken with professional guidance, monitoring, and support, and must be followed alongside a healthy diet. Do not compile your own program using over-the-counter vitamin and mineral supplements because certain nutrients can accelerate the degeneration process and these are often included in general multivitamin and mineral supplements. To find help in the U.S., contact the Trisomy 21 Research Foundation (see Useful Addresses, page 474).

SUMMARY

In summary, the aim of optimum nutrition is to give a person with Down's syndrome the best possible biochemical support, given their genetic uniqueness. This needs to be done with professional guidance. As one mystic says, Down's syndrome children are those who have given so much, who have served so completely in a previous life, that they come back in this life to be looked after. Who knows if this is true, but like the rest of us, they too deserve optimum nutrition.

Diet, crime, and delinquency

Anne was notorious for her anti-authoritarian attitudes and violence. She had lived in foster care since the age of 10, and had a history of assault and burglary, and bouts of severe depression and solvent abuse. Analyses showed abnormal glucose tolerance, and zinc, magnesium, and B-vitamin deficiencies. Her energy level was very low in the morning and she'd often have drops in energy during the day, leaving her depressed and edgy. Within three weeks on a low-sugar diet plus supplements, she had freed herself of drugs, was no longer depressed, had improved energy, and described how she had never felt so relaxed.

Crime and incidences of violent behavior are going up all over the world. Why? Could changes in diet be playing a part? When someone commits a crime what do you do? Punish them, remove them from society to prevent further crime, or try to understand the causes of deviant behavior in order to socially rehabilitate the offender? In the world of rehabilitation, one factor that is almost completely overlooked is nutrition.

Bernard Gesch came across Anne's case in the course of his work. A former probation officer, he is now director of the U.K.-based non-profit group Natural Justice, which investigates the root causes of crime. Gesch

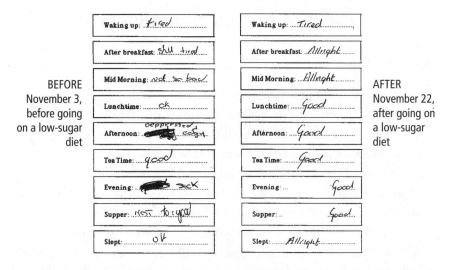

Fig 33. Handwriting and mood: before and after sugar. Reproduced with the kind permission of Natural Justice

believes that the criminal justice system falsely places all the emphasis on social issues, ignoring physical factors such as nutrition. "There are many chemicals around us that are known to affect behavior. Our environment is increasingly polluted. Our food supply has fundamentally changed. In the same way that we don't notice aging, how would we notice the effects of gradual changes to our diet and environment?" Yet the effects are there.

The fact is that all thoughts and consequently behavior are processed through the brain and nervous system, which are totally dependent on nutrition. Approximately half of all the glucose in the blood goes to power the brain, which is also dependent on a second-by-second supply of micronutrients—vitamins, minerals, and essential fatty acids. Antinutrients such as lead and cadmium fundamentally affect brain function. "What we're trying to do," says Gesch, "is introduce something new into the criminal justice system: that is, the existence of the human brain." His research, and that of others, has identified biochemical factors that influence behavior: exposure to neurotoxins, nutrient deficiencies, paradoxical reactions to given substances, and reactive hypoglycemia.

What's behind the crimes?

Sugar blues

In a remarkable pilot project known as SCASO (South Cumbria Alternative Sentencing Options), young offenders were required, as part of their sentence, to undergo nutritional rehabilitation. The participants underwent a series of tests for vitamin and mineral levels, toxic minerals, and blood-sugar balance, as well as dietary assessment. "The most common problems were glucose intolerance and zinc deficiency. Every single person we tested had abnormal glucose tolerance on a five-hour glucose tolerance test," says Gesch.[102] The importance of glucose control in relation to behavior is a consistent finding in the criminal population. In Finland Dr. Matti Virkkunen investigated 69 habitual offenders for glucose balance. Every single one had reactive hypoglycemia. A later study confirmed higher insulin activity during glucose tolerance tests among habitually violent offenders.[103]

In the U.S., Professor Stephen Schoenthaler at California State University has reported a 21 percent reduction in antisocial behavior, a 25 percent reduction in assaults, a 75 percent reduction in the use of restraints, and a 100 percent reduction in suicides when 3,000 inmates were placed on an experimental diet which reduced refined and sugary foods.[104] These results were confirmed in a double-blind study involving 1,382 detained juvenile offenders placed on a reduced sugar diet. There was a 44 percent reduction in antisocial behavior with most significant reductions among the serious offenders.[105]

A rebound low, otherwise known as reactive hypoglycemia, occurring after a rapid increase in blood-sugar levels from consuming sugar, sweets, or stimulants, is associated with extreme fatigue, depression, aggression, and attempted suicide. In other words, if you feel bad you're much more likely to behave badly. According to Gesch, "Of the forty to fifty people we worked with on SCASO we could create an effect within a week or two." His team taught the young offenders how to prepare simple and nutritious meals and develop an interest in food.

Heavy metals

One of the most insidious effects on behavior is that of unseen pollution. A worldwide consensus of research has shown that high lead levels correspond to low intellectual performance and antisocial behavior. The correlation between high lead and increased antisocial or delinquent behavior was found in an observational study of 1,000 children by R. Freeman and co-workers in New South Wales,[106] by Herbert Needleman and co-workers in the U.S. who found antisocial behavior correlated to high dentine lead levels in 2,146 children,[107] and by G. Thomson and colleagues at the University of Edinburgh education department, who found deviant behavior correlated with high blood lead levels.[108] Professor Richard Pihl from the Department of Psychology, McGill University in Montreal, Canada, found a correlation between high hair lead and cadmium in violent inmates compared to non-violent inmates.[109] Other researchers have confirmed an association between high lead and cadmium and deviant behavior.

The level of neurotoxins like lead, cadmium, copper, and mercury needed to produce an effect on behavior is around 1 percent of the level needed to produce physical symptoms. This indicates how sensitive that part of the brain involved with socialization is to environmental and nutritional changes.

Nutritional deficiencies

Zinc is an antagonist of heavy metals, and supplementing it has had favorable effects on behavior. Dr. Alex Schauss found significantly higher levels of lead, cadmium, and copper in violent, antisocial adults compared to non-offenders.[110] The effect of zinc on brain function is consistent with previous studies that have linked zinc deficiency to hyperactivity and learning and eating disorders.

Needless to say, nutritional deficiency is rife among young offenders. In the course of his well-known work with offenders, Professor Stephen Schoenthaler has found evidence of widespread folic acid, thiamine (vitamin B1), and vitamin C deficiencies. Even adding orange juice, which contains each of these nutrients, to the diets of detainees produced a staggering 47 percent reduction in antisocial behavior among juvenile offenders.[111]

Deficiencies in calcium, magnesium, zinc, selenium, and essential fatty acids have also been shown to correlate with increases in violence. The simple addition of a multivitamin and mineral supplement containing RDA levels of nutrients has been shown to have extremely positive effects on behavior in prison populations in the U.S., according to extensive research by Schoenthaler. In a recent study he compared the behavior of young offenders in the three months prior to and during supplementation, to those given a placebo, and showed an overall reduction in recorded offenses of 40 percent, with the subjects on supplements producing 22 percent fewer assaults on staff and a 21 percent reduction in violent and non-violent anti-social behavior when compared with the subjects on the placebo. Blood tests for vitamins and minerals showed that around one-third of the juveniles had low levels of one or more vitamins and minerals before the trial. Those whose levels had become normal by the end of the study demonstrated a massive improvement in behavior of between 70 and 90 percent.[112]

Recently, deficiencies in essential fats have started to be considered a real contributor to deviant behavior. Changes in modern diets have certainly reduced our intake of these essential fats and, if deficient during pregnancy, could have long-lasting effects on mental development and behavior (see Chapter 4). Recent research from Dr. Tomohito Hamazaki of Toyama University in Japan suggests that omega-3 fats help control anger and hostility. He reasoned that, under conditions of stress, from an evolutionary point of view, a certain level of aggression could have survival value, but too much aggression would have the opposite effect.

So, he decided to see what would happen to students, under the stress of exams, if given omega-3 fats, specifically 1.5 grams of DHA, or a placebo. He measured hostility at the start of the study and again, three months later, just before the exams. He measured hostility by showing the participants potentially emotionally charged cartoons, with speech bubbles for the characters. The students then filled in the bubbles. The second measure, just before the exams, showed a big increase, a 59 percent jump in hostile reactions, in those taking the placebo but no change at all in the students taking the omega-3 fats![113] Omega-3 fats, it seems, help you to keep your head when all about you are losing theirs.

Antisocial foods

The fourth factor proving to be significant is that of paradoxical reactions to foods. I. C. Menzies found that, in a study of 25 children with tension fatigue syndrome, all had disturbed sleep, 84 percent had abnormal EEG (brain wave patterns) and 72 percent had digestive problems. All consumed a diet unusually high in refined foods and chemical additives.[114]

Severe allergic reactions can produce Jekyll and Hyde changes in behavior, as has been well reported in hyperactive children with chemical or food intolerances[115] and juvenile offenders.[116] The same can be true for adults, as illustrated by this extraordinary case report by Dr. Alex Schauss.

A president of a large American company, with no previous history of arrest, goes for a drink at his local bar. For some reason he decides to have a glass of red wine, a drink he's never had before. Ten minutes later he pulls out a revolver and guns down a man walking past him. He shoots anyone trying to help this man and ends up injuring 22 people. Miraculously, none are killed, but many have serious wounds to their thighs, arms and torsos. A few hours later, in the local police station, he asks for a psychiatrist. When the psychiatrist arrives, the man asks: "Why am I here?"

Fortunately this man was able to afford the best psychiatrist, neurologists, and doctors. But none could find out what triggered this atrocious action. He could not even remember committing the crime, and was deeply horrified at having done so. Tests eventually showed he had a very imbalanced immune system and the common allergic symptoms of rhinitis and headaches.

The businessman was then tested for two months (by injection, sublingual drops, and ingestion) for sensitivity to various substances, including red wine—the likely offender. But, without anyone else's knowledge, he was simply being given placebos—non-reactive dummy substances. Then, again without anyone else's knowledge, he was given exactly the same wine he had drunk that fateful evening. Within 10 minutes he became increasingly violent and aggressive, grabbing the nurse present and tearing things apart in the laboratory. He was literally going through a Jekyll-and-Hyde like metamorphosis: the psychiatrists present classified him as acutely paranoid schizophrenic.

Twelve years before this incident, the man had moved to a very expensive block of flats in which a type of natural gas was used for heating and cooking. In the following years, most people left their apartments because of the health-damaging effects of the gas, even though they had no chance of getting their money back. Birds had been known to die because of exposure to the gas. This man had spent seven years in the flat. It is likely the gas considerably weakened his immune system, contributing to his aggressive reaction, which was probably to an amine in the wine.

Of the few studies so far conducted, all show dramatic reductions in recidivism rates among offenders maintained on low-sugar, high-nutrient diets. Although much harder to identify (and eliminate), it is certainly possible that the introduction of 3,500 new chemicals into the food supply could be contributing to deviant behavior. Suspect foods include wheat and milk, overconsumption of which has been reported in delinquent behavior.

According to Gesch, whose SCASO project encouraged whole foods and no refined sugar, "Seventy-five percent of our referrals were for violent offenses, many of whom were multiple offenders. Of those kept on the combined social and nutritional regime, none re-offended with a violent offense by the end of the 18-month pilot study."[117] The nutritional supplements used in the treament only cost between $6.49 and $16.23 a month, compared to the average cost of over $3,246.00 a month to keep someone in prison.

Crime: nourishment or punishment?

Of course, many offenders are suffering from undiagnosed or untreated mental illness such as manic depression or schizophrenia. Any of the most common biochemical imbalances (see Chapter 21), including pyroluria, neurotransmitter imbalances, and hormonal imbalances, can lead to aggressive and delinquent behavior.

One of the most promising treatments is the role of tryptophan in correcting serotonin deficiency, which leads to depression and, in some, aggressive and violent behavior.[118] Antidepressant drugs which block the reuptake of serotonin can also lead to aggressive behavior in some people (see Chapter 22), which shows the importance of this neurotransmitter in relation to antisocial behavior. So many of these biochemical imbalances could be nutritionally treated, if only they were checked for.

However, the focus within the criminal justice system is culpability, not testing for and correcting biochemical imbalances. If behavior is thought of purely as a psychological/social phenomena, then the blame rests on the individual and their relationship with society. Hence the current strategy of punishment, removal from society, and social rehabilitation. If brain function, and all the factors that affect brain function, are put into the equation, then issues around nutrition and environmental pollution have to be considered.

This will necessitate the establishment of diagnostic centers at each prison and hospital. Education is so often the key, and the establishment of prison nutrition clubs to promote awareness of good nutrition among patients, prisoners, and security personnel, backed up by the availability of food charts and literature, would do much to improve the awareness that's currently so sadly lacking. Perhaps even more pressing is the need for a research institute dealing with psychopathic, violent, and antisocial behavior.

After years of fundraising and campaigning, Natural Justice persuaded the Home Office to allow the first U.K. double-blind trial with young offenders in a maximum security prison in Aylesbury, giving them either a multinutrient containing vitamins, minerals, and essential fatty acids, or a placebo. The results, published in the *British Journal of Psychiatry*, showed a staggering 35 percent decrease in acts of aggression after only two weeks.[119] Since prison diets are, if anything, better than those most young offenders eat when not serving time, this shows just how important optimum nutrition is for reducing violent and deviant behavior. When the trial was over and the supplements were stopped, there was a 40 percent increase in offenses in the prison.

CHAPTER 32

Beating addictions

Chris, a heroin addict, was taken off heroin and given prescriptions for methadone, temazepam, diazepam, and Valium, to which he became addicted. He then tried a nutrition-based detox program, which includes a *purification phase* involving large amounts of niacin and other nutrients, plus daily saunas. "It's the easiest detox I've ever done. Having gone through the purification I understand why, after previous detoxes, I was still craving. In the beginning of the sauna program I would get flashbacks, but after two weeks I was feeling full of energy, and happy, which has stayed with me since I finished. I'm keeping on the vitamins. I've closed that chapter of my life without a doubt."

In the words of one of the first pioneers of the optimum nutrition approach, Dr. Roger Williams, "No one who follows good nutrition practice will ever become alcoholic." Addiction, whether it be to alcohol, tranquilizers, cigarettes, or heroin, is less likely to occur in those who are well-nourished, for a number of reasons. First, the use of stimulants, like caffeine, nicotine, or cocaine, is more attractive if you are constantly tired. Secondly, the use of relaxants such as alcohol or tranquilizers is more attractive if you suffer from anxiety. The more your brain chemistry is out of balance, the more out of balance it will become if you expose yourself to potentially addictive substances.

Of course, addiction is not only chemical. Psychological factors, as well as the drug abuse itself, are usually present in those who become addicted. Obviously, such psychological factors that predispose a person to addiction will need to be dealt with alongside nutritional intervention. However, whatever the cause, once a person is addicted, this has chemical and physiological effects. You can't just remove the addictive substance without inducing withdrawal symptoms, sometimes severe enough to cause death.

One in four people are addicted

Addiction affects every one of us. The use of addictive substances, from caffeine in tea and coffee, to alcohol and cigarettes, is part of everyday life for most. Take a look at the table below to get an idea of how many people currently suffer from addictions.

Number of people dependent/addicted (% of U.K. population)

Nicotine	15 million	(25%)
Caffeine	12 million	(20%)
Alcohol	4.6 million	(8%)
Tranquilizers	1.5 million	(2.5%)
Heroin	150,000	(0.25%)
Cocaine	16,000	(0.0003%)

Sources: Ash, Drug Scope, Alcohol Concern, Department of Health

Some of these substances are legal, some illegal. Some are prescribed by your doctor and some are self-prescribed. But all are addictive and harm mind and body to varying degrees.

The classic symptoms of addiction include depression or feelings of doom, nervousness and anxiety, craving for sweets or alcohol, irritability or rages, headaches, weight problems (either way), extreme fatigue or weakness, dizziness or feeling faint, morning nausea, blurred vision, transient muscle aches or joint pain, and insomnia and nightmares. If you have quite a few of these symptoms it may be time to do something about your addictions.

Why addiction?

Is it in the genes?

There is supporting evidence for a genetic factor in some people, predisposing them to addictions. Since the 1990s, evidence has been growing for a genetic link to alcoholism and possibly other addictions. The gene in question, the D2 dopamine-receptor gene, encourages the building of receptor sites for the pleasure-giving neurotransmitter dopamine. Some people have a variation of this gene that means less dopamine receptors, hence less pleasure.[120] These individuals are therefore more prone to lower moods and motivation. As a natural consequence, they then seek activities and substances that promote dopamine activity in the brain. Dr. Kenneth Blum, one of the pioneers in this research, calls this reward deficiency syndrome (see Chapter 28, page 321).

Such people are especially prone to overuse of stimulants (caffeine, nicotine, and cocaine), as well as alcohol. They are also more likely to seek stimulating activities, from daring sports to gambling.

Many addictive types are also histadelic—genetically preprogramed to overproduce high levels of histamine (see also page 250). This makes a person more prone to compulsive and obsessive behavior. Once nutrient-depleted, the high-histamine type often becomes seriously, sometimes suicidally depressed. Alcohol abuse can become a way of slowly killing yourself.

Both of these genetic factors run through families, so a history of addiction, depression, suicide, and mental illness of a compulsive/obsessive nature is a good clue, although, of course, behaviors can be inherited in addition to genes.

Empty calories lead to addiction

Genes are only one side of the equation. They don't determine behavior, just predispose it. By providing optimum nutrition for a person with reward deficiency syndrome or histadelia, their mood, energy, and general well-being can be so substantially improved that compensations using addictive substances no longer become necessary.

One study with mice shows how poor nutrition also predisposes addiction. The mice in this study were split into two groups: one was given a healthy diet, the other a junk food diet. Both had free access to water or alcohol. The junk food mice soon became alcoholic and died prematurely. The health food mice stayed teetotal and lived to a ripe old age.[121]

As the alcoholic mice become more and more nutrient deficient, they became less interested in food, and more interested in alcohol. Alcohol not only stops you absorbing, it also affects appetite. So bad nutrition not only leads to alcoholism, but alcoholism leads to bad nutrition. It's a vicious downhill spiral. The same link between junk food and addiction has also been recorded in humans.[122]

How addiction happens

Before looking at specific types of addiction, and how to break the habit, let's understand more about the chemical nature of addiction itself. Most addictive substances either promote more of a particular neurotransmitter, such as dopamine, or mimic a desirable brain chemical by docking onto its receptor sites.

Caffeine, for example, blocks the breakdown of dopamine and adrenalin, hence elevating circulating levels of these motivating neurotransmitters. Cocaine also blocks the breakdown, giving a more intense dopamine high. Heroin, on the other hand, looks like the brain's own opioids, instantly killing pain and inducing a euphoric state.

The sugar link

Most alcoholics and drug addicts have hypoglycemia. One way of raising your blood-sugar level is to smoke a cigarette, have a coffee, eat chocolate, drink alcohol, or take a drug, from marijuana to cocaine. A group of researchers in 1973 decided to test how many of 200 alcoholics had abnormal blood-sugar balance with a glucose tolerance test. No less than 97 percent came up positive.[123] The same is true for most other addicts.

Many people have learned to control their blood-sugar level by eating, drinking, and smoking substances that alter their body chemistry. There's also a synergy of these pharmacological agents in food and drink. High coffee consumption can precipitate alcoholism, because the shakiness from coffee can be controlled by alcohol. In animal studies, giving animals caffeine increases consumption of alcohol, confirming a complex interaction between these addictive psychoactive substances.[124]

Allergy or addiction?

Addictions have a lot in common with hidden allergies. Often the allergic substance becomes addictive, and if it isn't consumed, withdrawal symptoms set in, which can be relieved by consuming the allergen. This is why people often feel worse on a short fast, until the withdrawal phase is over, and then feel much better.

Allergy expert Dr. James Braly believes that people suffering from IgG hidden food allergies (see Chapter 12) are also prone to food addiction; that is, they are likely to become addicted to the very same foods that are causing the allergic reaction. Braly also believes that in turn, food addictions induced by food allergies play a key role in a predisposition to, and perpetuation of, alcohol and drug abuse.

This is because when alcoholics stop drinking, their brain chemistry is still imbalanced, and the cravings and other abstinence symptoms soon lead them elsewhere for a fix. "Two substitutes commonly seen at Alcoholics Anonymous meetings are pastries and coffee laced with sugar," explains Braly. "In order to reduce the risk of abusing alcohol and drugs, and to become sober and remain sober, a person must successfully address the problem of food allergy-induced food addiction as well."

It can, of course, also work the other way—recovering food addicts may turn to alcohol to help temporarily relieve the abstinence symptoms of food addiction. Braly and I both recommend alcohol abstinence when you're coming off a food allergen, not only because withdrawal often increases cravings for alcohol, but also because alcohol damages the gut, making it more leaky which, in turn, increases your allergic potential.

Mirroring the tendency to become addicted to food allergens, many people who regularly consume alcohol also become allergic to it, or to something in it. For example, many beer drinkers become allergic to brewer's yeast. Drs. William Philpott and Dwight Kalita found that 75 percent of tobacco smokers tested allergic to tobacco on skin tests.[125] I tested this when working in a medical allergy treatment center and failed to find a single smoker who wasn't allergic to tobacco on intradermal testing. This is why, with regular consumption, people often find they don't feel so good after alcohol, cigarettes, marijuana or whatever has become their drug of choice. Most allergies require a 5- to 10-day avoidance before a person becomes symptom-free. A similar length of time is often required for addictions.

Alcohol: the greatest anti-nutrient of them all

There are costs and benefits attributable to the drinks and leisure industries. On the one hand this sector of business employs over a million people and, in 2005, generated almost $22.72 billion in revenue for the government. On the other hand it has been estimated that 60 percent of suicides, 30 percent of divorces, 40 percent of domestic violence, and 20 percent of child abuse cases are associated with alcohol misuse.[126]

Pronounced nutritional deficiency states are well recorded in many drug addictions, but none so obviously as in addiction to alcohol. Alcohol is the greatest anti-nutrient of all. It is well proven to deplete almost every vitamin (vitamins A, B1, B2, B6, folic acid, B12, C, D, and E), mineral (calcium, magnesium, potassium, zinc, and selenium), amino acid (tryptophan, taurine, glutathione, etc.), essential fat (omega-3 and 6), as well as disturbing blood-sugar control.[127] Just reading the mountains of research on how alcohol destroys nutrients in the body is sobering!

Many of the symptoms and problems of alcohol abuse arise directly from these nutritional deficiencies. For example, tryptophan depletion leads to depression, while B-vitamin deficiencies make you anxious, unable to concentrate, and even crazy. B6 deficiency may account for some of the perceptual distortions that occur in both alcohol intoxication and withdrawal.

Even without alcohol these deficiencies can bring on mental illness, as illustrated by the story of one 61-year-old woman from New Zealand, diagnosed with schizophrenia.[128] She refused medication for four months, had the delusion she was dying from cancer, and neglected her nutrition. She was admitted to hospital and went into a coma. She was then given thiamine (vitamin B1), and responded in three hours.

As well as inducing deficiencies, alcohol reduces appetite and impairs absorption. When there is organic damage such as pancreatitis, cirrhosis, or hepatitis, appetite is further impaired, creating even more deficiencies. So, the first step in treating addiction is to prepare the person for withdrawal by correcting these deficiencies. Giving all essential nutrients in optimal amounts dramatically reduces craving for alcohol. In animal studies, rats given vitamin B1 cut their drinking by a staggering 80 percent.[129] Those given the amino acid glutamine cut their drinking by 34 percent.[130] The amino acid taurine, at 3g a day, reduces withdrawal symptoms.[131] There are also many nutrients that protect the liver from damage from alcohol. These include taurine, choline, glutamine, glutathione, and many others.

How to quit

Coming off booze without side effects

It is no surprise to find that a number of researchers report that megadoses of a cocktail of nutrients, given orally as supplements or intravenously, can virtually eliminate symptoms of withdrawal. Even the basics—that's a whole-food diet plus a multivitamin—kept 81 percent of alcoholics off booze six months after withdrawal, compared to 38 percent left to their own devices.[132]

Large amounts of specific nutrients can help. In 1974 Dr. Russel Smith in the U.S. gave 507 hard-core alcoholics 3–5g of niacin/vitamin C a day for a year.[133] At the end of the year 71 percent were sober. Drs. Abram Hoffer and Humphrey Osmond have reported on the combined use of niacin, B6 and vitamin C.[134] They reported a 75 percent success rate after a year, compared to 30 percent success from counseling alone.

However, the best results are achieved by providing high amounts of all the key nutrients, especially B vitamins, vitamin C, glutamine, taurine, tryptophan (although this can be difficult to access—see page 152), and essential fats. The extraordinary and sad fact is that most alcohol recovery units don't do this, so people both have to go through the agony of withdrawal without optimal nutrition support, and have a much greater chance of going back on the booze. For an up-to-date list of addiction treatment centers, I recommend viewing www.mentalhealthproject.com.

Heroin withdrawal made easier

Drs. Alfred Libby and Irwin Stone pioneered a detoxifying treatment for drug addicts using megadoses of vitamin C.[135] In one study involving 30 heroin addicts, they gave 30–85g a day and achieved a 100 percent success rate. Others have reported similar positive results using vitamin C combined with niacin.

Both heroin addiction and alcoholism increase acid levels in the body, causing a depletion of calcium and potassium. In 1973 Dr. Blackman decided to test what would happen if he neutralized this acidity. He gave 19 heroin addicts sodium bicarbonate, potassium bicarbonate, and calcium carbonate every half hour for two hours, followed by a two-hour break, repeating the cycle until withdrawal was over. All volunteers said the withdrawal symptoms were either completely eliminated or considerably reduced. Sixteen out of 19 reported no severe withdrawal symptoms. Of the others, symptoms lasted for no more than four hours. This research, however, has not been published, or followed up, so it remains speculative.

Once again, giving heroin addicts high levels of a cocktail of vitamins, minerals, amino acids and essential fats can dramatically reduce symptoms of withdrawal and increase chances of staying clean.

Quitting cigarettes

One of the most common and socially acceptable addictions is to nicotine in tobacco. The same principles apply here as with other addictions. An alkaline diet, with plenty of fruit and vegetables, or the use of alkaline salts certainly helps reduce craving, as do megadoses of vitamin C and niacin, among other nutrients. Most smokers are hypoglycemic, so a diet with complex carbohydrates, and no sugar, tea, and coffee is essential. Extra chromium, B6, and zinc also help to stabilize blood sugar. These nutritional factors, plus counseling to deal with the psychological and behavioral factors, plus gradual reduction of nicotine intake, are highly effective for those who wish to quit. Exactly how to do all this is explained in my book *How to Beat Stress and Fatigue* and on the website www.patrickholford.com; just click on "A to Z of Solutions" and you'll find the guidelines under "How to Quit Smoking."

Kicking addiction to prescription drugs

The sad truth is that many prescription drugs used to treat mental health problems are addictive. The most commonly prescribed antidepressant drugs, originally marketed as completely safe happy pills, were originally touted to benefit even those who didn't think they were depressed. Yet recently the U.S. authorities found that when people try to come off these drugs, even with a gradual reduction, at least 2 in every 100 people suffered abnormal dreams or pains resembling electric shocks, and 7 in every

100 experienced dizziness. They are now insisting that these drugs carry a new warning requiring doctors to monitor patients for any side effects that may indicate a physical dependency.

Most concerning of all is tranquilizer addiction. There are an estimated 1.5 million people addicted to tranquilizers in Britain. Coming off them is not only difficult, but without the right support it can be very dangerous, even fatal in some instances. The longer people are on these dangerous drugs the more forgetful, drowsy, and withdrawn they become. If they try to stop, they become anxious and can't sleep. They may experience tremors, tremendous irritability, headaches, even seizures. That's why it's vital to come off tranquilizers gradually, with support, and with the support of natural relaxants such as kava and valerian. The names of good organizations and information on how to do this are found on the website www.patrickholford.com; just click on "A to Z of Solutions" and you'll find it under "How to Quit Tranquillisers."

Are you a stimulant addict?

The most widespread addiction of all is to stimulants—tea, coffee, caffeinated drinks, sugar, chocolate, and cigarettes. To be in tip-top mental health, you need to address this issue too. The odd cup of tea or coffee is no big deal, but if you *need* these substances every day, or every hour, you are in trouble! Any trip through a mental health ward will show you that most people with mental health problems are stimulant addicts. Whether legal or illegal drugs, the see-saw between tranquilizers or alcohol and stimulants keeps your brain out of balance. Chapter 10 explains how to quit stimulants and what to eat and drink instead.

Why withdrawal and detoxification are different

Optimum nutrition during the first week of drug withdrawal can make all the difference, as the studies above have shown. Very large amounts of vitamin C, B vitamins, glutamine, and other amino acids should be given four times a day, under supervision. Calcium and magnesium are especially important because they can virtually eliminate the terrible cramping and nerve pain associated with opiate withdrawal. During this time 24-hour counseling support is essential.

One consistent and yet widely ignored finding is that withdrawal from a drug doesn't mean the person is decontaminated. Most drugs take months to completely leave the system, as residues are stored in body cells. Hence, high-level nutritional support in the months following withdrawal is vital for long-term success, until the addict is truly clean.

One particularly effective method of speeding up drug detoxification is the combined use of niacin, saunas, and water. Niacin helps eliminate toxins from cells. It is best taken 30 minutes before entering a sauna, on an empty stomach. The sauna needs to be set at 80°F. The participant then stays in the sauna for an hour, coming out if need be, while keeping very hydrated by drinking water. Some people experience some level of flashbacks so such an approach needs to be done under supervision. This needs to be done every day until the person feels significantly better, which can take from 5–25 days depending on the former level of intoxication.

Have you quit and still feel like s**t?

All this evidence really illustrates how, whatever might lead a person into addiction, once addicted they will have developed biochemical imbalances in the brain that need correcting. Even once a person has stopped abusing that substance, a number of symptoms may remain, including:

- Drug cravings
- Sugar and carbohydrate cravings
- Salt cravings
- Depression
- Anxiety
- Internal shakiness
- Trembling
- Restlessness
- Impulsivity
- Inability to concentrate

- Lack of energy/fatigue

- Hypersensitivity to noise, pain, and/or stress

- Irritability

- Sleep problems

- Memory problems

- Negative self-talk

- Sense of emptiness.

I believe that it is the presence of these symptoms that lead so many people to go back to their addiction. At Bridging the Gaps, an addiction treatment center in Winchester, Virginia, David and Marlene Miller (authors of the excellent book *Staying Clean and Sober*), working with Dr. James Braly, provide an intensive nutrition-based withdrawal program. Their results are probably the best in the world. With most addiction strategies, 20 percent of patients are reported to be still abstaining after a year. The clients of Bridging the Gaps report 80 percent abstinence after a year.

The reason, very simply, is that adding a nutrition-based approach causes most of the symptoms shown above to disappear, instead of piling up to drive the person back to their addiction. The approach used by the Millers and Dr. Braly, which involves a comprehensive intravenous nutrient mix of vitamins, minerals, and amino acids, given in a daily drip, for the patient's first month, produces results better than those achieved by diet and supplementation only.

Another treatment center that has reported great results, although it doesn't use intravenous nutrients, is the Health Recovery Center in Minneapolis, Minnesota, headed by Joan Matthews Larson, author of *Seven Weeks to Sobriety*.

So some highly successful strategies for dealing with addiction have been tested and proven to work. Sadly, very few addiction treatment centers, and none that I know of in Britain at this time, apply these strategies. Consequently, their success rates are poor. Many ignore the biochemical aspects of addiction and simply involve withdrawal and counseling. A radical rethink on the treatment of addiction is badly needed.

SUMMARY

In summary, if you are dealing with addiction:

- Get professional help and guidance.

- Deal with psychological issues with a psychotherapist.

- Increase your intake of nutrients, including a high-strength B complex plus niacin 500 mg, pantothenic acid (B5) 500 mg, vitamin B6 100 mg, folic acid 1 mg, vitamin C 3–10g a day spread throughout the day.

- Take L-glutamine powder, 5g am and pm, plus enough essential fats including GLA, EPA, and DHA, and minerals including calcium, magnesium, potassium, and zinc.

- Eat an extremely healthy diet that supports your brain (see Part 1).

- Come off your addictive drug slowly, replacing it with natural relaxants/stimulants as appropriate.

CHAPTER 33

Overcoming eating disorders

One of the greatest shortcomings of human logic is the unquestioned belief that psychological problems, whether involving behavior or intelligence, are influenced only by psychological factors, and that physical problems are influenced only by physical factors. This presupposes that mind and body are separate, that the energy of mind and of body are two different things. Ask a chemist, an anatomist, and a psychologist to define where the mind starts and the body ends and they will find that the two are intimately interconnected. The same is especially true of anorexia nervosa and bulimia, because they are behavioral disorders involving eating, a physiological event.

Anorexia—essentially, self-starvation—was first identified by Dr. William Gull in 1874. This is his treatment: "The patient should be fed at regular intervals, and surrounded by persons who could have moral control over them, relations and friends being generally the worst attendants." Today, treatment is often essentially the same, summed up as "drug them, feed them and let them get on with their lives" in an article in the *Guardian* describing treatment in "leading hospitals." The modern approach includes behavior therapy, that is, rewards and privileges, and drugs to induce compliance. The drugs include psychotropic drugs such as chlorpromazine, sedatives, and antidepressants. The diet is high carbohydrate, sometimes as much as 5,000 calories, with little regard to quality.

Bulimia is binge eating followed by self-induced vomiting or laxative use, and is probably a more common condition nowadays—although it may also be the easiest to hide, as bulimics may approach or exceed normal weight. Some anorexics are also bulimic. Some bulimics are not anorexic. It is still a food/weight compulsive/obsessive disorder, characterized by:

- Recurrent episodes of binge eating (rapid consumption of large amounts of food in a discrete period of time).

- A feeling of lack of control over eating behavior during the binges.

- The person regularly engages in self-induced vomiting, use of laxatives, diuretics, strict dieting, fasting, or exercise in order to prevent weight gain.

- A minimum average of two binge-eating sessions a week.

- Persistent overconcern with body shape and weight.

The zinc link

The idea that nutrition, or malnutrition, could play a part in the development and treatment of this condition did not really emerge until the 1980s, when scientists began to realize just how similar the symptoms and risk factors of anorexia and zinc deficiency were (see table on page 368). As early as 1973 two zinc researchers, K. Hambidge and A. Silverman, concluded that "whenever there is appetite loss in children zinc deficiency should be suspected."[136] In 1979, Rita Bakan, a Canadian health researcher, noticed that the symptoms of anorexia and zinc deficiency were similar in a number of respects and proposed that clinical trials be undertaken to test its effectiveness in treatment.[137] Meanwhile, David Horrobin, most renowned for his research into evening primrose oil, proposed that "anorexia nervosa is due to a combined deficiency of zinc and EFAs."[138] More recently, strong evidence has come to light that those with anorexia and bulimia may be more prone to tryptophan deficiency. Tryptophan is the building block for serotonin, the brain's happy neurotransmitter, which also helps control appetite.

Anorexia	Zinc deficiency
Symptoms	
Weight loss	Weight loss
Loss of appetite	Loss of appetite
Amenorrhea	Amenorrhea
Impotence in males	Impotence in males
Nausea	Nausea
Skin lesions	Skin lesions
Malabsorption	Malabsorption
Disperceptions	Disperceptions
Depression	Depression
Anxiety	Anxiety
Risk factors	
Female under 25	Female under 25
Stress	Stress
Puberty	Puberty

Zinc hypothesis confirmed

In 1980, when the zinc link had been reported, the first trial started at the University of Kentucky. The researchers discovered that 10 out of 13 patients admitted with anorexia and 8 out of 14 patients with bulimia were zinc deficient on admission. After vigorous feeding they became even more zinc deficient. Since zinc is required to digest and utilize protein, from which body tissue is made, they recommended that extra zinc, above that required to correct deficiency, should be given as the anorexic starts to eat and gain weight.[139]

There were two important research findings and the first case of an anorexic treated with zinc, which shed light on the importance of zinc. The first study, since confirmed, showed that animals deprived of zinc very rapidly developed anorexic behavior and loss of appetite, and that if these animals were force-fed a zinc-deficient diet to gain weight, they became seriously ill.[140] The second study showed that zinc deficiency damages the intestinal wall and therefore the absorption of nutrients including zinc, potentially leading to a vicious spiral of deficiency.[141]

Then, in 1984, Professor Derek Bryce-Smith, now patron of the Institute for Optimum Nutrition, reported the first case of anorexia treated with zinc. The patient was a 13-year-old girl, tearful and depressed, weighing 37 kg. She was referred to a consultant psychiatrist, but, despite counseling, three months later her weight was 31.5 kg (under 5 stone). Within two months of zinc supplementation at a level of 45 mg per day, her weight returned to 44.5 kg, she was cheerful again, and tests for zinc deficiency were normal.[142]

Meanwhile, the first double-blind trial with 15 anorexics was being carried out at the University of California. In 1987 the researchers reported: "Zinc supplementation was followed by a decrease in depression and anxiety. Our data suggest that individuals with anorexia nervosa may be at risk for zinc deficiency and may respond favorably after zinc supplementation."[143] By 1990, many researchers had found that over half of anorexic patients showed clear biochemical evidence of zinc deficiency.[144] In 1994 Dr. Carl Birmingham and colleagues carried out a double-blind controlled trial giving 100 mg of zinc gluconate or a placebo to 35 women with anorexia. They concluded that "the rate of increase in body mass of the zinc-supplemented group was twice that of the placebo group and this difference was statistically significant."[145] Sadly, many treatment centers still fail to supplement those suffering from anorexia with zinc.

Zinc: the chicken or the egg?

The evidence linking zinc and anorexia is now beyond question. In fact, a recent review of all the research concludes: "There is evidence that suggests zinc deficiency may be intimately involved with anorexia in humans: if not as an initiating cause, then as an accelerating or exacerbating factor that may deepen the pathology of anorexia."[146] The fact that high levels of zinc supplementation help to treat anorexia does not mean the cause of anorexia is zinc deficiency. Psychological issues may, and probably do, bring about change in the eating habits of susceptible people.

By avoiding eating, a young girl can repress the signs of growing up. Menstruation stops, breast size decreases and the body stays small. Starvation induces a kind of high by stimulating changes in important brain chemicals, which may help to block out difficult feelings and issues that are too hard to face. Many anorexics also choose to become vegetarian, and most vegetarian diets are lower in zinc, essential fats, and protein, according to a study at the Health Sciences Department of the British Columbia Institute of Technology in Burnaby, Canada, which analyzed the diets of vegetarian anorexics, versus non-vegetarian patients.[147]

Whether vegetarian or not, once the route of not eating is chosen and becomes established, zinc deficiency is almost inevitable, due to both poor intake and poor absorption. With it comes a further loss of appetite and even more depression, disperceptions, and the inability to cope with the stresses that face many adolescents, especially girls, growing up in the 21st century.

The optimum nutrition approach to help someone with anorexia, or bulimia, is best carried alongside work with a skilled psychotherapist. The nutritional approach emphasizes quality of food rather than quantity, including supplements to ensure vitamin and mineral sufficiency, and of course 45 mg of elemental zinc per day, halving this level once weight gain is achieved and maintained.

Low tryptophan: the appetite controller

Loss of weight and loss of muscle tissue is an indication of protein deficiency. This can be the result of either insufficient intake, or inadequate digestion, absorption, or metabolism. The amino acids valine, isoleucine, and tryptophan have been found to be low in people with anorexia. Supplementing valine and isoleucine helps to build muscle, while tryptophan is the building block of serotonin, a neurotransmitter that controls both mood and appetite.

Recent research has found striking differences in blood levels of tryptophan in anorexic patients.[148] Also, both starvation and excessive exercise have been shown to influence the availability of tryptophan in the blood of anorexic patients.[149] To date, the evidence is pointing towards a problem with how people with eating disorders respond to low tryptophan. In fact, the conversion of tryptophan into serotonin is both zinc- and B6-dependent. These three nutrients may all be needed for proper appetite control, as well as a balanced, happy mood.

The interplay between body and mind, or nutrients and behavior, is well illustrated by recent research at Oxford University's psychiatry department by Dr. Philip Cowen and colleagues which found, not surprisingly, that women on calorie-restricted diets develop lower levels of tryptophan and serotonin. However, recovered bulimics, when put on a diet free of tryptophan, rapidly become more depressed and overly concerned about their weight and shape, as well as more fearful of their loss of control over their eating.[150] In a similar trial that deprived both women with bulimia and healthy controls of tryptophan for one day, the bulimic women became more depressed and had a much greater desire to binge than the controls.[151]

All this research strongly suggests that those prone to anorexia or bulimia have a special need for tryptophan, and probably zinc and B6, and that when deprived of these nutrients they are more likely to develop unhealthy reactions, including loss of appetite control.

While supplementing tryptophan, or 5-hydroxytryptophan (5-HTP), plus zinc and B6, is the most direct way to address these imbalances in people with eating disorders, in the long run the goal must be to change the diet. Often, especially in those with anorexia, supplements, including concentrated fish oils, are more acceptable at first because unlike food they contain virtually no calories. However, as a person's nutrition improves, so their anxieties and compulsiveness become better and they can see the logic for making dietary changes.

The ideal diet should include easily assimilable foods containing good-quality protein such as quinoa, fish, soy, and spirulina or blue-green algae. Other good foods are ground seeds, lentils, beans, plus fruits and vegetables.

Fish and seeds are especially important because they contain essential fats. Since most people with eating disorders go out of their way to avoid fat, their diets are frequently low in these essential nutrients. Also, essential fats are vital for the body to both make serotonin and receive the serotonin signals that cross between one neuron and another.

The optimum nutrition approach, therefore, involves ensuring all these nutrients are provided in optimal amounts.

What's your binge food?

In the case of bulimia, what a person binges on is very revealing, either of food sensitivities or blood-sugar problems. The most common binge foods are sweet foods, wheat foods, or dairy foods. Both wheat and dairy products contain exorphins, chemicals that mimic (and can therefore block) pleasure-giving endorphins in the brain, and again, may influence behavior. Sweetened foods, of course, satisfy a low blood-sugar condition, and the cure is to eat foods that keep your blood-sugar level even. I have often asked people with bulimia to binge as much as they like for the next two weeks, but not on these foods. Often they report that their desire to binge at all is dramatically reduced. Once again, these foods, in certain people, may provoke a change in mood and behavior that sets them off on a slippery slope.

Don't think, however, that if a person is deficient, or has a biochemical uniqueness that makes them more prone to react strongly to the lack of a nutrient like zinc or tryptophan, this excludes psychological problems as part of the cause. Many people with anorexia are the bearers of a secret, a trauma, or a problem that needs to be resolved, and can be with the help and support of a psychotherapist. A good place to start is contacting the National Eating Disorders Association. See Useful Addresses, page 474, for contact details.

SUMMARY

In summary, I recommend the following for anyone who is dealing with an eating disorder:

- See a clinical nutritionist who can assess what you are deficient in and advise you accordingly.

- Their advice will probably be to take 30–50 mg of zinc, 100 mg of B6, 200 mg of 5-HTP, plus essential fats, either in capsules or in seeds and fish.

- See a psychotherapist with experience in helping people with eating disorders to make a full recovery.

CHAPTER 34

Fits, convulsions, and epilepsy

Epilepsy is a mysterious condition, characterized by occasional fits, technically called convulsions. It affects almost half a million people in Britain. The convulsions, which last for seconds or minutes, are thought to be caused by a temporary upset in the brain's chemistry, causing neurons to fire off faster than usual and in bursts.

Convulsions can be brought on by neurological problems such as a brain injury, a stroke, an infection, and less frequently, a tumor. High levels of stress and panic attacks can also trigger a convulsion. So too can heart disease, especially irregular heartbeats, and blood-sugar problems. Whatever the triggers, convulsions indicate that the brain is out of balance. An obvious place to start is to ensure an optimal intake of the brain's best friends—nutrients. The optimum nutrition approach can be highly effective, as Francis's story illustrates.

While teaching classes in Oxford, Francis had a bad car accident. This left him with severe headaches, poor memory and concentration, severe depression, but most of all, epilepsy. So bad was his epilepsy that he complained of what he called "epileptic storms," sometimes daily. During the night he would often have five or six fits, despite being on anti-epilepsy drugs. His memory had so deteriorated he could no longer teach, and being epileptic, he found it hard to get work. Naturally he became depressed.

After years under medical supervision he decided to try some alternatives and was referred to me. He promised to avoid tea, coffee, and sugar and we discussed how to eat a balanced diet, with plenty of fruit, vegetables, and whole grains—the optimum diet.

I wanted to give him every chance to change and included high levels of supplements, including B3, B5, and B6, choline, calcium, zinc, magnesium, and manganese as well as other nutrients. Magnesium and manganese have both been shown to help epilepsy, while B5 and choline have a specific effect on memory.

When he came back after one month, he had made tremendous changes to his diet and had reaped the rewards of his efforts. "I am amazed at how well I feel," he commented, and went on to tell me how he hadn't had a single muscle tremor or panic attack. Three months later, he had still only had one epileptic "storm." His brain is working better, his depression is completely gone, and he can sleep straight through the night, without any fits or muscle tremors. (Case gratefully supplied by Christopher Scarfe.)

Differences in the nutritional status of those with convulsions or epilepsy and those without has been demonstrated by many researchers. The key nutrients that have frequently been shown to be deficient are folic acid, the minerals manganese and magnesium, and essential fats.

Finding what helps

B vitamins

Folic acid, a vitamin that is often low in those with mental health problems, is depleted by convulsions. This suggests that it is somehow involved.[152] Ironically, anticonvulsant drugs such as phenytoin, primidone, and phenobarbital further deplete folic acid. Combining a drug such as phenytoin with folic acid works better than giving the drug alone. In one study, epileptics were given the drug with either folic acid or a placebo and after a year, only those on folic acid reported substantially less fits.[153] However, folic acid could be a double-edged sword. Some uncontrolled studies suggest that folate supplementation may create epileptic fits in a minority of people. Several controlled studies, however, have failed to confirm this observation, suggesting that this effect must be very rare.[154] With the guidance of your doctor, folic acid supplementation is well worth trying, although don't expect immediate results. Also worth supplementing is vitamin B6.

Unlike folic acid, high doses of vitamin B6 can produce almost immediate results. The first research to identify a role for B6 in the treatment of epilepsy in children took place in Japan in the 1980s. More than half the children with infantile spasms responded very well to B6 supplementation, although the doses used were very high and caused side effects in some of them.[155]

In a more recent study at the University of Heidelberg in Germany, 17 children were given high doses of vitamin B6 (300 mg/kg/day orally). Five out of the 17 had immediate relief within two weeks, while after four weeks all patients were more or less free of seizures. No serious adverse reactions were noted. Side effects were mainly gastrointestinal symptoms, and were reversible after reduction of the dosage.[156]

Magnesium, manganese, and zinc

The mineral manganese is completely essential for proper brain function and, to date, four studies have shown a correlation between low levels and the presence of epilepsy, suggesting that as many as one in three children with epilepsy have low manganese levels.[157–159] Supplementing manganese helped to reduce fits. In one study published in the *Journal of the American Medical Association*, one child who was found to have half the normal blood manganese levels didn't respond to any medication, but on supplementing manganese had fewer seizures and improved speech and learning.[160] Dr. Carl Pfeiffer was the first to report the successful treatment of epilepsy with manganese.[161] At the Institute for Optimum Nutrition we have frequently found that patients with convulsions or fits are manganese deficient and have no or fewer fits once supplementation is started.

Magnesium is another mineral well worth checking. Magnesium is also vital for proper nerve and brain function, and, once again, a number of researchers have found low levels in patients with epilepsy and reported fewer fits on supplementation.[162–163] In animals, magnesium injections have also been shown to instantly suppress convulsions.[164]

If a child is found to have low blood levels of magnesium, as many as 75 percent respond, with fewer fits, according to research from

Romania.[165] Supplementing this mineral is especially helpful to those with temporal lobe epilepsy. This is especially useful since people with this type of epilepsy rarely respond to conventional anticonvulsant drugs.[166] It is also possible that pregnant women, deficient in manganese, may be more likely to have children with epilepsy.

It is also well worth testing for zinc. Once again, zinc levels have been found to be lower in children with epilepsy,[167] and anticonvulsant drugs can further deplete this vital mineral. There is also some suggestion that too much copper and not enough zinc may increase the odds of having a seizure.[168] Ideally, we need to take in 10 times more zinc than copper. Zinc is also a valuable ally for vitamin B6, since it helps convert B6 (pyridoxine) into the active form of the vitamin, called pyridoxal phosphate. It is highly likely that the few children who have had adverse reactions to very high doses of vitamin B6 may not have done so if given B6 together with zinc.

In fact, most adverse reactions to vitamins or minerals arise when they are treated like drugs and given at very high doses without other nutrients, thereby completely ignoring the principle of synergy. For this reason I strongly recommend that any person who is experiencing fits, convulsions, or epilepsy see a nutritional therapist for a thorough nutritional workout.

This should involve both hair and blood analyzes for magnesium, manganese, and zinc, as well as folic acid. Levels of magnesium and folic acid are best tested in red blood cells. Depending on the results, a nutritional therapist can work out what combination of these nutrients, often in high doses, are worth trying, together with basic multivitamin supplementation.

The optimum nutrition approach involving an all-round good diet and supplements program is especially important since other nutrients have also been shown to have positive effects on mental health in those with epilepsy. These include vitamin B1,[169] selenium,[170] and vitamin E.[171]

Absolutely essential: the right fats

Imbalances in essential brain fats is one of the hottest areas of research. It is highly likely, with so many people deficient in essential fats, and especially omega-3 fats, that ensuring an optimal intake and balance of essential fats may help reduce the incidence of fits in epileptics.

The anticonvulsant properties of the two EFAs in a ratio 1:4, omega-3 to omega-6, have been demonstrated in epileptic rats. Three weeks of EFA supplementation resulted in up to 84 percent fewer rats having seizures, and up to a 97 percent reduction in the duration of seizures. The experimenters postulated that the anticonvulsant effects of EFAs may be related to the stabilization of neuronal membranes in the brain.[172]

It also works in humans. Researchers at the Kalanit Institute for the Retarded Child in Israel gave people with epilepsy 3g of omega-3 fats for six months and found a dramatic reduction in both the number and severity of epileptic seizures.[173]

Amino acids and phospholipids

Many of the *brain food* nutrients discussed in Part 1 may also be helpful for those with fits. This includes phospholipids such as phosphatidylcholine, and essential fats. Also potentially helpful are the brain's master tuners—SAMe and trimethylglycine (TMG). A close relative, dimethylglycine (DMG), produced remarkable results in one 22-year-old man with long-standing mental retardation, who had been having around 17 seizures per week despite anticonvulsant medication. Within one week of starting DMG, at 90 mg twice daily, his seizures dropped to just three per week. Two attempts to withdraw the DMG caused dramatic increases in seizure frequency.[174]

The amino acid taurine, which helps to calm down the nervous system, may also have a role to play. In animals studies low brain taurine concentrations have been found at the site of maximal seizure activity, and supplementing taurine was found to have a potent, selective, and long-lasting anticonvulsant effect.[175]

However, the most powerful relaxant amino acid has got to be GABA, the brain's peacemaker, because it acts directly as a neurotransmitter. One possible mechanism for explaining why anticonvulsant drugs work is that they block the activity of the excitatory neurotransmitter, glutamic acid, and thereby promote the inhibitory neurotransmitter, GABA. However, I would be cautious about supplementing GABA, and possibly large amounts of taurine, except under medical supervision. This is mainly because animal studies have shown that rats prone to petit mal (absence) seizures sometimes have too much of these amino acids.[176] Another brain-friendly nutrient, DMAE, while potentially helpful, should also be given with caution.

Vinpocetine, an extract of the periwinkle plant (*Vinca minor*) may also help, according to research in Russia.[177] This herbal extract does many useful things in the brain (see Chapter 14). It improves production of cellular energy in brain cells, and it widens blood vessels in the brain, thus improving transport of glucose and oxygen to the brain and their use once they get there. One theory is that epileptic fits may be caused by fluctuations in glucose or oxygen supplies to the brain, which might explain the positive effects of vinpocetine.

Check for allergies

As with so many types of mental health problems, it's well worth checking for allergies. One epileptic's fits were proven to be induced by certain foods. Without knowing which, they were given either a minute amount of their trigger foods or placebos, and only the foods brought on fits.[178] Professor William Rea from Texas, renowned for his special sealed hospital wing that is completely free of all allergens, environmental pollutants, and chemicals, designed specially for those with multiple allergies, has also found some epileptics stop having fits. One of his patients, a 29-year-old man with a four-year history of grand mal epilepsy as well as double vision, tachycardia, dizziness, edema, and spontaneous bruising, none of which had responded to the usual drugs, had complete relief after fasting for six days. When he was reintroduced to certain foods and chemicals he once more started having fits. For him, peanuts were the worst food.[179] Another powerful trigger substance for some people with epilepsy is the smell of rosemary oil, found in many essential oil blends.

SUMMARY

In summary, if you are prone to fits, convulsions, or epilepsy and haven't been checked out by a nutritional therapist, there is plenty of room for hope.

- Have your vitamin and mineral levels checked. If low in folic acid, B6, magnesium, manganese, or zinc, supplementation may well help.

- Make sure you are getting enough essential fats, from seeds, fish, and their oils.

- Other brain-friendly nutrients, including amino acids, choline, DMAE, taurine, and vinpocetine may help, but they are best taken under professional guidance.

PART 7

Mental Health
in Old Age

Age-related memory decline is not inevitable. Parkinson's disease and Alzheimer's disease can be prevented or even arrested with the right nutrition. This part reports on amazing discoveries in the treatment and prevention of these health problems, backed up by proper science and remarkable recoveries using nutritional therapy.

CHAPTER 35

Putting the brakes on Parkinson's disease

Parkinson's disease isn't just an affliction of old age. In the U.K. there are more than 120,000 sufferers, ranging from teenagers to the elderly. Nor is Parkinson's a disease of poverty, as the high-profile cases of Michael J. Fox, Muhammad Ali, and the late Katharine Hepburn attest. My first hands-on experience of the condition came through treating the late comic actor Terry-Thomas.

Whatever the age of the person with Parkinson's, the condition can be very tough to live with. People with Parkinson's disease first show symptoms of tremor, rigidity, unsteadiness, and slow movement (bradykinesia). The reason for these problems with muscular control and function has been attributed to a deficiency of the neurotransmitter dopamine.

Conventional treatment is based on drug therapy giving L-dopa, the direct precursor of dopamine, which is made from the amino acid phenylalanine, found in dietary protein (see Figure 34).

Other drugs are available which may increase the effectiveness of L-dopa, and there are surgical methods of helping control the tremors. There is also ongoing research in both areas. However helpful, drugs and surgery do run the risk of side effects. As such, so many people with Parkinson's opt for drugs only when they cannot function effectively enough without them. With the right nutritional support, this threshold may never be reached.

Thanks to the pioneering work of Dr. Geoffrey Leader and Lucille Leader, a doctor and nutritional therapist living in London, we now know that the right nutritional intervention can effectively improve the symptoms of Parkinson's disease. Harry's story is a case in point.

Harry was referred by his GP to Dr. Geoffrey Leader and Lucille Leader at their clinic in London (see Useful Addresses, page 474). He made repetitive movements, had tremors (made worse by stress), intractable constipation, and very low energy, and was very underweight. The Leaders arranged biochemical tests, which demonstrated that Harry was deficient in nutrients. They also found that he was eating foods that compromised the absorption of his L-dopa medication.

They recommended nutrients to address the deficiencies that were found, dealt successfully with the constipation, and worked out a suitable diet and a schedule for taking the L-dopa in relation to different foods, which would maximize the efficacy of Harry's drugs. This enabled him to take smaller doses of L-dopa, which in turn reduced its side effects, which included the distressing dyskinesia. The weight problem was addressed using a specific dietary strategy that was compatible with his drug regimen. They also helped Harry to keep his stress levels low by a special relaxation technique called autogenic training that also helps control the symptoms.

Within a few weeks, Harry was experiencing a feeling of wellbeing. His bowel function had normalized, his energy had improved, the dyskinesia was a thing of the past, and he was putting on weight. His body movements were more controlled.

Note: The full details of this integrated nutritional strategy are given in the Leaders' books, *Parkinson's Disease: The Way Forward* and *Parkinson's Disease: Reducing Symptoms with Nutrition and Drugs* (see Recommended Reading on page 471).

Many roads to dopamine deficiency

There is little doubt that dopamine deficiency is the major cause of the symptoms of Parkinson's, and most drug therapy aims to improve the

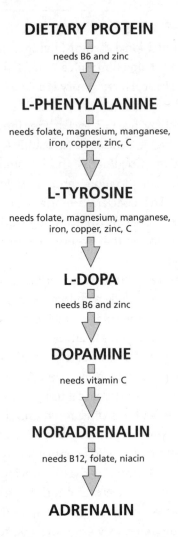

DIETARY PROTEIN

needs B6 and zinc

L-PHENYLALANINE

needs folate, magnesium, manganese,
iron, copper, zinc, C

L-TYROSINE

needs folate, magnesium, manganese,
iron, copper, zinc, C

L-DOPA

needs B6 and zinc

DOPAMINE

needs vitamin C

NORADRENALIN

needs B12, folate, niacin

ADRENALIN

Fig 34. How we make dopamine[1]. Adapted with permission from Dr. Geoffrey Leader and Lucille Leader, *Parkinson's Disease—The Way Forward* (see Recommended Reading, page 471).

body's ability to make dopamine from L-dopa. But, why do some people develop this impaired ability to make this key neurotransmitter? There are many answers to this question.

In some cases the neurons that produce dopamine don't work properly, sometimes because they lack the raw materials, or the enzymes that turn the building blocks, amino acids, into neurotransmitters. The neurons can die off or be damaged, for example by oxidants, or by environmental toxins such as pesticides and herbicides. Interestingly, researchers at the University of Miami have found levels of these chemicals to be higher in the brains of Parkinson's sufferers.[2] The incidence of Parkinson's is notably higher in rural areas where a lot of crop spraying takes place, and some pesticide combinations have shown a clear geographical correlation with incidences of the disease.[3-4] Deficiency of nutrients such as folic acid can also make these dopamine-producing brain cells more susceptible to damage.[5]

The balance of neurotransmitters, including dopamine, is controlled to a large extent by the process of methylation. Most people with Parkinson's have raised homocysteine levels,[6] which indicates disrupted methylation patterns. However, whether raised homocysteine is a cause or consequence of the disease is not yet clear, since L-dopa medication tends to raise homocysteine levels.[7] Deficiency in vitamin B6 has also been linked to an increased risk of Parkinson's, more so than folic acid or B12, the other key homocysteine-lowering vitamins; this suggests that B6 may play a specific part in preventing Parkinson's in addition to its homocysteine-lowering role.[8] Either way, I recommend testing for homocysteine and supplementing homocysteine-lowering nutrients accordingly (see Chapter 8).

In addition to faulty methylation, sometimes there is a problem in how the body detoxifies, a job primarily done by the liver, leaving neurons unprotected.[9] Then there are other factors such as prolonged stress and the likelihood of genetic predispositions.

Geoffrey and Lucille Leader figured that each of these pieces of the jigsaw puzzle could be made a lot better if sufferers followed a targeted optimum nutrition program. They started to test patients with Parkinson's disease and found that literally 100 percent of them had nutritional deficiencies based on tests that measure what is going on within cells. They also found that many people were deficient in stomach acid and digestive enzymes, leading to poor digestion, and had increased intestinal permeability, leading to faulty absorption of nutrients. Intestinal permeability is tested by drinking polyethylene glycol (PEG 400), a substance that shouldn't pass through the gut wall, and then measuring levels of PEG 400 in the urine. Using this test, people with Parkinson's disease may often show an increase in gut permeability or evidence of malabsorption. While there is no conclusive evidence yet that Parkinson's disease is caused by nutrient deficiencies, the Leaders have found that correcting these deficiencies often helps.

Brain toxins, oxidants, and the liver

All this faulty digestion and absorption places extra stress on the liver, the detoxification capital of the body. Since the brain's neurons can't protect themselves from toxins, they depend on the liver. A simple example of this is alcohol—once you drink more than your liver can detoxify, you get drunk, which is what happens when brain cells are exposed to this toxin. In excess, you lose muscular control and movements, including speech, slow down.

Problems with liver detoxification are often a hallmark of Parkinson's patients. One of the liver's best detox allies is the sulphur-containing amino acids, which have the ability to mop up undesirable toxins in a process called sulphation. Researchers have reported faulty sulphation in patients with Parkinson's, which can be helped by supplementing cysteine, methionine, and molybdenum and avoiding wine, coffee, certain cheeses, and chocolate, all known inhibitors of sulphation.[10] Eating foods rich in glucosinolates, such as broccoli, Brussels sprouts, cabbage, cauliflower, and kale, also helps the liver to detoxify.

The greatest toxins of all are oxidants, or free radicals. Giving antioxidants helps to prevent free-radical damage to brain cells and slows the progression of the disease. In a 7-year pilot study, 21 patients with early Parkinson's were given 3,000 mg of vitamin C and 3,200 IU of vitamin E daily. The need for drug therapy was delayed up to two to three years compared to those who did not receive the antioxidants.[11]

Along with its negative effect on neurons, Parkinson's also damages function in the mitochondria, which are the energy factories in our cells where energy conversion takes place. One of the most critical antioxidants for protecting mitochondria is coenzyme Q10 (CoQ10). The older you are, the more likely you are to be deficient. A study published in 2002 in the *Archives of Neurology* has determined that CoQ10 slows the progression of Parkinson's disease. Researchers at 10 different universities across the U.S. tested a total of 80 Parkinson's patients who were in the early stages of the disease and were not taking any medications for their condition. Participants took either a placebo, or 300, 600, or 1,200 mg of CoQ10

4 times a day for 16 months, or until their condition required more traditional medical treatment.

Halfway through the trial, there was already a marked difference between the four groups, with those participants given the 300 mg and 600 mg dosages noticing a lessening of their motor impairments, while those receiving the 1,200 mg dosage experienced a significant reduction in their loss of motor function. By the end of the study, those in the 1,200 mg group had a 44 percent slower rate of deterioration, while those in the 300 mg and 600 mg groups enjoyed a 20 percent slower rate of disease progression.

These nutrients are some but by no means all of the allies that can support liver function, thereby preventing brain damage from toxins. Dr. Jeffrey Bland from Gig Harbor, Washington, an expert in liver detoxification, has also found tremendous improvement by supporting liver function with nutritional supplementation, increasing the effectiveness of drugs, reducing symptoms, and boosting energy levels in those suffering from the early stages of Parkinson's in studies.[12]

Personalized nutrition works best

The best results with Parkinson's come from a total optimum nutrition approach. This involves both diet and supplements, helping to improve digestion, absorption, liver function, and the cell's ability to work properly and to produce dopamine, thus optimizing cellular metabolism and energy production.

As you can see in Figure 32 on page 382, the ability to make dopamine efficiently depends on many vitamins and minerals. This includes nutrients such as zinc, magnesium, and the B vitamins, especially B6 and folic acid. Researchers at the National Institute on Aging in the U.S. found that mice fed a folic-acid-deficient diet have a significantly greater risk of developing Parkinson's-like symptoms. One likely reason for this is that, without folic acid, the body produces too much homocysteine, a toxic substance that damages brain cells and so hinders dopamine production. Researchers at Boston University have found that a high homocysteine level is a strong, independent risk factor for the development of Alzheimer's disease.[13] In mice fed adequate amounts of folic acid, they were able to repair the damage in dopamine-producing neurons and counteract the adverse effects of homocysteine.[14]

The Leaders have found that the best approach involves a tailor-made nutritional program of diet and supplements, which may often reduce symptoms and make drugs more effective, thus optimizing dosage. They recommend many supplements based on patients' biochemical individuality, including vitamins, minerals, essential fats, amino acids, antioxidants, phospholipids, and brain-friendly herbs such as ginkgo.

As with so many mental health problems, controlling blood sugar and checking and correcting food allergies or intolerances can make a big difference. The most common allergy-provoking foods are the gluten grains (especially wheat, but also rye, oats, barley, and spelt) and dairy products. Managing stress is also important because we respond to stress by producing the stress hormones noradrenalin and adrenalin, which are made from dopamine. This is why the symptoms of Parkinson's often get worse when the sufferer is stressed.

Working with medication: what to eat when

The right diet is very important in such a strategy that tackles every piece of the jigsaw of Parkinson's. Movement problems can get worse when dense protein foods containing certain amino acids in high proportion are eaten too close to the times of taking L-dopa medication.[15] This is because L-dopa competes with the amino acids for absorption at the receptor sites in the intestine and at the blood-brain barrier, so less gets through. To make best use of the L-dopa, protein-rich foods containing the other amino acids should not be eaten at the same time as taking L-dopa medication, according to the following guidelines:

L-dopa medication and diet—what to eat when*

L-dopa is affected by protein-containing foods which contain significant amounts of the amino acids tyrosine, phenylalanine, valine, leucine, isoleucine, tryptophan, methionine, and histidine. Foods which contain these amino acids include eggs, fish, meat, poultry, dairy produce (not butter), legumes, green peas, spinach, soy, couscous, bulgur, coconut, avocado, asparagus, and gluten-containing grains (oats, rye, wheat, barley, spelt).

- Take L-dopa medication
  Wait ONE HOUR before eating any of the foods listed above.

- After eating any of the foods listed above, wait TWO HOURS, if possible, before taking L-dopa medication again.

*This dietary protocol has been developed and proven helpful by Dr. Geoffrey Leader and Lucille Leader and is reproduced with their kind permission.

With older types of the drug L-dopa, vitamin B6 caused its conversion to dopamine before reaching the brain. This was disastrous. Latterday L-dopa drugs contain a decarboxylase inhibitor, which inhibits premature carboxylation of L-dopa to dopamine. As such, vitamin B6, which helps turn L-dopa into dopamine, can be used safely together with the Parkinson's drugs Sinemet and Madopar.[16]

The drug selegiline is also often used for Parkinson's disease. In higher doses (above 30 mg), there is a risk of hypertension if a person eats foods rich in another amino acid—tyramine.[17] These include cheddar and other strong cheeses, ripe avocado, pepperoni, salami, soy sauce, old liver pâté, overripe bananas, brewer's yeast, broad beans, Chianti, overripe or canned figs, Vermouth, Drambuie, yeast extract (Marmite, etc.), miso soup, fish (pickled, salted, or smoked), caviar, chocolate (large quantities), or caffeine (large quantities). Some people are more susceptible to this dose-dependent side effect than others, and few react at a dose of 10 mg, which is commonly given for Parkinson's.[18]

While being careful to avoid these foods around medication, it is important to get enough protein from foods at other times. Good whole proteins include fish, soy products, and eggs. Many people choose to have their meal contain concentrated protein at night. This is because they do not need as much help with movement control at night as during the day when their L-dopa medication is necessary to see them through all their activities. Some people leave out L-dopa completely after the protein meal. Otherwise it is best to follow the time protocol for taking L-dopa with a protein-rich meal, as above.

It is also important to have a well-balanced diet throughout the day including fruits and vegetables, gluten-free whole grains, and plenty of fluids. A common problem in Parkinson's is constipation. Having a diet rich in fruits and vegetables and drinking plenty of water throughout the day makes a big difference, as can a few prunes, figs, or dried apricots with each meal, or psyllium husk capsules between meals with water.

SUMMARY

In summary, with the appropriate individualized nutritional management there's a good chance you can put the brakes on Parkinson's disease. It may alleviate symptoms and reduce the speed of increasing drug dosages. I recommend the following:

- See a nutritional therapist who can assess you for nutritional deficiencies, digestive problems, and liver function.

- Pursue a tailor-made nutritional strategy, including a specific diet regime that maximizes the effects of any medication.

- Check your homocysteine level and supplement homocysteine-lowering nutrients accordingly.

- Avoid environmental toxins and eat organic when possible.

- Do all you can to reduce your level of stress.

- Reduce auto-intoxication from constipation by eating six to eight prunes, figs, or apricots before each meal.

CHAPTER 36

Preventing age-related memory decline

We are on the threshold of a new disease. It isn't dementia, senility, or Alzheimer's, although for some it marks the beginning of that slippery slope. It's age-related memory and/or mood decline. It affects at least 1 in 4 people over the age of 60 and is accepted by most as an inevitable but undesirable consequence of aging.

Imagine this scenario: "Doctor, I'm 55 and there's little doubt that my memory isn't as sharp as it used to be. What can you recommend?" You're then asked a sequence of questions that conclude you don't have dementia or Alzheimer's, followed by "It's just what happens later in life." Of course, the drugs companies are well aware of this missed opportunity and are pushing for official classification of a disease. Age-related memory impairment affects many more people than Alzheimer's disease, although, it's certainly true, it is a much less severe condition, says Dr. Paul Williams of Glaxo Pharmaceuticals, adding, "We believe at least 4 million people in the U.K. suffer from this." Glaxo has been developing drugs to enhance memory and mental performance. In fact, most major players have already patented and developed smart drugs, discussed in Chapter 38, that will soon be prescribed in these scenarios. According to the drugs companies, memory decline is becoming a massive and widespread problem.

The good news is that there really is something you can do, and the place to start is optimum nutrition.

Boosting the aging brain

Vitamin-fueled vitality

The misconception that you get everything you need from a well-balanced diet becomes increasingly further from the truth as you age. First, for many people the ability to digest and absorb nutrients decreases. A common finding among older people is that hydrochloric acid production in the stomach declines, immediately affecting the ability to make use of protein, vitamins, and minerals. So too, for most of us at least, does exercise and/or general physical activity, and consequently appetite. Less food means fewer nutrients.

Circulation, at least for many, also becomes worse with age, so fewer nutrients make it from the gut to the brain. An underlying causer of many of the diseases of later life—cancer, heart disease, diabetes, and Alzheimer's—is inflammation. Increases in underlying inflammatory processes in the brain, which can ultimately lead to neuronal damage, can leave the brain in dire need of certain nutrients. The famous five are:

- B vitamins

- Antioxidants

- Trace elements

- Essential fats

- Phospholipids and other methylating nutrients

While Part 1 gave you the background on the general importance of all these nutrients for brain health, they really come into their own in later life, as the evidence now overwhelmingly shows. Many studies have shown that even supplementing a multivitamin containing moderate amounts of vitamins and trace elements can make a noticeable difference. And multivitamins don't just improve your mental performance; they also make you happier. One double-blind, placebo-controlled trial gave elderly people a B-complex supplement, containing 10 mg of B1, B2, and B6. That's about

10 times the RDA. Compared to those taking placebos, there was a definite improvement in mood.[19]

However, the most promising results of all lie in giving homocysteine-lowering nutrients, which include vitamins B2, B6, B12, folic acid, and TMG. This is especially effective for people with raised homocysteine levels, as both low levels of these nutrients and high levels of homocysteine are strongly predictive of memory decline.[20-21] The link between homocysteine and memory becomes even more persuasive when you consider the fact that, as a person's memory function gets worse, their homocysteine levels increase—and vice versa.

A study conducted by Jane Durga at Wageningen University in the Netherlands gave 818 people aged 50–75 either a vitamin containing 800 mcg of folic acid a day, or a dummy pill. That's almost three times the RDA and the equivalent of 2.5 pounds of strawberries a day—more than you can reasonably eat. Three years later, different aspects of intelligence were measured. On memory tests, the supplement users had scores comparable to people 5.5 years younger. On tests of cognitive speed, the folic acid helped users perform as well as people 1.9 years younger.[22]

What is badly needed, and under way, is a study giving not only folic acid, but also B6, B12 and possibly other homocysteine-lowering nutrients to participants with age-related memory decline. OPTIMA (the Oxford Project to Investigate Memory and Ageing), headed by Professor David Smith from Oxford University, is currently doing such a trial. The results will be available some time in 2009.

Antioxidant protection

The best vitamins for boosting your mood and memory are the antioxidants, which include A, C, and E, although the minerals selenium and zinc and the semi-essential nutrient CoQ10 have antioxidant properties too. These not only protect the brain from oxidation, but also improve the supply of oxygen, the brain's most critical nutrient. So too do B vitamins, especially folic acid and B12, deficiency of which results in anemia and an inability to efficiently transport oxygen to the brain, and vitamins B1, B2, and B3, which help the brain make use of oxygen in generating brain power in every cell.

The more antioxidants you have in your blood, the sharper your mind. That's what researchers at the University of Berne in Switzerland found when they tested 442 people aged 65–94 years. Those with the highest levels of vitamin C and beta carotene in their blood had the best scores on memory tests.[23] Other researchers in the U.S. have found a similar positive link between vitamin E and memory performance.[24]

The likely explanation for these associations is that antioxidants improve circulation, and reduce the risk for heart disease.[25] It is becoming more and more evident that Alzheimer's and heart disease share many of the same risk factors and mechanisms. As arteries become more and more inflamed and damaged, so too does the brain.

Antioxidants not only protect the brain from oxidation; they also reduce inflammation. Inflammation, often characterized by pain, redness, or swelling, but insidiously invisible in the brain, is how the body lets you know something is wrong. When the body exceeds its capacity to detoxify, for example when the liver is overloaded with alcohol, inflammation is the result. Improving liver function by increasing your intake of liver-friendly nutrients such as antioxidants, methylsulfonylmethane or MSM, glutathione, and cysteine helps lessen the burden on the brain.

In fact, there is a direct link between liver function and cognitive function. Investigating the reason for memory and concentration problems in alcoholics, a study of 280 patients with liver damage at the Johns Hopkins University School of Medicine in Baltimore found that this cognitive impairment results from liver damage rather than alcohol intake directly, as those with non-alcohol-related liver damage had similar reductions in cognitive function.[26]

While most multis give you small amounts of these antioxidants, there's a good case for upping your intake as you get older. As he approached old age, Dr. Linus Pauling upped his intake of vitamin C as high as 10g. Rats make the equivalent of 3g a day, while goats make 16g a day. We humans have lost the ability to make vitamin C, he argued, and suffer the consequences in old age.

I recommend as an optimum amount 3g of vitamin C when you're 40, 4g when you're 50, 5g when you're 60, and so on, divided into two daily doses. For vitamin E, the magic formula is 100 IUs for every decade. So, if you are 60 years old, that's 600 IUs (400 mg) a day.

Go for the smart fats

It's also worth upping your intake of essential fats, especially omega-3s. Simply eating three servings of oily fish (herring, salmon, mackerel, or tuna) a week halves your risk of a heart attack. As we are learning, cardio-vascular disease and memory decline are intimately connected.

Omega-3 fats are not only extremely powerful anti-inflammatory agents, which is one of the main mechanisms by which brain cells get damaged, they may also be involved in encoding memories. One theory of memories is that they are encoded in lipoproteins, built out of essential fats and phospholipids. In this respect, the omega-3 fat DHA may prove the most important. Mice on a DHA-deficient diet had 90 percent greater loss of brain connections compared to those fed the DHA-rich diet.[27] The changes resemble what is seen in the brains of people with Alzheimer's. On memory tests, those on the DHA-deficient diet took twice as long to perform a test of spatial memory. The test would be roughly equivalent to someone trying to remember where he parked his car. Another theory is that memories are encoded through RNA, the messenger molecule in charge of building new cells. Since brain cells are permanently being replaced and rebuilt, memory must be transmittable. If this theory is cor-rect, zinc is important to memory because it is essential for building RNA. Fish is not only a good source of omega-3 fats, it's also rich in both RNA and zinc.

As we'll see in the next chapter, amazing results have been achieved with Alzheimer's by supplementing omega-3 fish oils, and there's no rea-son not to assume that supplements can't sharpen your mind and mem-ory and prevent dementia from ever developing. Once you hit the age of 50, I recommend 1,000 mg of DHA/EPA a day. Most supplements provide 400–600 mg, so this means two fish oil capsules a day.

There is another advantage to eating fish. It's high in vitamin D and, for reasons not yet conclusively known, the better your vitamin D status, the better your mood and memory.[28] Apart from eating fish, make sure your multivitamin provides extra vitamin D in the order of 5 mcg.

Acetylcholine: memory key

As we learned in Chapter 5, acetylcholine is the mind and memory neuro-transmitter, helping you to learn new information. It is built out of choline, the most usable form of which is CDP choline (also known as citicholine), followed by phosphatidylcholine. These phospholipids also help to make membranes in the brain and therefore protect against declining numbers and efficiency of neurons.

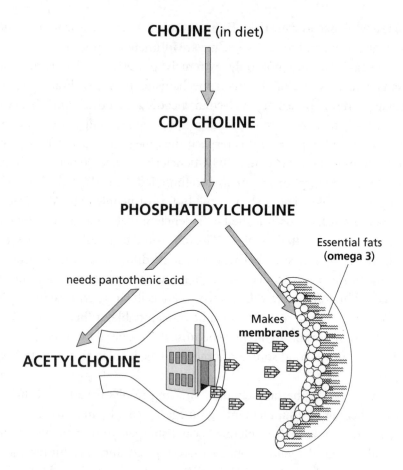

CHOLINE (in diet)

CDP CHOLINE

PHOSPHATIDYLCHOLINE

Essential fats
(omega 3)

needs pantothenic acid

Makes
membranes

ACETYLCHOLINE

Fig 35. How the brain makes phospholipids

As you get older the number of neurons and synapses you have decreases, which is why both memory and emotion become blunted. However, this doesn't need to happen if you can just get these phospholipids and essential fats into the brain.

As you can see from the figure above, what you want is to get phosphatidylcholine into the brain. While it would be logical to think that supplementing phosphatidylcholine would be the best way to do this, much of this breaks down into choline before it gets into the brain. The same is not true for citicholine. This is the most effective for increasing membrane building in the brain.[29] Since the phospholipids literally soak up essential fats, combining citicholine and phosphatidylcholine, plus essential fats, is like oysters for your brain. These can keep you as sharp as a pencil throughout life. They are also essential nutrients after a stroke.

Another phospholipid, phosphatidylserine, has well proven memory-boosting effects. In animal studies phosphatidylserine is especially good at reversing age-related memory decline. Research on rats, carried out by the Yakult Central Institute for Microbiological Research, found that 60 days of supplementing phosphatidylserine could improve some mental function in older rats with age-related memory decline to that of young rats.[30] Human studies have also shown that phosphatidylserine is effective in reversing memory decline (see Chapter 14).

Other acetylcholine helpers, such as DMAE, pyroglutamate, and pantothenic acid, are well worth supplementing on a daily basis. These are often found together in brain-food formulas.

Ginkgo: back in circulation

Another proven brain booster, especially in old age, is the herb ginkgo biloba. While studies on younger people haven't always proven its benefit, studies on older people, especially those with circulation problems, have shown very positive results. A review of 10 studies testing ginkgo's effects on people with circulation problems, carried out at the University of Limburg in the Netherlands, found significant improvement in memory, concentration, energy, and mood.[31] A more comprehensive double-blind, placebo-controlled trial in France found remarkable improvement in speed of cognitive processing of 60- to 80-year-olds, almost comparable to those of healthy young people, when given 320 mg a day.[32] Ginkgo biloba may also be helpful in elderly depression—it has been shown to increase serotonin receptor sites in elderly but not young rats, suggesting that it may block an age-related loss of serotonin receptors.[33]

A review of all the studies on ginkgo up to 2002 concluded that there is "promising evidence of improvement in cognition and function with ginkgo."[34] This review spawned tremendous medical interest in ginkgo in the context of dementia, and three further trials. The results of these, however, weren't so encouraging. Two failed to find a significant effect in people who had dementia,[35–36] while the third showed some improvement in elderly people who had not been diagnosed with dementia.[37] In this last study, 262 people aged 60 and older were given ginkgo at a dose of 160 mg a day, or a placebo, for six weeks. Those on ginkgo were found to have significantly improved memory function. So this herb may have a role to play in prevention, but does not seem to have a remarkable effect once a person actually has dementia.

Ginkgo contains two phytochemicals called ginkgo flavone glycosides and terpene lactones, which give it its remarkable healing properties. Ginkgo usually comes in capsule form and you should look for a brand that shows the flavonoid concentration, which determines strength. The recommended flavonoid concentration is 24 percent, of which one would take 30–50 mg up to three times a day. Ginkgo is sometimes also contained in brain-food formulas.

Stay cool, use it or lose it and keep fit

As we saw in Chapter 9, stress has an enormous impact on our memories, too. A mild dose of stress can actually stimulate memory and mental alertness, but long-term stress is definitely bad news: it puts too much of the hormone cortisol into circulation, and this literally damages the brain. Raised levels of cortisol have been linked to poorer memory and a shrinking of the brain's memory sorting center.

After only two weeks of the raised cortisol levels of stress, the dendrite arms of brain cells that reach out to connect with other brain cells start to shrivel up, according to research carried out at Stanford University in California by Robert Sapolsky, professor of neuroscience.[38] The good news is that such damage isn't permanent. Stop the stress and the dendrites grow back. One way to reduce your stress levels is to reduce your intake of sugar and stimulants. The more dependent on stimulants you are, and the more your blood-sugar levels fluctuate, the more you are likely to react stressfully to life's inevitable challenges.

With the right nutrition and the right attitude, age-related memory loss doesn't need to happen to you. You can build new brain cells at any age. Research clearly shows that healthy, well-educated elderly people can show no decline in mental function right up to death, and no increased rate of brain shrinkage even after 65. It's a use it or lose it situation.

It isn't only your brain you need to exercise. Physical exercise has a direct effect on mental powers, probably by improving circulation. Research published in the *Journal of Internal Medicine* found that regular walking improved memory and reduced signs of dementia.[39] The threshold for this positive effect was about 1,000 steps, or a little over a mile a day.

The steps you need to take to keep all your marbles are, in essence, the same as those needed to maximize your memory and mental alertness earlier in life. So, whether you are 20 or 60 years old, the time to act is now. However, if you are over 50 it's worth upping the amounts of these brain-friendly nutrients.

SUMMARY

In summary, staving off age-related memory decline means:

- Eat oily fish three times a week.
- Eat plenty of antioxidant-rich fruits and vegetables.
- Supplement a high-strength multivitamin and mineral.
- Check your homocysteine level and adjust your diet and life-style, and take homocysteine-lowering nutrients accordingly.
- Supplement between 3 and 8g of vitamin C a day, increasing your intake with age.
- Supplement 100 IU of vitamin E daily for each decade of your age.
- Supplement 2 fish oil capsules giving 1,000 mg of EPA/DHA.
- Supplement phospholipids (phosphatidylcholine and serine).
- Supplement a brain-food formula giving phospholipids, pyro-glutomate, DMAE, pantothenic acid, ginkgo biloba and/or vinpocetine.
- Keep fit.
- Keep learning new things.
- Reduce the stresses in your life.

If you do all this there is no reason why your memory and mental powers need decline with age. As Leonard Larson, president of the American Medical Association in 1960, said, "There are no diseases of the aged, but simply diseases among the aged."

CHAPTER 37

Preventing and arresting Alzheimer's

What is the point of a long life if you can't remember it—and what is more tragic than losing your mind before your body? Yet, this is exactly what is happening to 3 out of 10 people over the age of 70, who experience poor memory, concentration, and confusion. More, 1 in 10 of them are diagnosed with dementia, and out of these, most go on to develop Alzheimer's disease. That means a 50/50 chance of entering the last quarter of your life with your mind intact.

Yet, according to a number of top health experts, Alzheimer's is probably completely preventable. "It is time that medical science and practice takes nutrition seriously as one of the key factors that determines the health of the brain," says Professor David Smith, Deputy Head of Oxford University's Medical Sciences Division, whose research team believe they've found out how to identify those at risk—and reverse the risk with simple dietary changes. But you have to start young, says Professor Smith: "Most cases of Alzheimer's, possibly over 90 percent, are preventable. Only one in a hundred are caused by genes. For example, we have good reason to believe that many of those likely to develop Alzheimer's have raised homocysteine levels that can be reversed with large amounts of specific nutrients. We need to find out if these nutrients will slow the damage to the brain that is associated with high homocysteine." Professor Smith is currently conducting a three-year trial focusing on this hypothesis, to be completed in 2009. "If the trial is successful, then at least some Alzheimer's should be preventable by a simple nutritional intervention," he adds. So the good news is that it's highly likely that you can reverse the risk of Alzheimer's with diet and lifestyle changes.

❓ HOW SHARP ARE YOUR MIND AND MEMORY?

☐ Is your memory deteriorating?

☐ Do you find it hard to concentrate and often get confused?

☐ Do you sometimes meet someone you know quite well but can't remember their name?

☐ Do you often find you can remember things from the past but forget what you did yesterday?

☐ Do you ever forget what day of the week it is?

☐ Do you ever go looking for something and forget what you are looking for?

☐ Do your friends and family think you're getting more forgetful now than you used to be?

☐ Do you find it hard to add up numbers without writing them down?

☐ Do you often experience mental fatigue?

☐ Do you find it hard to concentrate for more than an hour?

☐ Do you often misplace your keys?

☐ Do you frequently repeat yourself?

☐ Do you sometimes forget the point you're trying to make?

☐ Does it take you longer to learn things than it used to?

Score 1 for each *yes* answer.

If your score is:

Below 5: You don't have a major problem with your memory—but you'll find that simple dietary changes and supplementing natural mind and memory boosters will sharpen you up even more.

5 to 10: Your memory definitely needs a boost—you are starting to suffer from brain drain. Certain dietary changes and supplements can make a big difference.

More than 10: You are experiencing significant memory decline and need to do something about it. As well as following these diet and supplement recommendations, we recommend you see a nutritional therapist.

At the Brain Bio Centre in Richmond, we've been pioneering a nutrition-based treatment for reversing the risk of both age-related memory decline and Alzheimer's. We're not only seeing big improvements in people with declining memory and mental alertness, but we're also seeing mild improvements in some people with Alzheimer's. None of our Alzheimer's patients are getting any worse. In Wales, Dr. Andrew McCaddon is seeing similar results in his patients, as you'll see on page 404.

Homocysteine and Alzheimer's

If you're at all concerned about your memory or that of a loved one, the key initial step is to test the blood homocysteine level, which correlates directly with the condition of your memory and your mental alertness and mood. A healthy *H score* is 7 or less. Anyone with a score of 15 or more is not only likely to have worsening mental alertness, but also at risk of Alzheimer's disease later in life.

Chris Kruger is a case in point. He felt very unwell—constantly tired and depressed, lacking any sex drive, and even worse, beset by a brain-dead feeling, with a worsening memory and concentration. After testing, we found his homocysteine score was a massive 119. Chris followed my Alzheimer's Prevention Plan for three months. His homocysteine level dropped to 19; after 6 months it had dropped to 11, and after 12 months, to 9. Now he cannot believe how well he feels. His memory and concentration are completely restored, his energy is so good he now exercises for an hour every day and his sex drive has returned. "You have saved my life, or, at least made it worth living again," he told me.

The fact that homocysteine is a reversible risk factor for Alzheimer's and is almost certainly a causative agent in the specific kind of brain degeneration that causes Alzheimer's (see below) is the single most important discovery in the prevention of this terrible disease. You'd think that such an important finding would be welcomed with open arms by the medical community and governments alike. But, the sad truth is that, with no patentable or profitable treatment, scientists are finding it hard to get their studies funded. And if they do get funding, it isn't always easy for them to publish in mainstream journals, since they are dominated by editors who believe the current dogmas. Many pharmaceutical companies are funding very poorly designed trials, often using only folic acid, or doses that are too low, almost as if they would like to slow down the progress of this break-through. After all, the discovery of the homocysteine link will ultimately be bad news for the pharmaceutical industry's profits from potentially competitive drugs such as statins and acetylcholinesterase inhibitors (Aricept). These drug categories generate billions in profits, and one can expect their market share will be well protected.

All this means that you are more likely to find out about this vitally important discovery from reading a book like this than from your doctor.

The first firm link

The first firm link between Alzheimer's and homocysteine was reported by British and Norwegian scientists at the Universities of Oxford and Bergen as long ago as 1998, when they discovered high levels of homocysteine in the blood of patients who, after death, were proven to have Alzheimer's by examination of the brain.[40] This research has been pioneered by Dr. Robert Clarke and Professor David Smith from Oxford University, and Professor Helga Refsum, now at the University of Oslo, as part of OPTIMA (the Oxford Project to Investigate Memory and Ageing). Since then, many different research groups have found high levels in those suffering with both age-related mental decline and Alzheimer's. More recently, a number of indicators of Alzheimer's-related degeneration in the brain have been shown to be directly linked to homocysteine levels.[41] For instance, as Alzheimer's progresses, the width of the hippocampus, a part of the brain in memory, shrinks. The width of the hippocampus is directly related to homocysteine levels.[42] Before you switch off, thinking "I don't have Alzheimer's so it isn't relevant to me," what has been discovered is that both the changes in the brain and rising homocysteine levels happen *before* any noticeable symptoms emerge. This opens up the possibility that you can pre-diagnose the risk for Alzheimer's by getting to grips with your homocysteine level, and lowering it if you need to to reverse that risk.

While these discoveries may provide an important clue to the prevention of Alzheimer's, they don't prove that high homocysteine actually causes Alzheimer's. Since cardiovascular disease, poor blood circulation to the brain, and silent strokes can be caused by high homocysteine, and high homocysteine is an indicator of low levels of B vitamins, methylation, and glutathione, all of which are associated with increased risk of Alzheimer's, how do you know that homocysteine actually causes Alzheimer's, rather than just predicting it?[43] Some researchers have argued that the high homocysteine score found in Alzheimer's sufferers is simply showing the person has these conditions, rather than proving this kind of direct link.

A recent study from the School of Medicine at the University of California, Davis, is a case in point. Comparing 43 patients with Alzheimer's to 37 without, the team found a stronger association between a high homocysteine score and cardiovascular disease across both groups, than between a high homocysteine score and Alzheimer's. They also found that participants with low levels of vitamin B6 in their blood were more likely to have high homocysteine levels.[44] The researchers concluded that "elevated plasma homocysteine in patients with Alzheimer's appears related to vascular disease and not Alzheimer's." In addition, "low vitamin B6 status is prevalent in patients with Alzheimer's. It remains to be determined if elevated homocysteine and/or low vitamin B6 status directly influences Alzheimer's pathogenesis or progression."

This is another of those chicken-or-egg situations that is starting to be unraveled. However, the evidence to date strongly favors the position that homocysteine, independent of vascular disease, is a major risk factor for Alzheimer's. Of course, if you have both high homocysteine and vascular disease, or both dementia and vascular disease, then you are even worse off.[45]

Does high homocysteine cause Alzheimer's?

So, the big question is which comes first—a high homocysteine level or Alzheimer's? Doctors from the Department of Neurology at the Boston University School of Medicine wanted to determine whether homocysteine precedes mental decline, or occurs as a result of dementia-related B vitamin deficiencies.

Their study looked at 1,092 people who had an average age of 76 and did not have dementia (loss of memory, concentration, and judgement, sometimes accompanied by emotional disturbance and personality changes). These people had already taken part in another study measuring their homocysteine levels eight years earlier. Researchers again measured their homocysteine, and then kept track of their mental health over the next eight years. During that time, 111 developed dementia, and 83 of them were diagnosed with Alzheimer's. The findings revealed that the higher the homocysteine levels preceding any symptoms of mental decline, the greater the risk of later developing dementia. In those with a homocysteine score of more than 14 units, the risk of Alzheimer's almost doubled.[46] They concluded that "an increased homocysteine level is a strong, independent risk factor for the development of dementia and Alzheimer's disease." This strongly suggests that optimum nutrition could, at the very least, halve your risk of developing Alzheimer's in later years by lowering homocysteine.

More recently, evidence has emerged that even before there is evidence of declining mental function in so-called healthy elderly individuals, high homocysteine also predicts physical degeneration in certain parts of the brain.[47–48] These findings are being echoed by research around the world.[49]

In Scotland, researchers have found that reduced mental performance in old age is strongly associated with high homocysteine and low levels of vitamins B12 and folate. They studied people who had taken part in the Scottish Mental Surveys of 1932 and 1947, which surveyed childhood intelligence. And they found that while homocysteine was higher and mental performance weaker in the older group, the most mentally agile of either group had the highest levels of B vitamins and lowest levels of homocysteine. In the older group, high homocysteine accounted for a 7–8 percent decline in mental performance.[50]

Homocysteine doesn't cause just mental deterioration, it also predicts physical deterioration. Research at the University of California has found that physical performance in older people, using tests of body strength, coordination, manual dexterity, and gait, also declines as homocysteine levels decline.[51]

Whichever way you cut it, the accumulating evidence is pointing to a consistent pattern. The higher your H score and the lower your B vitamin status, the greater your chances of declining memory, poor concentration and judgement, lowered mood, physical degeneration, and poor circulation to the brain. But, can you reverse the process? This is the million dollar question.

To answer it, I'd like to tell you about the work of a family doctor in Wales, Dr. Andrew McCaddon. He started researching homocysteine more than a decade ago and has pioneered research in the area of Alzheimer's treatment. It all began in 1990, when he met a 59-year-old patient with a nine-year history of memory problems due to early-onset familial Alzheimer's disease. His patient had low B12 levels in the blood, but normal B12 absorption. Dr. McCaddon noticed that other affected family members also had low vitamin B12 levels in their medical records.

In 1992, he published a hypothesis describing how this deficiency might contribute to Alzheimer's, but he needed to test his theory.[52] Since B12 and folic acid are necessary for converting homocysteine to methionine, he predicted that these patients would have elevated blood levels of homocysteine. That is exactly what he found.[53] He also found that a person's homocysteine level was the best predictor of decline in cognitive function.[54] Since this early research, McCaddon has gone on to prove that homocysteine levels increase as cognitive function declines—a finding now consistently being reported by other research groups.[55] He then started giving patients large amounts of B vitamins. This is what happened:

> 66 In the beginning, we gave B12 and folic acid to patients with high homocysteine levels, but we didn't really get much improvement. We realized that in Alzheimer's and in vascular dementia, there's a lot of oxidative stress, which also impacts homocysteine and methylation. So we started to give N-acetyl cysteine as well, which the brain uses to make glutathione, the brain's primary antioxidant. That's when I started to see a difference.
>
> To date, I have six cases of people diagnosed with Alzheimer's who have not got worse. Often they report an

improvement in general well-being and other aspects of mental health. For example, one lady has a clear improvement in her drawing ability.

Another example is Mrs R. She developed cognitive impairment 10 years ago. Her husband became seriously concerned five years ago after she had gone shopping and couldn't find her way back home. He helplessly watched her get worse. When she came to see me, I tested her homocysteine level, which was very high, and gave her B12, folic acid, and N-acetyl cysteine.

Within six months she became calmer and started sleeping properly. When she went out, she knew where she was going. Her underlying personality is now back. She's friendly, she can cope, and her behavior is good. In the words of her husband, "We can sit, have tea and cookies, watch TV and talk. I've got my wife back." Her short-term memory isn't great, but she hasn't gotten any worse. This is exactly what we are seeing consistently—a halting of the course of the disease. People don't get worse. 🙷

Dr. McCaddon's research has not only shown that the right amount and form of vitamins can arrest the Alzheimer's process in the small number of people treated so far, it has also shown that people with Alzheimer's may not use B12 properly, despite showing apparently normal levels in the blood. [56–57] One way round this B12 blockage is to give a special form of B12, either methylcobalamine or glutathionalcobalamine.[58]

How homocysteine damages the brain

Exactly how high homocysteine—and the inevitable B vitamin and SAMe deficiencies that always accompany it—might contribute to the kind of brain damage seen in Alzheimer's is a subject of heated debate in scientific circles around the world.

In Japan, Dr. Matsu Toshifumi and colleagues at Tohoku University conducted brain scans on 153 elderly people and checked them against each individual's homocysteine level. The evidence was clear—the higher the homocysteine, the greater the damage to the brain.[59] They also confirmed that high homocysteine levels were strongly correlated with low folic acid levels.

There's also evidence that homocysteine and its derivatives can activate certain receptors on the surface of nerve cells that result in the cell's death.[60–61] Another possible explanation is that homocysteine damages the microscopic blood vessels supplying critical brain regions, reducing blood supply and again, resulting in nerve cell death.[62] A research group at the Baylor University Metabolic Disease Center in Dallas, Texas, led by Dr. Teodoro Bottiglieri—one of the world's leading experts in the connection between folate and mental illness—proposes that low levels of folate (leading to raised homocysteine) directly causes brain damage that triggers dementia and Alzheimer's. Their research has found that a third of those with both dementia and high homocysteine scores (above 14 units) are deficient in folate.[63] Dr. David Snowdon at the University of Kentucky has also confirmed from autopsies that the lower the levels of serum folic acid, the greater the brain damage that person suffered.[64]

Alzheimer's sufferers also have less SAMe in their brains, as well as higher levels of homocysteine in their blood. SAMe, derived from the methylation of homocysteine, is the brain's single most important methyl donor, helping produce and activate all sorts of neurotransmitters, including the memory enhancer acetylcholine—declining levels of which are another hallmark of Alzheimer's and a likely reason for declining memory.[65]

Homocysteine—the story so far

So where are we with the H factor in relation to Alzheimer's? In summary, what we already know is that:

- People with Alzheimer's consistently have high homocysteine, and low B12 and folate levels.[66–67]

- High homocysteine, as well as low folate and B12 status, predict risk of developing Alzheimer's and age-related memory problems.[68]

- High homocysteine is associated with more rapid progression of the disease.[69]

- Homocysteine levels correlate with degree of brain damage and, as homocysteine levels increase, memory declines.

- High homocysteine can both damage the brain, and damage arteries, leading to poor blood supply to the brain.

- Early case studies show that giving increased amounts of homo-cysteine-lowering nutrients seems to arrest the progression of Alzheimer's.

What we don't yet know is the degree to which dementia and Alzheimer's are preventable by lowering homocysteine with optimum nutrition, or the degree to which dementia and Alzheimer's can be arrested or even reversed with optimum nutrition.

There are three research groups investigating these questions by giving people with age-related cognitive decline, or Alzheimer's, combinations of nutrients. The first group is the Alzheimer's Disease Co-operative Study in the U.S., which is giving Alzheimer's patients large amounts of B vitamins. OPTIMA (see page 401) has started a trial of B vitamins in people with age-related cognitive decline, and, on a smaller scale, Dr. Andrew McCaddon continues his research. It will take some time before we know what the ideal combination and amount of homocysteine-lowering nutrients is, both for prevention and treatment of people with Alzheimer's. OPTIMA is giving 800 mcg of folic acid, 500 mcg of B12 and 20 mg of B6 (that's more than 20 times the RDA), while the U.S. trial is using 5,000 mcg of folic acid, 1,000 mcg of B12 and 50 mg of vitamin B6.

Knowing all this, you'd be crazy not to test your homocysteine level, and if it's high, change your diet and lifestyle and take homocysteine-lowering supplements, supplementing the amounts shown in Chapter 8.

The current vogue in medicine is just to recommend folic acid. But while it's been described in the *British Medical Journal* as "the leading contender for panacea of the 21st century," folic acid alone is far less effective than the right nutrients in combination. The amount you need also depends on your current homocysteine level. One study found that homocysteine scores reduced by 17 percent on high-dose folic acid alone; 19 percent on vitamin B12 alone; 57 percent on folic acid plus B12; and 60 percent on folic acid, B12, and B6.[70] All this was achieved in three weeks. However, even better results would have been achieved by including TMG, the best methyl donor to supplement, even better than SAMe (see page 72). This is because only it can immediately donate a methyl group to homocysteine, thus detoxifying it.

In a study in New Zealand, the homocysteine scores of patients with chronic kidney failure and very high homocysteine levels were reduced by a further 18 percent when 4g of TMG was given, along with 50 mg of vitamin B6 and 5,000 mcg of folate, compared to patients taking just B6 and folate.[71] At the Brain Bio Centre we achieve, on average, over 70 percent reductions in high homocysteine scores in eight weeks with the combination of these nutrients plus an optimal diet.

Some companies produce combinations of these nutrients (see Product and Supplement Directory, page 486). These are the most cost-effective supplements for restoring a healthy homocysteine level.

Memory-boosting foods

Of course, the key B vitamins are also found in food, along with many other brain-friendly nutrients. A study led by Professor Maria Corrada at the University of California, Irvine, collected data on 579 men and women aged 60 and over who participated in the Baltimore Longitudinal Study of Aging. The people in this study had kept track of what they ate and what supplements they took. Nine years later, Corrada's team looked at the number of people who developed Alzheimer's (57) and the differences in their intake of nutrients, from diet and supplements, compared to those who didn't develop the disease. Compared with those who developed the disease, study participants with the highest folate had a 55 percent reduced risk of developing Alzheimer's.[72]

The vital keys to keeping your mind and memory sharp are to have a high dietary intake of B vitamins, found in whole foods, especially beans and greens (the best food sources of folate); lots of antioxidants, found in fruit and vegetables; a daily source of omega-3 fats, found in fish particularly, and seeds; and phospholipids, found in eggs. This Mediterranean-style diet has been shown to substantially reduce the risk of developing Alzheimer's.[73]

Eating fish just once a week, for instance, reduces the risk of developing Alzheimer's by 60 percent, according to a recent study by Dr. Martha Morris and colleagues from Chicago's Rush Institute for Healthy Aging. They followed 815 people, aged 65–94 years, for 7 years and found that dietary intake of fish was strongly linked to the risk of developing Alzheimer's. The strongest link, they found, was the amount of the omega-3 DHA, which is abundant in certain fish. The more DHA the person consumed, the lower their risk of developing Alzheimer's. The lowest amount of DHA per day that offered some protection was 100 mg. The level of the omega-3 EPA a person took in did not affect Alzheimer's risk, however, below 30 mg a day. The ongoing Hordaland Health Survey in Norway, involving more than 18,000 men and women since 1992, has also found that the higher the oily fish intake, the lower the risk of developing dementia or Alzheimer's. This certainly implies that three servings of oily fish a week help protect your brain.

But what about supplements of essential fats? Can they prevent or reverse this condition? The truth is that we don't yet know. One randomized trial found a small effect of omega-3 on very mild dementia.[74] This is encouraging but not conclusive. However, I would personally recommend taking a basic supplement of omega-3 fish oil providing 400 mg of combined EPA and DHA as a likely optimal intake, as well as eating oily fish three times a week as an insurance policy.

A study published in the *Journal of the American Medical Association* found that the risk of developing Alzheimer's was 67 percent lower in those with a high dietary intake of vitamin E, found in fish, and seeds, and their oils, versus those with a low intake. A recent study involving 4,000 people age 65 or older found a 78 percent reduction in the risk of developing Alzheimer's in those supplementing both vitamin E and C. Taking one and not the other didn't reduce the risk. The best results were achieved with 1,000 mg of vitamin C and 1,000 IU of vitamin E.

Use your body—and don't lose your mind

With the right nutrition and the right attitude, age-related memory loss doesn't need to happen to you. You can build new brain cells at any age. Research clearly shows that healthy, well-educated elderly people can show no decline in mental function right up to death, and no increased rate of brain shrinkage even after 65. As we saw in the last chapter, there is also plenty of evidence that keeping both your mind and body active will help to prevent decline in mental function. For example, researchers at the Albert Einstein College of Medicine in New York have tested the link between leisure activities and the risk of memory loss in the elderly. They studied 469 people over the age of 75 over a period of five years, and found that reading, playing cards and board games, doing crossword puzzles, playing musical instruments, and dancing were all associated with a reduced risk of dementia, memory loss, and Alzheimer's. Overall, the study participants who did these kinds of activities about four days a week were two-thirds less likely to get Alzheimer's compared with those who did these activities once a week or less.

But it's not just your brain that needs a workout. Physical exercise has a direct effect on mental powers, probably for a number of reasons. First, since brain and body are made up of the same stuff, and we know that exercise keeps your body healthy, it stands to reason that exercise will keep your brain healthy too. Also, people at greater risk of cardiovascular disease are at greater risk of Alzheimer's. Secondly, part of the benefit of exercise is likely to be because exercise reduces stress. Thirdly, exercise increases blood flow to the brain, bringing more oxygen and nutrients.[75–76] And lastly, there is evidence that being overweight increases the risk of Alzheimer's, so part of the positive effect of exercise is likely to be that it helps you keep to a healthy weight.

The importance of keeping fit was highlighted in a five-year study of 5,000 Canadian men and women over the age of 65, published in 2001. Those who had high levels of physical activity, compared to those who rarely exercised, halved their risk of Alzheimer's disease.[77] Another study, from 1995, found that regular walking improved memory and reduced signs of dementia. About 1,000 steps, or a little over a mile a day, was the minimum distance required to achieve the positive effect.[78]

But the most convincing evidence for the value of exercise comes from a six-year study, published in 2006, of 1,740 elderly people. Those who exercised three or more times a week had a 30–40 percent lower risk for developing dementia, compared with those who exercised fewer than three times per week.[79]

Exercise also prevents physical deterioration of the brain. Our brains become less dense and lose volume as we age and with that loss of density and volume comes mental decline. Researchers at the University of Illinois used MRI scans to examine the brains of 55 elderly people. When they compared their scans with their level of physical exercise they found that the people who exercised more and were more physically fit had the densest brains.[80] So the old saying "Use it or lose it" takes on greater significance in this context. Basically, if you don't use your body, you're at risk of losing your mind.

Exercise is not only protective against Alzheimer's, it can also lift your mood. In fact, it's more effective than antidepressants for mild depression, as we've seen. Depression is a common problem among Alzheimer's patients. A 2003 study at the University of Washington in Seattle showed that exercise significantly improved the mood and physical health of depressed Alzheimer's patients and meant they were less likely to need to be moved into a nursing home.[81]

SUMMARY

Here are my 10 top tips to keep your memory and mind sharp and minimize your risk of ever developing Alzheimer's:

- Eat fish and seeds high in essential omega-3 fats. Have wild or organic salmon, herring, sardines, or mackerel three times a week; sprinkle ground flaxseeds on your cereal; and snack on pumpkin seeds.

- Eat eggs, high in the *smart fats* phospholipids. The best eggs are omega-3-rich eggs, from chickens fed flaxseeds. Lecithin, which you can buy in health food stores in either capsules or granules, is high in phospholipids. Sprinkle 2 teaspoons on your cereal. Some brain-food supplements provide phosphatidylcholine, the most important phospholipid.

- Eat complex carbohydrates such as oat-based cereals, oatmeal cookies, whole-wheat pasta and brown basmati rice.

- Eat vitamin, mineral, and antioxidant-rich foods such as berries, and dark green, leafy, and root vegetables such as kale, spinach, watercress, carrots, sweet potatoes, broccoli, Brussels sprouts, green beans, or peppers. Also consider taking an antioxidant supplement, providing vitamins A, C, and E, as well as coenzyme Q10, lipoic acid, glutathione, or N-acetyl cysteine.

- Avoid hydrogenated (solidified) fats found in junk food, and burned fats such as are found in fried food, as well as sugar and excess caffeine and alcohol.

- Take a high-strength multivitamin, with vitamins E and C, and at least 20 mg of vitamin B6, 10 mcg of B12, and 250 mcg of folic acid.

▶

- Test your homocysteine level. If it's above 6 also supplement a homocysteine formula. If it's above 7, take 2 a day. If it's above 9 take 4 a day, and if your homocysteine level is above 15 take 6 a day. Retest yourself two months later, and reduce your supplements accordingly.

- Use your brain. Play games, puzzles, and crosswords frequently. Learn a new language. Keep learning throughout your life.

- Keep physical. If walking is your exercise, walk a mile a day. Ideally, take up an exercise that helps develop yogic breathing, such as yoga, t'ai chi or psychocalisthenics. Dancing to music helps to improve memory.

- Make sure you get enough light. Spend some time outdoors most days. Use full-spectrum lighting. Have a sunny holiday in the winter.

Dig deeper by reading *The Alzheimer's Prevention Plan: 10 Proven Ways to Stop Memory Decline and Reduce the Risk of Alzheimer's* by Patrick Holford, Shane Heaton, and Deborah Colson.

CHAPTER 38

Smart drugs and hormones

I'm a purist. **I believe in nutrients** that are part of our evolutionary design, tried and tested over thousands of years. But what if there were drugs or hormones that were safe and did enhance mental performance, or help restore or retain it? What if there were drugs and hormones that could reverse mental decline above and beyond the positive effects of nutrients? The truth is there are and, especially in situations of memory decline in old age, they are well worth considering.

What are smart drugs?

Over a hundred smart drugs have already been developed, and once age-related memory decline becomes a classified disease there is no doubt that such drugs will become very widely used in society. Some have also been shown to enhance mental abilities in those without diagnosed memory problems. This raises the important question of whether some of these drugs fit the category of natural highs in the sense of improving mental ability without a downside, or whether their use should be restricted to those with cognitive problems.

For the pharmaceuticals industry, the advantage of these drugs is that they are not nutrients but in most cases man-made substances—that is, they can be patented and hence are more profitable. The disadvantage of such man-made chemicals is that they are alien to the human body. They may not produce a perfect fit in enzyme systems and while creating the desired effect in the short term, may, in the long term, unbalance the brain's sensitive chemistry. In any case, with many of these new smart drugs, the long-term effects are still unknown, so it is best to proceed with caution.

Smart drugs tend to fall into one of three categories:

- Drugs which block the breakdown of neurotransmitters, thereby keeping more of these information molecules in circulation. These include Deprenyl, Aricept, and huperzine A.

- Drugs which mimic or improve the action of neurotransmitters. These include piracetam, Hydergine, and Dilantin.

- Hormones that influence brain function. These include DHEA, pregnenolone, progesterone, and melatonin.

These are by no means the only smart drugs and hormones, but they are among the most interesting, well researched, and widely taken, with a track record of relative safety. They therefore have a potential role in restoring an active memory and mind, if not promoting it.

More mileage from your neurotransmitters

Deprenyl, also called selegiline, is part of a group of drugs called monoamino-oxidase inhibitors, or MAOIs for short. They work as antidepressants by preventing neurotransmitters from being broken down. Most of these drugs, however, are MAO-A inhibitors, and as such are associated with potentially dangerous side effects. Deprenyl, on the other hand, does not cause this effect, since it is an MAO-B inhibitor.[82]

Deprenyl is particularly effective at stopping the breakdown of dopamine, a deficiency of which is associated with Parkinson's disease. It is mainly prescribed for the treatment of both Parkinson's and Alzheimer's disease. Some people recommend taking it to prevent these diseases and as a general stimulant to mental functioning, even when no symptoms are present. In animals it has also been shown to extend lifespan.[83] Deprenyl has a better track record in terms of toxic effects than a number of MAOI drugs, which can have unpleasant side effects.

Research by the National Institutes of Health in the U.S. has shown that 10 mg of Deprenyl does significantly improve memory, attention span, and learning in people with Alzheimer's.[84] To what extent it makes a difference in normal people is a subject of controversy. If you want to experiment, start with 1–2 mg and build up to 5 mg. If you experience insomnia, lower the dose. Deprenyl is available on prescription as Eldepryl, while the liquid form (Deprenyl citrate) can be ordered by post.

Aricept (donepezil) is a drug widely prescribed for people with Alzheimer's. It works by inhibiting the enzyme acetylcholinestase, which breaks down acetylcholine, hence keeping more of this important memory neurotransmitter in circulation. There are other drugs that do this such as Cognex (tacrine), but most have very unpleasant side effects. Aricept is perhaps the best drug in this class, but it is neither side-effect free nor recommended for those without serious memory problems. A better bet is the plant product *Huperzia serrata*.

Huperzia serrata, a moss used for centuries in China, contains an alkaloid called huperzine A, which is also a powerful and highly selective acetylcholinesterase inhibitor, working like the anti-Alzheimer's drug Aricept to keep more acetylcholine in circulation. *Huperzia serrata* has been reported to have fewer side effects than such drugs and may work in a more natural way. It also protects against the toxic effects of glutamate (such as MSG). The recommended daily dose is 200 mcg.

Nootropics: your brain's best friends?

Piracetam is one of a number of new drugs called nootropics, which are related to the amino acid pyroglutamate. Over 150 studies have been published on piracetam, which has been shown to have a broad effect on enhancing mental performance. Numerous studies have shown improvements in memory, concentration, coordination, and reaction time.[85] The drug is also being used with reasonable success in the treatment of Alzheimer's, although it is more effective in the early stages of memory decline.

One such study tested the effects of piracetam on 18 people aged 50 and older, with demanding jobs and above-average IQs, who were basically fully functional except that they were having problems retaining and recalling memory. They were extensively tested for cognitive function and assigned to the piracetam or placebo group, without them or the researchers knowing who was on the real thing. On retesting those taking piracetam, they had significantly improved on a number of cognitive tests. These people were then put on a placebo, while those previously on a placebo were given piracetam. Again, the piracetam group improved dramatically while those on the placebo did not.[86] Another double-blind placebo trial involved 162 French people aged 55 and over with age-related memory decline who had sought help from their doctor. With the group taking piracetam, it proved effective after six weeks.[87] These are just a couple of several convincing studies that have led to piracetam being widely prescribed. Nootropil, one brand of piracetam, has registered sales of over a billion dollars in recent years.

So, how does piracetam work? It seems to promote memory retention, improve acetylcholine transmission and reception, reduce the effects of stress, and speed up reaction time. Part of its mode of action is that it improves communication across the corpus callosum, which connects the two hemispheres of the brain, hence improving the link between our analytical and relational thinking processes, most helpful for storing and finding memories.

Piracetam is, by all accounts, very safe and has no side effects at effective doses. It usually comes in 800 mg capsules, and the recommended dose is three to six capsules per day (2,400–4,800 mg). Since positive effects may only occur at higher doses, my recommendation is to start with 4,800 mg for two weeks, then reduce the dose to 2,400 mg or whatever level continues to be effective. Piracetam is far more effective if given with choline. Piracetam is available on prescription in the U.S., or without prescription from overseas.

Hydergine is the most widely used and thoroughly tested prescription drug for improving brain function. It is ergoloid mesylate, an extract of the ergot fungus that grows on rye and was discovered in the 1950s by Albert Hoffman, who is better known for his discovery of that other ergot-based drug, LSD. The way it works is by improving circulation to the brain and protecting against oxidant damage. It also seems to improve the production of neurotransmitters, especially dopamine, noradrenalin, and acetylcholine, and stabilizes the brain's glucose metabolism. In 1994 researchers from the University of California reviewed the results of 47 trials testing Hydergine for its effects on reversing memory loss in those with dementia. The majority of these studies proved effective, although it was little help to those with Alzheimer's.[88]

There is also some evidence that Hydergine improves memory in healthy people. In a U.K. study, 12 volunteers without cognitive problems were given cognitive tests before and after receiving 12 mg of Hydergine for two weeks. The results showed significant improvement in their alertness and cognitive abilities.[89] The usual dose for Hydergine is 9 mg, given as 3 mg three times a day. It appears to be non-toxic although there are rare reports of nausea and headaches that do not occur at lower doses.

Dilantin (phenytoin), which first became popular as an anti-seizure drug, has been found to improve concentration, response time, mental performance, and mood. It seems to normalize the electrical activity of the brain and may be especially helpful for those who have difficulty focusing. It was made popular by stockmarket mogul Jack Dreyfus, known as the "lion of Wall Street."

Later in life Dreyfus suffered from crippling anxiety and depression and described his brain as a "bunch of dry twigs." Fearful or angry thoughts set the twigs alight, so to speak, and he couldn't stop these negative thoughts spreading like wildfire. Then he discovered Dilantin, which he described as "gentle rain" keeping his excessive thoughts under control. He went on to fund substantial research that has proven that Dilantin can be very helpful for those people who are unfocused, easily distracted, short-tempered, impulsive, and obsessive. It has now been used for years and is free from side effects, at least at a low dose, and non-addictive and doesn't have the sedating effects of tranquilizers. The recommended dose is 100 mg, one to three times a day. It is available on prescription.

A smarter hormone

One step closer to nature is the use of smart hormones. These are naturally occurring hormones that have an effect on performance. In this category come melatonin, pregnenolone, and DHEA. In the U.S., these natural hormones are sold over the counter to deal with anything from jetlag to life extension. In the U.K. and most other countries they are only available on prescription.

DHEA and pregnenolone are naturally occurring hormones but that certainly doesn't make them harmless. As you can see from Figure 36, they can, if needed, be turned into estrogen and testosterone. Pregnenolone can also be turned into progesterone and adrenal hormones. So they can have a powerful effect on the balance of sex hormones, as well adrenal hormones which are involved in the stress response. Low levels of estrogen, progesterone, and adrenal hormones are all associated with declining memory.

Both DHEA and pregnenolone levels tend to decrease with age and the simplistic view is that supplementing them will stop the aging process. The trouble is, having more than you need means the body has to work hard to get rid of the excess. For these hormones, more is not necessarily better. While potentially useful for those with adrenal exhaustion, blood-sugar problems and hormonal imbalances, they are not recommended for supplementation except under the guidance of a health practitioner. Before and after tests should be carried out to determine whether or not there is a deficiency, in which case correcting it is likely to improve mental functioning. The older you are, the more likely you are to have low levels of DHEA and pregnelonone. For this reason, many older people in the U.S. supplement up to 25 mg of pregnenolone or 15 mg of DHEA a day. More than this is unwise without proper testing. DHEA and pregnenolone should be taken in the morning, before breakfast.

Melatonin became famous as the answer to jetlag. It is a hormone produced by the pineal gland, the master gland of the endocrine system, which conducts the orchestra of other hormone-producing glands that control blood-sugar levels, stress reactions, sex hormones, calcium balance, and other critical processes in the body.

The pineal gland also acts as a biological clock, secreting melatonin during the night. Long-distance traveling upsets this system and can result in jetlag symptoms—fatigue, fuzzy thinking, insomnia, and headaches. By taking melatonin in the evening in the new time zone, many people experience a substantial reduction in these symptoms.[90] More controversial is the recommendation to take melatonin for depression, for memory enhancement, or for extending lifespan. Given at the wrong time of day it can worsen mental functioning, creating the equivalent of jetlag. Taken at night it tends to promote calmness and sleep. However, it appears to work only if you have low levels of melatonin.[91–92]

Of all the smart hormones, it's melatonin I recommend using with the most caution, except possibly for seasonally affected depression (SAD) and short-term use in correcting jetlag. In these situations, 1.5–3 mg in the evening may be worth experimenting with, under the guidance of a health practitioner. Some people supplement 25 mg of melatonin a day, in the evening, and report benefits, but this certainly doesn't suit everybody and I would urge caution.

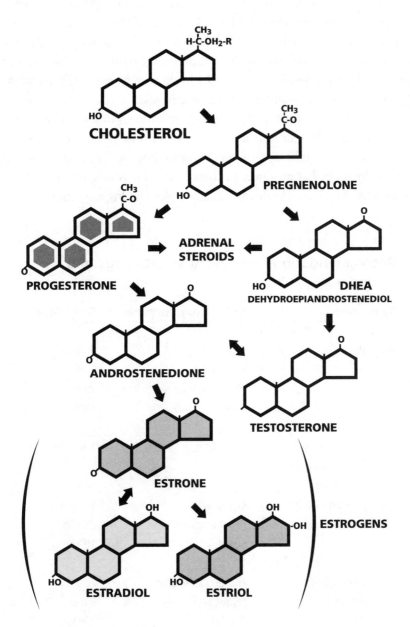

Fig 36. The hormone family tree

But do you need them?

As attractive as smart drugs and hormones might seem, my recommendation is not to take them, at least not in the first instance. In many cases, the combination of mind- and memory-enhancing nutrients as discussed in the last two chapters, does the trick. However, if these steps alone do not produce the effect you are after, and you suffer from the symptoms described below, you may wish to experiment with the following smart drugs and hormones. I recommend you do so with the guidance of your doctor or a suitably qualified health practitioner.

My recommendation under any circumstance is to start with no more than one smart drug or hormone, at the lower dose (with the exception of piracetam), and build up gradually, noting how you respond, and stopping at the dose that produces the best results for you. Then add others as required. Please check with your doctor before taking any smart drug.

Recommendations for taking smart drugs and hormones

Symptoms	Smart drug/hormone	Daily dose
Poor memory	Piracetam	2,400–4,800 mg
	Hydergine	3–6 mg
	Pregnenolone	25 mg
	DHEA	15 mg
Poor focus, obsessive and excess thoughts	Dilantin	100–300 mg
Lack of brain energy, mental slowdown	Deprenyl	1–10 mg
	Pregnenolone	25 mg
	DHEA	15 mg
Pronounced memory loss, dementia	*Huperzia serrata*	200 mcg
	Hydergine	9 mg
	Piracetam	4,800 mg

	Pregnenolone	25 mg
	DHEA	15 mg
Alzheimer's	Deprenyl	10 mg
	Huperzia serrata	200 mcg
	Piracetam	4,800 mg
	Pregnenolone	25 mg
	DHEA	15 mg

PART 8

Action Plan for Mental Health

CHAPTER 39

Finding help

The maxim that ricochets throughout this book is "Treat the cause, not the symptom." Most drug treatments fail to do this. Major tranquilizers may sedate a person to the point where they are less of a problem to themselves or others, but they're not addressing the cause. The same can be said for antidepressants. If you are depressed because your serotonin levels are low, then the causes of this need to be addressed.

Treating the cause, not the symptoms, is easier to say than do, especially in the area of mental health. Often there are many causes. And often there are subtle interplays between psychological problems and physical/chemical problems. A psychological problem can change our behavior around nourishing ourselves, or misusing mind-altering substances, leading to a chemical imbalance in the brain that makes the psychological problem worse.

I never cease to be amazed at the mind-body link, at what the body says about our minds. The person with a backache who needs to stand up for themselves. A person with sinus problems who can't breathe, and needs to make space in their life for themselves. A person with digestive problems who is fed up with their life and job.

Digging a bit deeper, there's the subject of this book—how our nutrition and biochemical imbalances affect how we think and feel. Depression, anxiety, and memory problems are all linked to what we eat. But, of course, the link isn't obvious. Often it's only after years of faulty nutrition that mental health symptoms emerge.

That's why I strongly recommend that anyone with mental health issues see both a professional nutritional therapist or doctor specializing in this area, who can assess all the possible underlying physical/chemical causes, and a professional psychotherapist who can delve into underlying psychological issues that may have a bearing on how you think and feel. Rarely can one person be a master of both domains. If you are suffering from a more serious mental health problem you will also be seeing a doctor or psychiatrist. This is your team to help you get back on the road, firing on all cylinders. And as you've seen here, there are many thousands of people with a vast range of conditions who have managed just that.

Finding a nutritional therapist

The good news is that help is widely available throughout Britain, and in many other countries. Nutritional therapists, well qualified to assess these areas of imbalance, are available in most cities and major towns. Since 1984, at the Institute for Optimum Nutrition, we've been training an army of nutritional therapists who can help you tune up your body and brain so you can experience your full potential. Not all nutritional therapists or dietitians have experience in the cutting edge of mental health and nutrition, so it's worth asking them if they can help you.

You can find your nearest nutritional therapist or doctor specializing in this area by visiting www.foodforthebrain.org. If you can come to London, you can visit our Brain Bio Centre clinic at the Institute for Optimum Nutrition in Richmond.

Finding a psychotherapist

Psychotherapists and counselors are also widely available all over Britain and other countries. The training to be a psychotherapist takes longer than that for counselors. That said, there are many great and well-qualified counselors. Again, it is well worth asking them whether they feel they can help you with the problem you are dealing with. Some have experience with more profound mental health issues than others.

There are different types of psychotherapy. Three often promising approaches are cognitive-behavior therapy, which helps change the way you think and therefore feel; interpersonal therapy, which works on communication in relationships; and problem-solving therapy, dealing with underlying issues that may be contributing to your problems. Then there's the transpersonal approach. This is a conceptual approach to psychological issues that includes the spiritual and therefore considers the deeper-meaning issues that often underlie chronic depression, anxiety, and schizophrenia. Often, breakdowns are, at one level, spiritual crises and it is good to work with a psychotherapist or counselor who has this level of understanding. When you're looking for a therapist you can ask them whether they have a transpersonal approach. In the U.K., two of the best transpersonal training colleges are the Psychosynthesis and Education Trust and the College of Counselling, Psychotherapy, and Education. They also have referral services. Details for finding a psychotherapist trained psychosynthesis in the U.S. are given in Useful Addresses on page 474.

Halfway houses and hospitals

If you are more seriously in need of help, you may be hospitalized in the short term, then possibly recommended to a number of halfway houses, often run by local charities.

Hospitals seldom follow the directions of nutritional therapists. Often, the best strategy for an optimum nutrition program is to have a person's daily supplements packaged into individual packets and given every day. Sometimes there is resistance to this, which is why your nutritional therapist must work with your psychiatrist to give you the best possible treatment. What's more, hospital diets usually include wheat, sugar, dairy produce, and large amounts of tea and coffee, none of which is going to aid recovery.

We badly need suitable alternatives to hospitalization. The alternatives may range from halfway houses to treatment in the home under the guidance of a home health aide and nutritional therapist. Parents or relatives can also give support in following an optimum nutrition strategy.

Right now there are few options available for halfway houses amenable to administering the optimum nutrition approach. The good news is that there are initiatives in some areas to get such halfway houses set up. The

Food for the Brain Foundation's website (www.foodforthebrain.org) gives an up-to-date list of what is available.

A halfway house takes years of effort to establish. The usual population of patients at any one time will vary from 6–20. Plans must be made for proper food, non-allergic housing, daily care and exercise, and discharge of patients. The houses should be organized as not-for-profit units and should receive help from government bodies or annual donations from benefactors. In the U.S., the insurance companies should pay for this care as they do for hospital care, especially since this approach is so much cheaper in the long run, as it helps get people back into the community. Some voluntary help can be used to ease the great financial burden.

I believe the future of mental healthcare will be best served by having doctors working closely with nutritional therapists and psychotherapists, with halfway houses offering people a chance to rebalance their psyche, their body and brain, with healthy eating, exercising, and psychological support. Once achieved, most people can find their way back into the world and lead a meaningful existence.

CHAPTER 40

The brain-friendly diet in a nutshell

The starting point for tuning up your brain is to follow an optimum nutrition diet and take daily supplements. Even if you have no mental health problem as such, this regime can increase your mental energy, improve your mood, and sharpen your mind. Here are the ten golden rules to follow to make sure your diet is maximizing your mental health:

- Eat whole foods—whole grains, lentils, beans, nuts, seeds, fresh fruit, and vegetables—and avoid refined, white, and overcooked foods.

- Eat five or more servings of fruits and vegetables per day. Choose dark green, leafy and root vegetables such as watercress, carrots, sweet potatoes, broccoli, Brussels sprouts, spinach, green beans, or peppers, raw or lightly cooked. Choose fresh fruit such as apples, pears, berries, melon, or citrus fruit. Have bananas in moderation. Dilute fruit juices and only eat dried fruits infrequently in small quantities, preferably soaked.

- Eat four or more servings per day of whole grains such as brown basmati rice, millet, rye, oats, whole wheat, corn, or quinoa as cereal, breads, and pasta.

- Avoid any form of sugar, and foods with added sugar.

- Combine protein foods with carbohydrate foods by eating cereals and fruit with nuts or seeds, and ensuring you eat starch foods (potato, bread, pasta, or rice) with fish, lentils, beans, or tofu.

- Eat coldwater carnivorous fish. A serving of herring, mackerel, organic or wild salmon, or fresh sardines two or three times a week (or fresh, not canned, tuna once a month), provides a good source of omega-3 fats—or good vegetable protein sources, including beans, lentils, quinoa, tofu (soy) and seed vegetables such as corn. If eating animal protein, choose lean meat or preferably fish, organic whenever possible.

- Eat eggs—preferably free-range, organic, and high in omega-3s.

- Eat seeds and nuts. The best seeds are flax, hemp, pumpkin, sunflower, and sesame. You get more goodness out of them by grinding them first and sprinkling on cereal, soups, and salads.

- Use cold-pressed seed oils. Choose an oil blend containing flaxseed oil or hemp oil for salad dressings and cold uses, such as drizzling on vegetables instead of butter.

- Minimize your intake of fried food, processed food, and saturated fat from meat and dairy products.

CHAPTER 41

Brain-friendly supplements

The brain uses about a third of all nutrients taken in from food. If you follow the brain-friendly diet described in the last chapter you will be maximizing your intake of nutrients from your food. In addition, there is great benefit to be had by taking the following supplements on a daily basis to ensure optimum nutrition for your mind.

- Supplement a multivitamin and mineral that gives you at least 25 mg of all the B vitamins, 10 mcg of B12, 100 mcg of folic acid, 200 mg of magnesium, 3 mg of manganese, and 10 mg of zinc.

- Supplement fish oil for omega-3 fats and borage or evening primrose oil for omega-6 fats.

- Supplement a brain-food formula providing phosphatidylcholine and phosphatidylserine, plus other brain-friendly nutrients such as DMAE and pyroglutamate.

- Add a tablespoon of lecithin granules, or a heaping teaspoon of phosphatidylcholine lecithin to your cereal every day.

- Consider supplementing some free-form amino acids, or individual amino acids if you have a related mental health problem.

In addition, you may choose to add the supplemental recommendations in chapters whose content specifically applied to you. Ensure that these recommended amounts of the specified nutrients are included in your daily supplement program. See the Product and Supplement Directory on page 486. Wherever possible we recommend consultation with a qualified practitioner, who can run the appropriate tests, rather than self-supplementation.

Last word

This book is about an idea whose time has come. Such ideas tend to go through three stages.

First, the powers that be say it is not true and not important. This denial of the importance of optimum nutrition for the mind was the hallmark of the 1980s, and it only began to be shattered with the advent of our research on vitamins and IQ.

During stage two, they say it's true, but it's not important. That's where we are now. No one in their right mind can deny the overwhelming evidence, presented in this book, that optimizing your nutrient intake can both prevent and reverse mental health problems, as well as improve mental performance and emotional balance.

Finally, they say it's true, and it's important—but it's not new! I can't wait for this day, when children with ADHD are first treated nutritionally and supported psychologically before any stimulant drug is doled out. Or, in fact, the day when schools support children's development with healthy food. I welcome the day when GPs explain the simple diet, supplement, and lifestyle changes that we already know are at least, if not more effective, then certainly less dangerous than today's antidepressant drugs. I anticipate the day when those diagnosed with schizophrenia are thoroughly investigated for biochemical imbalances and helped, through personalized nutrition and counseling support, to come back to life, instead of being imprisoned in the chemical straitjacket of the major tranquilizers. I also look forward to the day when the role of nutrition in mental health is on the curriculum of every medical school and every school of psychotherapy.

Humanity as a whole is having a hard time adapting to this extraordinary period of rapid change. The future is coming at us like a freight train. Time is compressing, demands are increasing. We are being stretched to our limits as a species. We need all the help we can get. Optimum nutrition isn't a luxury. It's a necessity if you want to stay healthy and happy and keep your mind intact in the 21st century.

Wishing you the best of health.

Patrick Holford

References
and Resources

References

Part 1: Food for Thought (Chapters 1–8)

1. Institute for Optimum Nutrition, *ONUK Survey*, 2004. See www.ion.ac.uk
2. F. Matthews and C. Brayne, "The incidence of dementia in England and Wales: Findings from the five identical sites of the MRC CFA Study," *PLos Med*, Vol 2(8), 2005, p. e193. See www.plosmedicine.org for free access to the article
3. House of Commons Education and Skills Committee, "Special educational needs: Third report of session 2005–06," Vol 1, p. 9
4. G. Baird et al., "Prevalence of disorders of the autism spectrum in a population cohort of children in South Thames: The Special Needs and Autism Project (SNAP)," *Lancet*, Vol 368(9531), 2006, pp. 210–5
5. U.S. National Center for Health Statistics, *Health, United States, 2004*, NCHS, Hyattsville, Maryland, 2004
6. World Health Organization, *The World Health Report 2001—Mental Health: New Understanding, New Hope*. See www.who.int/whr/2001/
7. D. Benton and G. Roberts, "Effect of vitamin and mineral supplementation on intelligence of school children," *Lancet*, Vol 1(8578), 1998, pp. 140–3
8. T.H. Crook et al., "Effects of phosphatidylserine in Alzheimer's disease," *Psychopharmacol Bull*, Vol 28, 1992, pp. 61–6
9. Survey by Dr. Bernard Rimland. See www.autism.com/ari
10. C. Birmingham et al., "Controlled trial of zinc supplementation in anorexia nervosa," *Int J Eat Disord*, Vol 15 (3), 1994, pp. 251–5
11. A. Hoffer, "Chronic schizophrenic patients treated ten years or more," *J Orthomolecular Medicine*, Vol 9, 1994, pp. 7–37 and *Vitamin B3 and Schizophrenia: Discovery, Recovery, Controversy*, Quarry Press (2000)
12. W. Poldinger et al., "A functional-dimensional approach to depression: serotonin

deficiency and target syndrome in a comparison of 5-hydroxytryptophan and fluvoxamine," *Psychopathology*, Vol 24(2), 1991, pp. 53–81

13. B. Gesch, "Influence of supplementary vitamins, minerals and essential fatty acids on the antisocial behavior of young adult prisoners," *Brit J Psychiatry*, Vol 181, 2002, pp. 22–8

14. J. Durga et al., "Folate and the methylenetetrahydrofolate reductase: Mutation correlate with cognitive performance," *Neurobiol Aging*, Vol 27(2), 2006, pp. 334–43

15. B. Nemets et al., "Addition of omega-3 fatty acid to maintenance medication treatment for recurrent unipolar depressive disorder," *Am J Psychiatry*, Vol 159, 2002, pp. 477–9

16. A. Schauss, "Nutrition and behavior: complex interdisciplinary research," *Nutr Health*, Vol 3(1–2), 1984, pp. 9–37

17. D. Benton, "The impact of the supply of glucose to the brain on mood and memory," *Nutr Rev*, Vol 59(1 Pt 2), 2001, p. S20–1

18. R. Dykman and R.T. Pivik, *Pediatric Academic Society*, Vol 5, 2002, pp. 453

19. T. Jones et al., "Enhanced adrenomedullary response and increased susceptibility to neuroglycopenia: Mechanisms underlying the adverse effects of sugar ingestion in healthy children," *J Pediatr*, Vol 126(2), 1995, pp. 171–7

20. M. Haapalahti et al., "Food habits in 10–11-year-old children with functional gastrointestinal disorders," *Eur J Clin Nutr*, (58)7, 2004, pp. 1016–21

21. R.G. Walton et al., "Adverse reactions to aspartame: Double blind challenge in patients from a vulnerable population," *J Biol Psychiatry*, Vol 34(1–2), 1993, pp. 13–17

22. K.A. Wesnes et al., "Breakfast reduces declines in attention and memory over the morning in schoolchildren," *Appetite*, Vol 41, 2003, pp. 329–31

23. S. E. Carlson et al., "Long-term feeding of formulas high in linolenic acid and marine oil to very low birth weight infants: phospholipid fatty acids," *Pediatr Res*, Vol 30, 1991, pp. 404–12

24. P. Willatts et al., "The role of long-chain polyunsaturated fatty acids in infant cognitive development," *Prostaglandins Leukot Essent Fatty Acids*, Vol 63(1–2), 2000, pp. 95–100

25. A. Ghys et al., "Red blood cell and plasma phospholipid arachidonic and docosahexaenoic acid levels at birth and cognitive development at 4 years of age," *Early Hum Dev*, Vol 69(1–2), 2002, pp. 83–90

26. M. Morris, "Docosahexaenoic acid and Alzheimer disease," *Arch Neurol*, Vol 63, 2006, pp. 1545–50

27. *New Scientist*, 26 June 1995

28. D. Horrobin, "Essential fatty acids, prostaglandins and schizophrenia," *Proceedings of the World Congress of Psychiatry*, October 1989

29. D. Horrobin et al., "Essential fatty acids in plasma phospholipids in schizophrenia," *Biol Psychiatry*, Vol 25, 1989, pp. 562–8

30. C. Bates et al., "Fatty acids in plasma phospholipids and cholesterol esters from identical twins concordant and discordant for schizophrenia," *Schizophr Res*, Vol 6(1), 1991, pp. 1–7

31. H. Kaiya et al., "Essential and other fatty acids in plasma in schizophrenics and normal individuals from Japan," *Biol Psychiatry*, Vol 30(4), 1991, pp. 357–62

32. K.S. Vaddadi et al., "A double blind trial of essential fatty acid supplementation in patients with tardive dyskenesia," *Psychiatric Res*, Vol 27, 1989, pp. 313–23

33. K.S. Vaddadi, "Use of gamma-linolenic acid in the treatment of schizophrenia and tardive dyskinesia," *Prostaglandins Leukot Essent Fatty Acids*, Vol 46(1), 1992, pp. 67–70

34. A. Glen et al., "Essential fatty acids and alcoholism," in D. Horrobin (ed), *Omega-6 Essential Fatty Acids: Pathopsysiology and Roles in Clinical Medicine*, Alan Liss (1990), pp. 321–2

35. A. Glen et al., "The role of essential fatty acids in alcohol dependence and tissue damage," *Alcoholism Clin Exp Res*, Vol 11, 1987, pp. 37–41

36. A. Glen et al., "Possible pharmacological approaches to the prevention and treatment of alcohol-related CNS damage: results of a double blind trial of essential fatty acid," in Edwards et al. (eds), *Pharmacological Treatments for Alcoholism*, Croon Helm (1985), pp. 331–50

37. Skinner et al., 1989, "Repeated automated assessment of abstinent male alcoholics: essential fatty acid supplementation and age effects," *Alcohol Alcoholism*, Vol 24, pp. 129–39

38. A. Glen et al., "Essential fatty acids in the treatment of the alcohol dependence syndrome," in Birch and Lindlay (eds), *Alcoholic Beverages*, Elsevier (1985), pp. 203–21

39. F.M. Corrigan et al., "Essential fatty acids in Alzheimer's disease," *Ann N Y Acad Sci*, Vol 640, 1991, pp. 250–2

40. G. Pyapali et al., "Prenatal dietary choline supplementation," *Journal of Neurophysiology*, Vol 79(4), pp. 1790–6 and W.H. Meck et al., *Neuroreport*, Vol 8, 1998, 1997, pp. 2831–5

41. R.J. Wurtman and S.H. Zeisel, "Brain choline: Its sources and effects on the synthesis and release of acetylcholine," *Aging*, Vol 19, 1982, pp. 303–13

42. S.L. Ladd et al., "Effect of phosphatidylcholine on explicit memory," *Clin Neuropharmacol*, Vol 16(6), 1993, pp. 540–9

43. D. Smith, "Prevention of dementia: A role for B vitamins?," *Nutr Health*, Vol 18(3), 2006, pp. 225–6

44. J. Selhub et al., "Association between plasma homocysteine concentrations and extracranial carotid-artery stenosis," *N Engl J Med*, Vol 332(5), 1995, pp. 286–91

45. T. Crook et al., 1991, "Effects of phosphatidylserine in age-associated memory impairment," *Neurology*, Vol 41(5), pp. 644–9

46. S. Suzuki et al., "Oral administration of soybean lecithin transphosphatidylated phosphatidylserine improves memory impairment in aged rats," *J Nutr*, Vol 131, 2001, pp. 2951–6

47. T. Crook et al., "Effects of phosphatidylserine in age-associated memory impairment," *Neurology*, Vol 41 (5), 1991, pp. 644–9

48. J. Gindin et al., "The effect of plant phosphatidylserine on age-associated memory impairment and mood in the functioning elderly," *Geriatric Institute for Education and Research, and Department of Geriatrics, Kaplan Hospital, Rehovot, Israel*, 1995

49. M. Maggioni et al., "Effects of phosphatidylserine therapy in geriatric subjects with depressive disorders," *Acta Psychiatr Scand*, Vol 81, 1990, pp. 265–70

50. W. Dimpfel et al., "Source density analysis of functional topographical EEG: Monitoring of cognitive drug action," *Eur J Med Res*, Vol 1(6), 1996, pp. 283–90

51. W. Dimpfel et al., "Efficacy of dimethylaminoethanol (DMAE) containing vitamin-mineral drug combination on EEG patterns in the presence of different emotional states," *Eur J Med Res*, Vol 8(5), 2003, pp. 183–91

52. W. Dean, J. Morgenthaler, S. Fowkes, *Smart Drugs II: The next generation*, Smart Publication, 1993. Case reproduced with their kind permission

53. S.Y. Chung et al., "Administration of phosphatidylcholine increases brain acetylcholine concentration and improves memory in mice with dementia," *J Nutr*, Vol 125, 1995, pp. 1484–9

54. S.H. Ferris et al., "Senile dementia. Treatment with Deanol," *J Am Geriatr Soc*, Vol 25, 1977, pp. 241–4

55. R. Alfin-Slater, reported at the International Congress of Nutrition in Kyoto, Japan, 1975

56. M. Kratz, "Dietary cholesterol, atherosclerosis and coronary heart disease," *Handb Exp Pharmacol*, Vol 170, 2005, pp. 195–213

57. S.Y. Chung et al., "Administration of phosphatidylcholine increases brain acetylcholine concentration and improves memory in mice with dementia," *J Nutr*, Vol 125(6), 1995, pp. 1484–9

58. D.J. Canty and S.H. Zeisel, "Lecithin and choline in human health and disease," *Nutr Rev*, Vol 52(10), 1994, pp. 327–39

59. W. Poldinger et al., "A functional-dimensional approach to depression: serotonin deficiency and target syndrome in a comparison of 5-hydroxytryptophan and fluvoxamine," 1991

60. J.B. Deijen et al., "Tyrosine improves cognitive performance and reduces blood pressure in cadets," *Brain Research Bulletin*, Vol 48 (2), 1999, pp. 203–9

61. I.S. Shiah and N. Yatham, "GABA functions in mood disorders: an update and critical review," *Nature Life Sciences*, Vol. 63(15) 1998, pp. 1289–1303

62. K.A. Smith et al, "Relapse of depression after rapid depletion of tryptophan," *Lancet*, Vol. 349, 1997, pp. 915–19

63. J.B. Deijen et al., "Tyrosine improves cognitive performance and reduces blood pressure in cadets," 1999

64. H. Pilch et al., "Piracetam elevates muscarinic cholinergic receptor density in the frontal cortex of aged but not of young mice," *Psychopharmacology*, Vol 94(1), 1988, pp. 74–8

65. D. Benton and G. Roberts, "Effect of vitamin and mineral supplementation on intelligence of school children," *Lancet*, Vol 1(8578), 1988, pp. 140–3

66. A. Lucas, R. Morley and T. Cole, "Randomized trial of early diet in preterm babies and later intelligence quotient," *BMJ*, Vol 317, 28 November 1998, pp. 1481–7

67. D. Benton et al., "The impact of long-term vitamin supplementation on cognitive functioning," *Psychopharmacology (Berl)*, Vol 117(3), 1995, pp. 298–305

68. D. Benton et al., "Thiamine supplementation mood and cognitive functioning," *Psychopharmacology (Berl)*, Vol 129(1), 1997, pp. 66–71

69. S. Loriaux et al., *Psychopharmacology*, Vol 87, 1985, pp. 390–5

70. M. Morris et al., "Dietary niacin and the risk of incident Alzheimer's disease and of cognitive decline," *J Neurol Neurosurg Psychiatry*, Vol 75(8), 2004, pp. 1093–9

71. G. Shor-Posner et al., "Impact of vitamin B6 status on psychological distress in a longitudinal study of HIV-1 infection," *Int J Psychiatry Med*, Vol 24(3), 1994, pp. 209–22

72. B. Rimland et al., "The effect of high doses of vitamin B6 on autistic children: A double-blind crossover study," *Am J Psychiatry*, Vol 135(4), 1978, pp. 472–5

73. S.I. Pfeiffer et al., "Efficacy of vitamin B6 and magnesium in the treatment of autism: A methodology review and summary of outcomes," *J Autism Dev Disord*, Vol 25(5), 1995, pp. 481–93

74. W. McGuiness, Food For the Brain conference, 1–2 October 2006

75. P. Godfrey et al., *Lancet*, Aug 18, 1990, pp. 392–5

76. M.J. Taylor et al., "Folic acid as ultimate in disease prevention: folate also improves mental health," *BMJ*, Vol 328(7442), 2004, pp. 768–9

77. T. Bottiglieri et al., "Homocysteine, folate, methylation, and monoamine metabolism in depression," *J Neurol Neurosurg Psychiatry*, Vol 69(2), 2000, pp. 228–32

78. A. Coppen et al., "Enhancement of the antidepressant action of fluoxitine by folic acid: a randomized: Placebo controlled trial," *J Affect Disord*, Vol 60(2), 2000, pp. 121–130

79. J. Durga et al., "Folate and the methylenetetrahydrofolate reductase: Mutation correlate with cognitive performance," 2006

80. M. Carney, "Serum folate values in 423 psychiatric patients," *Brit Med Journal*, Vol 4, 1967, pp. 512–16

81. R. Carmel et al., "The frequently low cobalamin levels in dementia usually signify treatable metabolic, neurologic and electrophysiologic abnormalities," *Eur J Haemotol*, Vol 54(4), 1995, pp. 245–53

82. Swiecicki et al., *Psychiatria Polska*, Vol 26(5), 1992, pp. 399–409

83. M. Louwman et al., "Signs of impaired cognitive function in adolescents with marginal cobalamin status," *Am J Clin Nutr*, Vol 72, 2000, pp. 762–9

84. J. Greenblatt et al., *Progress in Neuro-Psychopharmacology and Biological Psychiatry*, Vol 18(4), 1994, pp. 647–60

85. G. Milner, *Brit J Psychiat*, Vol 109, 1963, pp. 294–9

86. K. Suboticanec et al., "Vitamin C status in chronic schizophrenia," *Biol Psychiatry*, Vol 28, 1990, pp. 959–66

87. H. Vandercamp, *Int J Neuropsychiatry*, 22 July 1965

88. G.A. Eby and K.L. Eby, "Rapid recovery from major depression using magnesium treatment," *Med Hypotheses*, Vol 67(2), 2006, pp. 362–70

89. P. Alexander, "Serum calcium and magnesium in schizophrenia: relationship to clinical phenomena and neuroleptic treatment," *Br J Psychiatry*, Vol 133, 1978, pp. 143–9

90. C. Pfeiffer and B. Barnes, *International Journal Environmental Studies*, Vol 17, 1981, pp. 43–7

91. C. Pfeiffer and D. Bacchi, "Copper, zinc, manganese, niacin and pyridoxine in the schizophrenias," *Journal of Applied Nutrition*, Vol 27(223), 1975, pp. 9–39

92. B. Aston, *Orthomolecular Psychiatry*, Vol 9, 1980, pp. 237–49

93. J.G. Penland, presentation at Experimental Biology 2005 meeting, San Diego, 4 April 2005

94. A.K. Borjel et al., "Plasma homocysteine levels, MTHFR polymorphisms, and school achievement in a population sample of Swedish children," *Homocysteine Metab*, Vol 1, 2005, p. 4

95. H. Refsum et al., "Folate, vitamin B12, homocysteine, and the MTHFR polymorphism in anxiety and depression: The Hordaland Homocysteine Study," *Arch Gen Psychiatry*, Vol 60, 2003, pp. 618–26

96. D. Smith, "Homocysteine, B vitamins, and cognitive deficit in the elderly," *Am J Clin Nutr*, Vol 75, 2002, pp. 785–6

97. C. Sugden, "One-carbon metabolism in psychiatric illness," *Nutr Res Rev*, Vol 19, 2006, pp. 117–36

98. H. Refsum et al., "The Hordaland Homocysteine Study: A community-based study of homocysteine, its determinants, and associations with disease" *J Nutr*, Vol 136, 2006, pp. 1731S–40S

Part 2: Protecting Your Brain (Chapters 9–12)

1. S. Johnson, "Micronutrient accumulation and depletion in schizophrenia, epilepsy, autism and Parkinson's disease?," *Med Hypotheses*, Vol 56(5), 2002, pp. 641–5

2. S. Beratis et al., 2001, "Factors affecting smoking in schizophrenia," *Compr Psychiatry*, Vol 42(5), pp. 393–402

3. Z. Xu et al., "Fetal and adolescent nicotine administration: effects on CNS serotonergic systems," *Brain Res*, Vol 914(1/2), 2001, pp. 166–78

4. A. Corvin et al., "Cigarette smoking and psychotic symptoms in bipolar affective disorder," *British Journal of Psychiatry*, Vol 179, 2001, pp. 35–8

5. M. Ramirez-Lassepas "Stroke and the aging of the brain and the arteries," *Geriatrics*, Vol 53 Suppl 1, 1998, S44–8

6. A.J. Perkins et al., "Association of antioxidants with memory in a multiethnic elderly sample using the Third National Health and Nutrition Examination Survey," *Am J Epidemiol*, Vol 150(1), 1999, pp. 37–44

7. W.J. Perrig et al., "The relation between antioxidants and memory performance in the old and very old," *J Am Geriatr Soc*, Vol 45(6), 1997, pp. 718–24

8. R.T. Matthews et al., "Coenzyme Q10 administration increases brain mitochondrial concentrations and exerts neuroprotective effects," *Proc Natl Acad Sci*, Vol 95(15), 1998, pp. 8892–7

9. C.W. Shults et al., "Coenzyme Q10 levels correlate with the activities of complexes I and II/III in mitochondria from parkinsonian and nonparkinsonian subjects," *Ann Neurol*, Vol 42(2), 1997, pp. 261–4

10. S.N. Mattson et al., "Teratogenic effects of alcohol on brain and behavior," *Alcohol Res Health*, Vol 25(3), 2001, pp. 185–91

11. L.J. Launer et al., "Smoking, drinking and thinking: the Zutphen Elderly Study," *Am J Epidemiol*, Vol 143(3), 1996, pp. 219–27

12. J. Saxton et al., "Alcohol, dementia, and Alzheimer's disease: comparison of neuropsychological profiles," *J Geriatr Psychiatry Neurol*, Vol 13, 2000, pp. 141–9

13. T. den Heijer et al., "Alcohol intake in relation to brain magnetic resonance imaging findings in older persons without dementia," *Am J Clin Nutr*, Vol 80, 2004, pp. 992–7

14. H. Refsum et al., "The Hordaland Homocysteine Study: A community-based study of homocysteine, its determinants, and associations with disease," *J Nutr*, Vol 136, 2006, pp. 1731S–40S

15. R.M. Sapolsky, "Why stress is bad for your brain," *Science*, Vol 273(5276), 1996, pp. 749–50

16. J.D. Bremner, "Does stress damage the brain?," *Biol Psychiatry*, Vol 45(7), 1999, pp. 797–805

17. C. Kirschbaum et al., "Stress- and treatment-induced elevations of cortisol levels associated with impaired declarative memory in healthy adults," *Life Sci*, Vol 58(17), 1996, pp. 1475–83

18. J.W. Newcomer et al., "Decreased memory performance in healthy humans induced by stress-level cortisol treatment," *Arch Gen Psychiatry*, Vol 56(6), 1999, pp. 527–33

19. F. Giubilei et al., 2001, "Altered circadian cortisol secretion in Alzheimer's disease: clinical and neuroradiological aspects," *J Neurosci Res*, Vol 66(2), 2001, pp. 262–5

20. L.E. Carlson et al., "Relationships between dehydroepiandrosterone sulfate (DHEAS)

and cortisol (CRT) plasma levels and everyday memory in Alzheimer's disease patients compared to healthy controls," *Horm Behav* 35(3), 1999, pp. 254–63

21. O.M. Wolkowitz et al., "Dehydroepiandrosterone (DHEA) treatment of depression," *Biol Psychiatry*, Vol 41(3), 1997, pp. 311–8

22. A.G. Shauss, "Nutrition and behavior," *Journal of Applied Nutrition*, Vol 35(1), 1983, pp. 30–35 and MIT Conference Proceedings on Research Strategies for Assessing the Behavioural Effects of Foods and Nutrients, 1982

23. D. Benton et al., "Mild hypoglycemia and questionnaire measures of aggression," *Biol Psychol*, Vol 14(1–2), 1982, pp. 129–35

24. A. Roy et al., "Monoamines, glucose metabolism, aggression toward self and others," *Int J Neurosci*, Vol 41(3–4), 1988, pp. 261–4

25. A.G. Schauss, *Diet, Crime and Delinquency*, Parker House (1980)

26. M. Virkkunen, "Reactive hypoglycemic tendency among arsonists," *Acta Psychiatr Scand*, Vol 69(5), 1984, pp. 445–52

27. M. Virkkunen and S. Narvanen, "Tryptophan and serotonin levels during the glucose tolerance test among habitually violent and impulsive offenders," *Neuropsychobiology*, Vol 17(1–2), 1987, pp. 19–23

28. J. Yaryura-Tobias and F. Neziroglu F, "Violent behavior, Brain dysrhythmia and glucose dysfunction. A new syndrome," *J Ortho Psych*, Vol 4, 1975, pp. 182–5

29. M. Bruce and M. Lader, "Caffeine abstention and the management of anxiety disorders," *Psychol Med*, Vol 19, 1989, pp. 211–14

30. W. Wendel and W. Beebe, "Glycolytic activity in schizophrenia," in *Orthomolecular Psychiatry, treatment of schizophrenia*, (eds) D. Hawkins and L. Pauling (1973), W.H. Freeman, San Francisco

31. R. Prinz and D. Riddle, "Associations between nutrition and behavior in 5 year old children," *Nutr Rev*, Vol 43, suppl., 1986

32. L. Christensen, "Psychological distress and diet—effects of sucrose and caffeine," *J Appl Nutr*, Vol 40(1), 1988, pp. 44–50

33. D. Fullerton et al., "Sugar, opionoids and binge eating," *Brain Res Bull*, Vol 14(6), 1985, pp. 273–80

34. L. Christensen, "Psychological distress and diet"

35. M. Colgan and L. Colgan, "Do nutrient supplements and dietary changes affect learning and emotional reactions of children with learning difficulties? A controlled series of 16 cases," *Nutr Health*, Vol 3, 1984, pp. 69–77

36. J. Goldman et al., "Behavioural effects of sucrose on preschool children," *J Abnormal Child Psychol*, Vol 14(4), 1986, pp. 565–77

37. M. Lester et al., "Refined carbohydrate intake, hair cadmium levels and cognitive functioning in children," *Nutr Behav*, Vol 1, 1982, pp. 3–13

38. S. Schoenthaler et al., "The impact of low food additive and sucrose diet on academic performance in 803 New York City public schools," *Int J Biosocial Research*, Vol 8(2), 1986, pp. 185–95

39. M. Virkunnen, "Reactive hypoglycemia tendency among habitually violent offenders," *Nutr Rev*, Vol 44(suppl), 1986, pp. 94–103

40. S. Schoenthaler, "The effect of vitamin-mineral supplementation on juvenile delinquency among American schoolchildren: a randomized, double-blind placebo-controlled trial," *Int J Biosocial Res*, Vol 5(2), 1983, pp. 888–98

41. L. Lien et al., "Consumption of soft drinks and hyperactivity, mental distress, and conduct problems among adolescents in Oslo, Norway," *Am J Public Health*, Vol 96, 2006, pp. 1815–20

42. F.G. Epstein, "Mechanisms of disease," *N Eng J Med*, Vol 334(6), 1996, pp. 374–81

43. N.J. Richardson, P.J. Rogers et al., "Mood and performance effects of caffeine in relation to acute and chronic caffeine deprivation," *Pharmacology, Biochemistry and Behavior*, Vol 52(2), 1995, pp. 313–20

44. K. Gilliland and D. Andress, "Ad lib caffeine consumption, symptoms of caffeinism, and academic performance," *American Journal of Psychiatry*, Vol 138(4), 1981, pp. 512–4

45. See full references at http://www.doctoryourself.com/caffeine_allergy.html

46. S. Davies, Editorial, *J Nut Med*, Vol 2(3), 1991, pp. 227–47

47. C. Patterson, *An Alternative Perspective—Lead Pollution in the Environment*, Commission of Natural Resources Research Council, U.S. National Acadamy of Sciences (1980)

48. H.L. Needleman and C. A. Gatsonis, "Low level lead exposure and the IQ of children," *JAMA*, Vol 263(5), 1990, pp. 673–78

49. Q. Yule and R. Lansdown et al., "The relationship between blood lead concentrations, intelligence and attainment in a school population: a pilot study," *Dev Med Child Neurol*, Vol 23(5), 1981, pp. 567–76

50. G. Winneke, "Neuropsychological studies in children with elevated tooth-lead concentrations. I. Pilot study," *Int Arch Occup Environ Health*, Vol 51(2), 1982, pp. 169–83

51. H.L. Needleman et al., "The long-term effects of exposure to low doses of lead in childhood. An 11-year follow-up report," *N Engl J Med*, Vol 332, 1990, pp. 83–8

52. P. Shattock, presentation, Food for the Brain Conference, London, 1 October 2006

53. M.R. Geier and D.A. Geier, "Thimerosal in childhood vaccines, neurodevelopment disorders and heart disease in the United States," *J Am Physicians Surg*, Vol 8(1), 2003, pp. 6–11

54. V.K. Singh et al., "Abnormal measles-mumps-rubella antibodies and CNS autoimmunity in children with autism," *J Biomed Sci*, Vol 9, 2002, pp. 359–64

55. H.S. Singer et al., "Antibrain antibodies in children with autism and their unaffected siblings," *J Neuroimmunol*, Vol 178(1–2), 2006, pp. 149–55

56. P. Ashwood et al., "Immune activation of peripheral blood and mucosal CD3+ lymphocyte cytokine profiles in children with autism and gastrointestinal symptoms," *J Neuroimmunol*, Vol 173(1-2), 2006, pp. 126–34

57. J.J. Bradstreet et al., "Detection of Measles Virus Genomic RNA in Cerebrospinal Fluid of Children with Regressive Autism: a Report of Three Cases," *Journal of American Physicians and Surgeons*, Vol 9 (2), 2004, pp. 38–45

58. P. Holford and C. Pfeiffer, *Mental Health and Mental Illness—The Nutrition Connection*, ION Press (1996). Also see www.mentalhealthproject/features for feature on copper and schizophrenia

59. P. Hahn et al., "Disruption of ceruloplasmin and hephaestin causes iron overload and retinal degeneration with features of age related macular degeneration," *PNAS*, Vol 101(38), 2004, pp. 13850–5

60. A. Bush et al., "Rapid induction of Alzheimer A beta amyloid formation by zinc," *Science*, Vol 265, 1994, pp. 1464–7

61. M. Morris et al., "Dietary copper and high saturated and trans fat intakes associated with cognitive decline," *Arch Neurology*, Vol 63, 2006, pp. 1085–8

62. S. Davies et al., "Age-related decreases in chromium levels in 51,665 hair, sweat, and serum samples from 40,872 patients—implications for the prevention of cardiovascular disease and type II diabetes mellitus," *Metabolism*, Vol 46(5), 1997, pp. 469–73, and unpublished data on toxic element accumulation with age

63. R. Goyer, "Nutrition and metal toxicity," *Am J Clin Nutr*, Vol 61 (3Suppl), 1995, pp. 646S–50S

64. R. Goyer and M.G. Cherian, "Ascorbic acid and EDTA treatment of lead toxicity in rats," *Life Sci*, Vol 24(5), 1979, pp. 433–8

65. E.J. O'Flaherty, "Modeling normal aging bone loss, with consideration of bone loss in osteoporosis," *Toxicol Sci*, Vol 55(1), 2000, pp. 171–88

66. N.I. Ward et al., *J Nutr Med*, Vol 10, 1990, pp. 415–31

67. T. Randolph, "Allergy as a causative factor of fatigue, irritability and behavior problems of children," *J Pediatr*, Vol 31, 1947, p. 560

68. A. Rowe, "Allergic toxemia and fatigue," *Ann Allergy*, Vol 17, 1959, p. 9

69. F. Speer, ed., "Etiology: Foods," in *Allergy of the Nervous System*, Charles Thomas (1970)

70. M. Campbell, "Neurologic manifestations of allergic disease," *Ann Allergy*, Vol 31, 1973, p. 485

71. K. Hall, "Allergy of the nervous system: a review," *Annals of Allergy*, Vol 36, 1976, pp. 49–64

72. V. Pippere, "Some varieties of food intolerance in psychiatric patients," *Nutr Health*, Vol 3(3), 1984, pp. 125–36

73. C. Pfeiffer and P. Holford, *Mental Illness and Schizophrenia: The Nutrition Connection*, Thorsons (1989)

74. T. Tuormaa, *An Alternative to Psychiatry*, The Book Guild (1991)

75. J. Egger et al., "Controlled trial of oligoantigenic treatment in the hyperkinetic syndrome," *Lancet*, 9 March 1985, pp. 540–5

76. J. Egger et al., "Is migraine a food allergy? A double-blind controlled trial of oligoantigenic diet treatment," *Lancet*, 15 October 1983, pp. 865–9

77. W. Philpott and D. Kalita, *Brain Allergies*, Keats Publishing (1980)

78. D.S. King, "Can allergic exposure provoke psychological symptoms? A double-blind test," *Biol Psychiatry* 16(1), 1981, pp. 3–19

79. B. Feingold, "Dietary management of behavior and learning disabilities," in *Nutrition and Behavior*, S.A. Miller (ed), Franklin Institute Press, (1981), p. 37

80. J. McGovern et al., *Ann Allergy*, Vol 47, 1981, p. 123

81. E. Young et al., "A population study of food intolerance," *Lancet*, Vol 343, 1994, pp. 1127–9

82. British Society for Allergy and Environmental Medicine, *Effective Allergy Practice* (1984)

83. National Dairy Council, *Adverse Reactions to Food: Topical Update* (1994). Available from the National Dairy Council, 5–7 John Princes Street, London W1M 0AP

84. J.R. Cade et al., "Autism and Schizophrenia: Intestinal disorders," *Nutr Neurosci*, Vol 2, 1999, pp. 57–72

85. M. Hadjivassilou, "Idiopathic cerebellar ataxia associated with celia disease," *Neurology*, Vol 56, 1991, pp. 385–8

86. J. Braly, presentation, Food for the Brain Conference, London, 1 October 2006

87. S. Størsrud et al., "Adult celiac patients do tolerate large amounts of oats," *Eur J Clin Nutr*, Vol 57, 2003, pp. 163–9

88. L. Högberg et al., "Oats to children with newly diagnosed celiac disease: A randomized double blind study," *Gut*, Vol 54, 2004, pp. 649–54

89. H. Arentz-Hansen et al., "The molecular basis for oat intolerance in patients with celiac disease," *PloS Med.* See http://medicine.plosjournals.org/perlserv?request=get-document&doi=10.1371/journal.pmed.0010001

Part 3: Improving Your IQ, Memory, and Mood (Chapters 13–18)

1. A.L. Kubala and M.M. Katz, "Nutritional factors in psychological test behavior," *J Genet Psychol*, Vol 96, 1960, pp. 343–52

2. D. Benton and G. Roberts, "Effect of vitamin and mineral supplementation on intelligence of school children," *Lancet*, Vol 1(8578), 1988, pp. 140–3

3. S.J. Schoenthaler et al., "Controlled trial of vitamin-mineral supplementation: Effects on intelligence and performance," *Person Individ Diff*, Vol 12(4), 1991, pp. 351–2

4. J. Yudkin, *Daily Telegraph*, 22 February 1988

5. J. Yudkin, "Intelligence of children and vitamin-mineral supplements: The DRF study. Discussion, conclusions and consequences," *Pers Indiv Differ*, Vol 12, 1991, pp. 363–5

6. D. Benton, "Micro-nutrient supplementation and the intelligence of children," *Neuroscience and Biobehavioral reviews Rev*, Vol 25, 2001, pp. 297–309

7. J.G. Penland, presentation, Experimental Biology meeting, San Diego, California, 2–6 April 2005

8. J. Durga et al., "Folate and the methylenetetrahydrofolate reductase mutation correlate with cognitive performance," *Neurobiol Aging*, Vol 27(2), 2006, pp. 334–43

9. W. Snowden, *Person Individ Diff*, Vol 22(1), 1997, pp. 131–4

10. A.K. Borjel et al., "Plasma homocysteine levels, MTHFR polymorphisms and school achievement in a population sample of Swedish children," *Homocysteine Metab*, Vol 1, 2005, p. 4

11. P. Willatts et al., "Effect of long-chain polyunsaturated fatty acids in infant formula on problem solving at 10 months of age," *Lancet*, Vol 352(9129), 1998, pp. 688–91

12. C. Agostoni et al., "Developmental quotient at 24 months and fatty acid composition of diet in early infancy: a follow up study," *Arch Dis Child*, Vol 76(5), 1997, pp. 421–4

13. L. Horwood et al., *Pediatrics*, Vol 101, January 1998, pp. 1–13

14. C. Lanting et al., *Lancet*, Vol 344(13), 12 Nov 1994, pp. 9–22

15. D. Benton et al., "Mild hypoglycemia and questionnaire measures of agression," *Biol Psychol*, Vol 14(1–2), 1982, pp. 129–35

16. M. Colgan and L. Colgan, "Do nutrient supplements and dietary changes affect learning and emotional reactions of children with learning difficulties? A controlled series of 16 cases," *Nutr Health*, Vol 3, 1984, pp. 69–77

17. J. Goldman et al., "Behavioural effects of sucrose on preschool children," *J Abnormal Child Psychol*, Vol 14(4), 1986, pp. 565–77

18. M. Lester et al., "Refined carbohydrate intake, hair cadmium levels and cognitive functioning in chldren," *Nutr Behav*, Vol 1, 1982, pp. 3–13

19. S. Schoentahler et al., "The impact of a low food additive and sucrose diet on academic performance in 803 New York City public schools," *Int J Biosocial Res*, Vol 8(2), 1986, pp. 185–95

20. C.S. Wallace, W.T. Greenough et al., "Increases in dendritic length in occipital cortex after 4 days of differential housing in weanling rats," *Behav Neural Biol*, Vol 58(1), 1992, pp. 64–8

21. R.M. Sapolsky, "Why stress is bad for your brain," *Science*, Vol 273(5276), 1996, pp. 749–50

22. J.P. Jones, H.S. Swartzwelder et al., "Choline availability to the developing rat fetus alters adult hippocampal long-term potentiation," *Brain Res Dev Brain Res*, Vol 118(1–2), 1999, pp. 159–67

23. F. Safford and G.I. Krell (eds), *Gerontology for Health Professionals: A practice guide*, NASW Press (1997), p. 282

24. S.L. Ladd et al., "Effect of phosphatidylcholine on explicit memory," *Clin Neuropharmacol*, Vol 16(6), 1993, pp. 540–9

25. W. Dimpfel et al., "Source density analysis of functional topographical EEG: monitoring of cognitive drug action," *European Journal of Medical Research*, Vol 1(6), 1996, pp. 283–90

26. T.H. Crook et al., "Effects of phosphatidylserine in Alzheimer's disease," *Psychopharmacol Bull*, Vol 28, 1992, pp. 61–6

27. H. Pilch and W.E. Muller, "Piracetam elevates muscarinic cholinergic receptor density in the frontal cortex of aged but not of young mice," *Psychopharmacology*, Vol 94(1), 1988, pp. 74–8

28. D. Ward and J. Morgenthaler, *Smart Drugs and Nutrients*, B&J Publications, 1990, pp. 42–3

29. S. Grioli et al., "Pyroglutamic acid improves the age associated memory impairment," *Fundam Clin Pharmacol*, Vol 4(2), 1990, pp. 169–73

30. Judy Shabert et al., *The Ultimate Nutrient—Glutamine*, Avery Publications (1990)

31. T. Ziegler et al., "Safety and metabolic effects of L-glutamine administration in humans," *J Parenter Enteral Nutr*, Vol 14(4supp), 1990, pp. 137S–46S

32. L. Young et al., "Patients receiving glutamine-supplemented intravenous feedings report an improvement in mood," *J Parenter Enteral Nutr*, Vol 17, 1993, pp. 422–7

33. J. Liu, T.M. Hagen, B.N. Ames et al., "Memory loss in old rats is associated with brain mitochondrial decay and RNA/DNA oxidation: Partial reversal by feeding acetyl-L-carnitine and/or R-alpha-lipoic acid," *Proc Natl Acad Sci U S*, Vol 99(4), 2002, pp. 2356–61

34. J. Kleijnin and P. Knipschild, "Ginkgo biloba," *Lancet*, Vol 340(8828), 1992, pp. 1136–9

35. P.L. Le Bars, "A placebo-controlled, double-blind, randomized trial on an extract of Ginkgo Biloba for dementia," *JAMA*, Vol 278(16), 1997, pp. 1327–32

36. I. Hindmarch et al., "Efficacy and tolerance of vinpocetine in ambulant patients suffering from mild to moderate organic psychosyndromes," *Int Clin Psychopharmacol*, Vol 6(1), 1991, pp. 31–43

37. R. Balestreri et al., "A double-blind placebo controlled evaluation of the safety and efficacy of vinpocetine in the treatment of patients with chronic vascular senile cerebral dysfunction," *J Am Geriatr Soc*, Vol 35(5), 1987, pp. 425–30

38. Z. Subhan and I. Hindmarch, "Psychopharmacological effects of vinpocetine in normal healthy volunteers," *Eur J Clin Pharmacol*, Vol 28(5), 1985, pp. 567–71

39. A.B. Scholey et al., "Acute, dose-dependent cognitive effects of Ginkgo biloba, Panax

ginseng and their combination in healthy young volunteers: Differential interactions with cognitive demand," *Hum Psychopharmacol*, Vol 17, 2002, pp. 35–44

40. D.O. Kennedy et al., "Ginseng: Potential for the enhancement of cognitive performance and mood," *Pharmacol Biochem Behav*, Vol 75, 2003, pp. 687–700

41. Fusheng Yang et al., "Curcumin inhibits formation of amyloid B oligomers and fibrils, binds plaques, and reduces amyloid in vivo," *J Biol Chem*, Vol 280(7), 2005, pp. 5892–901

42. S.M. Loriaux et al., "The effects of nicotinic acid and xanthinol nicotinate on human memory in different categories of age. A double blind study," *Psychopharmacology (Berl)*, Vol 87(4), 1985, pp. 390–5

43. H.L. Newbold, *Meganutrients for Your Nerves*, Berkeley Books (1985)

44. S. Tsujimaru et al., "Vitamin B12 accelerates re-entrainment of activity rhythms in rats," *Life Sci*, Vol 50(24), 1992, pp. 1843–50

45. R.T. Bartus et al., "Profound effects of combining choline and piracetam on memory enhancement and cholinergic function in aged rats," *Neurobiology of Aging 2*, 1981, pp. 105–111

46. S. Ferris et al., "Combination of choline/piracetam in the treatment of senile dementia," *Psychopharmacology Bulletin*, Vol 18, 1982, pp. 94–8

47. P. Holford et al, Optimum Nutrition UK (ONUK) Survey, Institute for Optimum Nutrition, October 2004 (www.ion.ac.uk)

48. G. Milner, "Ascorbic acid in chronic psychiatric patients: A controlled trial," *Brit J Psychiat*, Vol 109, 1963, pp. 294–9

49. R. Jaffe and O. Kruesi, "The biochemical-immunology window: a molecular view of psychiatric case management," *Int Clin Nut Rev*, Vol 12(1), 1992, pp. 9–26

50. A. Dubini et al., "Do noradrenaline & serotonin differentially affect social motivation and behavior?," *European Neuropsychopharmacology*, Vol 7(Suppl), 1997, pp. S49–S55

51. G.R. Heninger, "Serotonin, sex, psychiatric illness," *Proc Natl Acad Sci*, Vol 94(4), 1997, pp. 823–4

52. K.A. Smith et al., "Relapse of depression after rapid depletion of tryptophan," *Lancet*, Vol 349, 1997, pp. 915–9

53. J. Shepherd, "Effects of estrogen on cognition, mood and degenerative brain diseases," *J Am Pharm Assoc (Wash)*, Vol 41(2), 2001, pp. 221–8

54. K.A. Smith et al., "Relapse of depression after rapid depletion of tryptophan," *Lancet*, Vol 349, 1997, pp. 915–9

55. R. Wurtman and J. Wurtman, "Carbohydrates and depression," *Scientific American*, Vol 260(1), 1989, pp. 68–75

56. P. Holford et al., "The effects of a low glycemic load diet on weight loss and key health risk indicators," *J Orthomol Med*, Vol. 21(2), 2006, pp. 71–8

57. I. von Sano, "L-5-Hydroxytryptophan (L-5-HTP) therapie," *Folia Psychiatrica et Neurologica Japonica*, Vol 26(1), 1972, pp. 7–17

58. T. Nakajima et al., "Clinical evaluation of 5-Hydroxytryptophan as an antidepressant," *Folia Pychiatrica et Neurologica*, Vol 32(2), 1978, pp. 225ff

59. E.H. Turner et al. "Serotonin a la carte: Supplementation with the serotonin precursor 5-hydroxytryptophan," *Pharmacol Ther*, Vol 109(3), 2006, pp. 325–38

60. W. Poldinger et al., "A functional-dimensional approach to depression: serotonin deficiency and target syndrome in a comparison of 5-hydroxytryptophan and fluvox-

amine," *Psychopathology*, Vol 24(2), 1991, pp. 53–81

61. A. Woggon and J. Schoef, "The treatment of depression with L-5-Hydroxytryptophan versus Imipramine," *Arch Psychiat Nervenkr*, Vol 224, 1977, pp. 175–86

62. T. Nakajima et al., "Clinical evaluation of 5-Hydroxy-L-Tryptophan as an antidepressant drug," *Folia Psychiatrisa et Neurologica Japonica*, Vol 32(2), 1978, pp. 223–30; H. M. van Praag et al., "A pilot study of the predictive value of the probnecid test in application of 5-Hydroxytryptophan as antidepressant," *Psychopharmacologica (Berl)*, Vol 25, 1972, pp. 14–21; M. Kaneko et al., "L-5-HTP treatment and serum 5-HT level after L-5-HTP loading on depressed patients," *Neuropsychobiology*, Vol 5, 1979, pp. 232–40; L.J. van Heile, "L-5-Hydroxytryptophan in depression: the first substitution therapy in psychiatry?," *Neuropsychobiology*, Vol 6, 1980, pp. 230–40; and I. von Sano, "L-5-Hydroxytryptophan (L-5-HTP) therapie," *Folia Psychiatrica et Neurologica Japonica*, Vol 26(1), 1972, pp. 7–17

63. E.H. Turner et al., "Serotonin a la carte: supplementation with the serotonin precursor 5-hydroxytryptophan"

64. H. Beckmann et al., "DL-phenylalanine versus imipramine: a double-blind controlled study," *Arch Psychiatr Nervenkr*, Vol 227(1), 1979, pp. 49–58

65. H.C. Sabelli et al., "Clinical studies on the phenylethylamine hypothesis of affective disorder: urine and blood phenylacetic acid and phenylalanine dietary supplements," *J Clin Psychiatry*, Vol (2), 1986, pp. 66–70

66. J. Mouret et al., "L-tyrosine cures, immediate and long term, dopamine-dependent depressions. Clinical and polygraphic studies," *C R Acad Sci III*, Vol 306(3), 1988, pp. 93–8 (in French)

67. J.B. Deijen et al., "Tyrosine improves cognitive performance and reduces blood pressure in cadets after one week of a combat training course," *Brain Research Bulletin*, Vol 48(2), 1999, pp. 203–9

68. S.F. McTavish et al., "Lack of effect of tyrosine depletion on mood in recovered depressed women," *Neuropsychopharm*, Vol 30(4) 2005, pp. 786–91

69. T. Audhya., "Advances in measurement of platelet catecholamines at sub-picomole level for diagnosis of depression and anxiety," *Clin Chem*, Vol 51(6) supplement, 2005, E-128

70. T. Audhya, "Advances in measurement of platelet catecholamines at sub-picomole level for diagnosis of depression and anxiety," *Clin Chem*, Vol 51(6) supplement, 2005, E-128

71. T. Audhya, *J Nutr Health* (awaiting publication)

72. H. Cass, "SAMe—the master tuner supplement for the 21st century," published on www.naturallyhigh.co.uk (2001)

73. B.L. Kagan et al., "Oral S-adenosylmethionine in depression: a randomized, double-blind, placebo-controlled trial," *Am J Psychiatry*, Vol 147(5), 1990, pp. 591–5

74. P.G. Janicak et al., "Parenteral S-adenosyl-methionine (SAMe) in depression: literature review and preliminary data," *Psychopharmacol Bull*, Vol 25(2), 1989, pp. 238–42

75. G.M. Bressa, "S-adenosyl-methionine as antidepressant: meta-analysis of clinical studies," *Acta Neurologica Scandinavian*, Vol 154(supp), 1994, pp. 7–14

76. J.R. Hibbeln, "Fish consumption and major depression," *Lancet*, Vol 351, 1998, p. 1213

77. M.B. Raeder et al., "Associations between cod liver oil use and symptoms of depression: The Hordaland Health Study," *J Affect Disord*, 18 December 2006 [Epub ahead of print]

78. M. Peet and R. Stokes, "Omega 3 fatty acids in the treatment of psychiatric disorders drugs," Vol 65(8), 2005, pp. 1051–9

79. B. Nemets et al., "Addition of omega-3 fatty acid to maintenance medication treatment for recurrent unipolar depressive disorder," *Am J Psychiatry*, Vol 159, 2002, pp. 477–9

80. S. Frangou et al., "Efficacy of ethyl-eicosapentaenoic acid in bipolar depression: randomized double-blind placebo-controlled study," *Brit J Psychiatry*, Vol 188, 2006, pp. 46–50

81. G.W. Lambert et al., "Effect of sunlight and season on serotonin turnover in the brain," *Lancet*, Vol 360(9348), 2002, pp. 1840–2

82. L. Craft et al., "The benefits of exercise for the clinically depressed," *Prim Care Companion J Clin Psychiatry*, Vol 6, 2004, pp. 104–111

83. N.A. Singh, "A randomized controlled trial of high versus low intensity weight training versus general practitioner care for clinical depression in older adults," *J Gerontol A Biol Sci Med Sci*, Vol 60, 2005, pp. 768–76

84. S. Leppamaki et al., "Drop-out and mood improvement: A randomized controlled trial with light exposure and physical exercise," *BMC Psychiatry*, Vol 4(1), 2004, p. 22

85. K. Martiny et al., "Adjunctive bright light in non-seasonal major depression: Results from clinician-rated depression scales," *Acta Psychiatr Scand*, Vol 112(2), 2005, pp. 117–25

86. L. Swiecicki et al., "Platelet serotonin transport in the group of outpatients with seasonal affective disorder before and after light treatment, and in remission (in the summer)," *Psychiatr Pol*, Vol 39(3), 2005, pp. 459–68

87. G.E. Abraham, "Nutritional factors in the etiology of the premenstrual tension syndromes," *J Reprod Med*, Vol 28(7), 1983, pp. 446–64

88. M.G. Brush and M. Perry, "Pyridoxine and the premenstrual syndrome," *Lancet*, Vol 1(8442), 1985, p. 1399

89. G.E. Abraham and M.D. Lubran, "Serum and red cell magnesium levels in patients with premenstrual tension," *Am J Clin Nutr*, Vol 34, 1981, pp. 1264–6

90. A. Nicholas, "Traitement du syndrome premenstrual et de la dysmenorrhee par l'ion magnesium," in J. Durlach (ed), *First Int Sympos on Magnesium Deficiency in Human Pathology*, Springer Verlag, 1983, pp. 261–3

91. D.F. Horrobin, "The role of essential fatty acids and prostaglandins in the premenstrual syndrome," *J Reprod Med*, Vol 28(7), 1983, pp. 465–8

92. G.A. Colditz et al., "The use of estrogens and progestins and the risk of breast cancer in postmenopausal women," *N Engl J Med*, Vol 332(24), 1995, pp. 1589–93

93. E. Barrett-Connor et al., "Bioavailable testosterone and depressed mood in older men: the Rancho Bernardo Study," *J Clin Endocrinol Metab*, Vol 84(2), 1999, pp. 573–7

94. O.M. Wolkowitz et al., "Dehydroepiandrosterone (DHEA) treatment of depression," *Biol Psychiatry*, Vol 41(3), 1997, pp. 311–18

95. NOP Poll, May 2001, *Panorama*, BBC, U.K.: see http://news.bbc.co.uk/hi/english/audiovideo/programmes/panorama/tranquillisers/newsid_1325000/1325909.stm

96. National Institute for Health and Clinical Evidence, "Insomnia—newer hypnotic drugs." See http://www.nice.org.uk/page.aspx?o=ta077

97. Netdoctor.co.uk, "Zimovane." See www.netdoctor.co.uk/medicines/100002841.html

98. I.S. Shiah and N. Yatham, "GABA functions in mood disorders: An update and critical

review," *Life Sciences*, Vol 63(15), 1998, pp. 1289–1303

99. G. Warnecke, "Psychosomatic dysfunctions in the female climacteric: clinical effectiveness and tolerance of kava extract WS 1490," *Fortschr Med*, Vol 109(4), 1991, pp. 119–22

100. H.P. Volz and M. Kieser, "Kava-kava extract WS 1490 versus placebo in anxiety disorders—A randomized placebo-controlled 25-week outpatient trial," *Pharmacopsychiatry*, Vol 30, 1997, pp. 1–5

101. T.F. Munte et al., "Effects of Oxazepam and an extract of kava root (*Piper methysticum*) on event-related potentials in a word-recognition task," *Neuropsychobiology*, Vol 27(1), 1993, pp. 46–53

102. H. Woelk et al., "Double blind study: Kava extract versus benzodiazepines in treatment of patients suffering from anxiety," *Z Allg Med*, Vol 69, 1993, pp. 271–7

103. D. Lindenberg et al., "Kavain in comparison with Oxazepam in anxiety disorders: a double blind study of clinical effectiveness," *Fortschr Med*, Vol 108, 1990, pp. 49–50

104. See www.patrickholford.com/kavaconcerns. For more in-depth information on kava, see Hyla Cass and Terrence McNally, *Kava: Nature's Answer to Stress, Anxiety, and Insomnia*, Prima Publishing (1998)

105. F.N. Pitts and J.N. McClure, "Lactate metabolism in anxiety neurosis," *New Engl J Med*, Vol 277, 1967, pp. 1328–36

106. M.J. Sateia and P. D. Nowell, "Insomnia," *Lancet*, Vol 364(9449), 2004, pp. 1959–73

107. M.M. Ohayon, "Interactions between sleep normative data and sociocultural characteristics in the elderly," *J Psychosom Res*, Vol 56(5), 2004, pp. 479–86

108. L. Shilo et al., "The effects of coffee consumption on sleep and melatonin secretion," *Sleep Med*, Vol 3(3), 2002, pp. 271–3

109. I.S. Shiah, and N. Yatham, "GABA functions in mood disorders: An update and critical review," *Life Sci*, Vol 63(15), 1998, pp. 1289–303

110. S. Young, "The clinical psychopharmacology of tryptophan," *Nutr and the Brain*, Vol 7, 1986, pp. 49–88

111. T.C. Birdsall, "5-Hydroxytryptophan: a clinically-effective serotonin precursor," *Altern Med Rev*, Vol 3(4), 1998, pp. 271–80

112. O. Bruni et al., "L -5-Hydroxytryptophan treatment of sleep terrors in children," *Eur J Pediatr*, Vol 163(7), 2004, pp. 402–7

113. A. Brzezinski et al., "Effects of exogenous melatonin on sleep: a meta-analysis," *Sleep Med Rev*, Vol 9(1), 2005, pp. 41–50

114. M. Spinella, *The Psychopharmacology of Herbal Medicine*, MIT Press (2001)

115. M. Dorn, "Valerian versus oxazepam: efficacy and tolerability in nonorganic and nonpsychiatric insomniacs—a randomized, double-blind clinical comparative study," *Forsch Komplementärmed*, Vol 7, 2000, pp. 79–81

116. E.U. Vorbach et al., "Treatment of insomnia: Effectiveness and tolerance of a valerian extract," *Psychopharmakotherapie*, Vol 3,1996, pp. 109–15

117. C. Stevinson and E. Ernst, "Valerian for insomnia: A systematic review of randomized clinical trials," *Sleep Med*, Vol 1, 2000, pp. 91–9

118. G.D. Jacobs et al., "Cognitive behavior therapy and pharmacotherapy for insomnia: A randomized controlled trial and direct comparison," *Arch Intern Med*, Vol 164(17), 2004, pp. 1888–96

119. M.J. Sateia and P.D. Nowell, "Insomnia"

120. P. Montgomery and J. Dennis, "Physical exercise for sleep problems in adults aged

60+" *Cochrane Review,* The Cochrane Library, Issue 4, 2005

121. L. Yal, "Brain music in the treatment of patients with insomnia," *Neurosci Behav Physiol,* Vol 28, 1998, pp. 330–5

122. I. Olszewska and M. Zarow, "Does music during dental treatment make a difference?" See http://www.silenceofmusic.com/pdf/dentists.pdf

Part 4: What Is Mental Illness? (Chapters 19–22)

1. World Health Organization, *The World Health Report 2001—Mental Health: New Understanding, New Hope,* WHO, 2001. Available at www.who.int/whr/2001/

2. WHO, *The World Health Report 2001*

3. WHO, *The World Health Report 2001*

4. R. Hall et al., "Physical illness manifesting as psychiatric disease," *Arch Gen Psychiatry,* Vol 37, 1980, pp. 989–95

5. D.G. Robinson, M.G. Woerner, M. McMeniman, A. Mendelowitz and R.M. Bilder, "Symptomatic and functional recovery from a first episode of schizophrenia or schizoaffective disorder," *American Journal of Psychiatry,* Vol 161, 2004, pp. 473–479.

6. World Health Organization. *International pilot study of schizophrenia,* Geneva: World Health Organization, 1973. 427 pp.

7. World Health Organization. *Schizophrenia: an international follow-up study,* Chichester (United Kingdom): Wiley, 1979. 438 pp.

8. A. Jablensky, N. Sartorius, G. Ernberg, M. Anker, A. Korten et al. "Schizophrenia: manifestations, incidence and course in different cultures. A World Health Organization ten-country study," *Psychol Med Monogr Suppl,* Vol 20, 1992, pp. 1–97

9. See www.hgi.org.uk/archive/psychosis.htm and J. Griffin and I. Tyrrell, *Dreaming Reality,* HG Publishing, 2004

10. British National Formulary, tricyclic antidepressant side effects

11. D. Healey et al. "Association between suicide attempts and selective serotonin reuptake inhibitors: systematic review of randomized controlled trials," *BMJ,* Vol 330, 2005, pp. 396–404

12. L. Watkins, conference report, annual meeting of the American Psychosomatic Society in Denver, Colorado, 4 March, 2006

13. Interview in *100% Health* newsletter, No 22, September 2004

14. J. Burne, "Antidepressants and suicide," *Medicine Today,* December 2001. Available at www.medicine-today.co.uk

15. See *Guardian* article "Murder, suicide: A bitter aftertaste for the 'wonder' depression drug" at www.guardian.co.uk/Archive/Article/0,4273,4201752,00.html

16. National Institute for Health and Clinical Excellence, "Depression—management of depression in primary and secondary care." See www.nice.org.uk/page.aspx?o=cg023

17. J. Biederman and S.V. Faraone, "Attention-deficit hyperactivity disorder," *Lancet,* Vol. 366(9481), 2005, pp. 237–48

18. L. Mintowt-Czyz, "Alert over Ritalin causing manic symptoms," *Evening Standard,* 22 August 2006

19. N.D. Volkow et al., "Therapeutic doses of oral methylphenidate significantly increase extracellular dopamine in the human brain," *J Neuroscience,* Vol 21(RC121), 2001, pp.

1–5

20. J. Baizer, *Annual Meeting of the Society for Neuroscience*, 11 November 2001
21. DoH, *Department of Health, U.K., Prescription Cost Analysis*
22. M. Lader, "Dependence on benzodiazapenes," *J Clin Psychiatr*, Vol 44, 1983, pp. 121–7
23. National Institute for Health and Clinical Excellence, "Insomnia—newer hypnotic drugs." See www.nice.org.uk/page.aspx?o=ta077
24. Netdoctor.co.uk, "Zimovane." See www.netdoctor.co.uk/medicines/100002841.html
25. A. Holbrook, "Treating insomnia," *BMJ*, Vol 29, 2004, pp. 1198–9
26. C. Nystrom, "Effects of long-term benzodiazepine medication. A prospective cohort study: Methodological and clinical aspects," *Nord J Psychiatry*, Vol 59(6), 2005, pp. 492–7
27. A. Hirst and R. Sloan, "Benzodiazepines and related drugs for insomnia in palliative care," *Cochrane Database of Systematic Reviews* 2001, Issue 4. Art. No. CD003346. DOI: 10.1002/14651858.CD003346
28. W.M Glazer, "Olanzapine vs haloperidol for treatment of schizophrenia," *JAMA*, Vol 291(9), 2004, pp. 1064–5
29. See http://news.bbc.co.uk and search under "tranquillisers"
30. A. Sohler and C. Pfeiffer, "A direct method for the determination of manganese in whole blood: patients with seizure activity have low blood levels," *Orthomolecular Psychiatry*, Vol 18, 1979, pp. 275–80
31. Robin Pagnamenta, "Eli Lilly was concerned by Zyprexa side effects from 1998," *The Times*, 23 January 2007
32. D. Healy et al., "Lifetime suicide rates in treated schizophrenia: 1875–1924 and 1994–1998 cohorts compared," *B J Psychiatry*, Vol 188, 2006, pp. 229–30
33. R. Whitaker, *Mad in America: Bad Science, Bad Medicine, and the Enduring Mistreatment of the Mentally Ill*, Perseus Publishing (2001)
34. M.R. Zonfrillo, J.V. Penn and H.L. Leonard, "Pediatric psychotropic polypharmacy," *Psychiatry*, Vol 2(8), 2005, pp. 14–19

Part 5: Solving Depression, Manic Depression, and Schizophrenia (Chapters 23–26)

1. A. Tylee and P. Ghandi, "The importance of Somatic Symptoms in Depression in Primary Care," *Journal of Clinical Psychology*, Vol 7(4), 2005, pp. 167–76. Also see NICE Guideline for Depression www.nice.org <http://www.nice.org>
2. A.L. Miller, "St. John's Wort: Clinical effects on depression and other conditions," *Alt Med Rev*, Vol 3(1), 1998, pp. 18–26
3. H. Woelk, "Comparison of St. John's Wort and imipramine for treating depression: randomized controlled trial," *BMJ*, Vol 321(7260), 2000, pp. 536–9
4. K. Linde, "St. John's Wort for depression: an overview and meta-analysis of randomized clinical trials," *BMJ*, Vol 313(7052), 1996, pp. 253–8
5. U. Schmidt and H. Sommer, "St. John's wort extract in the ambulatory therapy of depression. Attention and reaction ability are preserved," *Fortschr Med*, Vol 111(19), 1993, pp. 339–42 (in German)
6. S. Bratman, *Beat Depression with St. John's Wort*, Prima Publishing (1997)
7. H. Winterhoff et al., Nervenheilkunde 12, 1993, pp. 341–5

8. M. McLeod et al., "Effectiveness of chromium in atypical depression: A placebo-controlled trial," *Biol Psychiatry*, Vol 53(3), 2003, pp. 261–4

9. A. Nierenberg et al., "Clinical and demographic features of atypical depression in outpatients with major depressive disorder: Preliminary findings from STAR*D," *J Clin Psychiatry*, Vol 66(8), 2005, pp. 1002–11

10. J. Davidson et al., "Effectiveness of chromium in atypical depression: A placebo-controlled trial," *Biol Psychiatry*, Vol 53(3), 2003, pp. 261–4

11. J. Docherty et al., "A double-blind, placebo-controlled, exploratory trial of chromium picolinate in atypical depression," *J Psychiatr Pract.* Vol 11(5), 2005, pp. 302–14

12. P.G. Weston, "Magnesium as a sedative," *Am J Psychiatr*, Vol 78, 1921, pp. 637–8

13. G.A. Eby et al., "Rapid recovery from major depression using magnesium treatment," *Med Hypotheses*, Vol 67(2), 2006, pp. 362–70

14. I. Cernak et al., "Alterations in magnesium and oxidative status during chronic emotional stress," *Magnes Res*, Vol 13, 2000, pp. 29–36

15. C. Sugden, "One-carbon metabolism in psychiatric illness," *Nutr Res Rev*, Vol 19, 2006, pp. 117–136

16. M. Fava et al., "Folate, vitamin B12 and homocysteine in major depressive disorder," *Am J Pysch*, Vol 154, 1997, pp. 426–8

17. Bottiglieri et al., "Homocysteine, folate, methylation, and monoamine metabolism in depression," *J Neurol Neurosurg Psychiatr*, Vol 69(2), 2000, pp. 228–32

18. P.S. Godfrey et al., "Enhancement of recovery from psychiatric illness by methylfolate," *Lancet*, Vol 336, 1990, pp. 392–5

19. J.E. Alpert and M. Fava, "Nutrition and depression: the role of folate," *Nutr Rev*, Vol 55(5), 1997, pp. 145–9

20. H. Tiemeier et al., "Vitamin B12, folate, and homocysteine in depression: the Rotterdam Study," *Am J Psychiatr*, Vol 159(2), 2002, pp. 2099–101

21. A. Coppen and J. Bailey, "Enhancement of the antidepressant action of fluoxetine by folic acid: A randomized, placebo controlled trial," *J Affect Disord*, Vol 60, 2000, pp.121–30

22. M.J. Taylor et al., "Folate for depressive disorders: Systematic review and meta-analysis of randomized controlled trials," *J Psychopharmacol*, Vol 18(2), 2004, pp. 251–6

23. E.H. Reynolds et al., "Methylation and mood," *Lancet*, Vol 2(8396), 1984, pp. 196–8

24. B. Nemets et al., "Addition of omega-3 fatty acid to maintenance medication treatment for recurrent unipolar depressive disorder," *Am J Psychiatry*, Vol 159, 2002, pp. 477–9

25. E.C. Suarez, "Relations of trait depression and anxiety to low lipid and lipoprotein concentrations in healthy young adult women," *Psychosom*, Vol 61(3), 1999, pp. 273–9

26. T. Partonen et al., "Association of low serum total cholesterol with major depression and suicide," *British Journal of Psychiatry*, Vol 175, 1999, pp. 259–62

27. J.E. Alpert and M. Fava, "Nutrition and depression: the role of folate," *Nutr Rev*, Vol 55(5), 1997, pp.145–9

28. D. Nettle and H. Keenoo, "Schizotypy, creativity and mating success in humans," *Proceedings of the Royal Society B*, November 2005, DOI:10.1098/rspb.2005.3349

29. L. Craft and F. Perna, "The benefits of exercise for the clinically depressed," *Prim Care Companion J Clin Psychiatry*, Vol 6(3), 2004, pp. 104–11

30. N.A. Singh, "A randomized controlled trial of high versus low intensity weight training versus general practitioner care for clinical depression in older adults," *J Gerontol A Biol*

Sci Med Sci, Vol 60(6), 2005, pp. 768–76

31. D. Kritz-Silverstein et al., "Cross-sectional and prospective study of exercise and depressed mood in the elderly: the Rancho Bernardo study," *Am J Epidemiol*, Vol 153(6), 2001, pp. 596–603

32. G. Brown et al., "Social support, self-esteem and depression," *Psychol Med*, Vol 16(4) 1986, pp. 813–31

33. W. Lauder et al., "A comparison of health behaviors in lonely and non-lonely populations," *Psychol Health Med*, Vol 11(2), 2006, pp. 233–45

34. F. Barg et al, "A mixed-methods approach to understanding loneliness and depression in older adults," *J Gerontol B Psychol Sci Soc Sci*, Vol 61(6), 2006, pp. S329–39

35. S. Leppamaki et al., "Drop-out and mood improvement: A randomized controlled trial with light exposure and physical exercise," *BMC Psychiatry*, Vol 4(1), 2004, p. 22

36. K. Martiny et al., "Adjunctive bright light in non-seasonal major depression: Results from clinician-rated depression scales," *Acta Psychiatr Scand*, Vol 112(2), 2005, pp. 117–25

37. L. Swiecicki et al., "Platelet serotonin transport in the group of outpatients with seasonal affective disorder before and after light treatment, and in remission (in the summer)," *Psychiatr Pol*, Vol 39(3), 2005, pp. 459–68

38. D. Healy, "The myth of 'mood stabilising' drugs," *New Scientist*, 15 April 2006, p. 38

39. A. Corvin et al., "Cigarette smoking and psychotic symptoms in bipolar affective disorder," *British Journal of Psychiatry*, Vol 179, 2001, pp. 35–8

40. G.N. Schrauzer et al., "Lithium in scalp hair of adults, students and violent criminals. Effects of supplementation and evidence for interactions of lithium with vitamin B12 and with other trace elements," *Biol Trace Elem Res*, Vol 34(2), 1992, pp. 161–76

41. A. Coppen et al., "Plasma folate and affective morbidity during long-term lithium therapy," *Br J Psychiatry*, Vol 141, 1982, pp. 87–9

42. A.L. Stoll et al., "Omega 3 fatty acids in bipolar disorder: a preliminary double-blind, placebo-controlled trial," *Arch Gen Psychiatry*, Vol 56(5), 1999, pp. 407–12

43. G. Chouinard et al., "A pilot study of magnesium hydrochloride (Magnesiocard) as a mood stabiliser for rapid cycling bipolar affective disorder patients," *Prog Neuropsychopharmacol Biol Psychiatry*, Vol 14(2), 1990, pp. 171–80

44. A. Heiden et al., "Treatment of severe mania with intravenous magnesium sulphate as a supplementary therapy," *Psychiatry Res*, Vol 89(3), 1999, pp. 239–46

45. C.J. Schorah et al., "Plasma vitamin C concentrations in patients in a psychiatric hospital," *Hum Nutr Clin Nutr*, Vol 37C, 1983, pp. 447–52

46. Z.A. Leitner and I.C. Church, "Nutritional studies in a mental hospital," *Lancet*, Vol 1, 1956, pp. 565–7

47. J.W. Maas, *Arch Gen Psychiatry*, Vol 4, 1961, p. 109

48. G. Milner, "Ascorbic acid supplementation in chronic psychiatric patients: A controlled trial," *Br J Psychiatry*, Vol 109, 1963, pp. 294–9

49. G.J. Naylor et al., "Tissue vanadium levels in manic depressive psychosis," *Physiological Medicine*, Vol 14, 1984, pp. 767–72

50. D.A. Dick, "Plasma vanadium concentration in manic-depressive illness," *Psychol Med*, Vol 12(3), 1982, pp. 533–7

51. B.J. Kaplan et al., "Effective mood stabilization in open trials with a chelated mineral supplement: an open-label trial in bipolar disorder," *J Clin Psychiatry*, Vol 62(12),

2001, pp. 936–44

52. D.P. Cole et al., "Slower treatment response in bipolar depression predicted by lower pre-treatment thyroid function," *American Journal of Psychiatry*, Vol 159, 2002, pp. 116–21

53. G.D. Honey et al., *Proceedings of the National Academy of Sciences*, Vol 96, 1999, pp. 13418–23

54. D.F. Horrobin et al., "Fatty acid levels in the brains of schizophrenics and normal controls," *Biol Psychiatry*, Vol 30, 1991, pp. 795–805

55. D.F. Horrobin et al., "The membrane hypothesis of schizophrenia," *Schizophrenia Research*, Vol 13, 1994, pp. 195–207

56. P.E. Ward et al., "Niacin skin flush in schizophrenia: a preliminary report," *Schizophr Res*, Vol 29, 1998, pp. 269–74

57. S.H. Shah et al., "Unmedicated schizophrenic patients have a reduced skin response to topical niacin," *Schizophr Res*, Vol 43, 2000, pp. 163–4

58. C. Hudson, B.M. Ross et al., "Clinical subtyping reveals significant differences in calcium-dependent phospholipase A2 activity in schizophrenia," *Biol Psychiatry*, Vol 46(3), 1999, pp. 401–5

59. O. Christensen and E. Christensen, "Fat consumption and schizophrenia," *Acta Psychiatr Scand*, Vol 78, 1988, pp. 587–91

60. "50 patients given efas got better," A. Glen, personal communication, due for publication

61. K.S. Vaddadi et al., "A double-blind trial of essential fatty acid supplementation in patients with tardive dyskinesia," *Psychiatry Res*, Vol 27(3), 1989, pp. 313–23

62. M. Peet and D.F. Horrobin, "A dose-ranging exploratory study of the effects of ethyl-eicosapentaenoate in patients with persistent schizophrenic symptoms," *J Psychiatr Res*, Vol 36(1), 2002 pp. 7–18

63. W.S. Fenton et al., "A placebo-controlled trial of omega-3 fatty acid (ethyl eicosapentaenoic acid) supplementation for residual symptoms and cognitive impairment in schizophrenia," *Am J Psychiatry*, Vol 158(12), 2001, pp. 2071–4

64. D. Shtasel et al., *Psychiatric Services*, Vol 46(3), March 1995, p. 293

65. G. Milner, *Brit J Psychiat*, Vol 109, 1963, pp. 294–9

66. K. Suboticanec et al., *Biol Psychiatry*, Vol 28, 1990, pp. 959–66 (see also Part 1, reference 85)

67. T. Arinami et al., "A functional polymorphism in the promoter region of the dopamine D2 receptor gene is associated with schizophrenia," *Hum Mol Genet*, Vol 6(4), 1997, pp. 577–82

68. S.J. Lewis et al., "A meta-analysis of the MTHFR C677T polymorphism and schizophrenia risk," *Am J Med Genet B Neuropsychiatr Genet*, Vol 135(1), 2005, pp. 2–4

69. H. Grundt et al., "Reduction in homocysteine by n-3 polyunsaturated fatty acids after 1 year in a randomized double-blind study following an acute myocardial infarction: no effect on endothelial adhesion properties," *Pathophysiol Haemost Thromb*, Vol 33 (2), 2003, pp. 88–95

70. B. Regland et al., "Homocysteinemia is a common feature of schizophrenia," *J Neural Transm Gen Sect*, Vol 100(2) 1995, pp. 165–9

71. D.C. Goff et al., "Folate, homocysteine, and negative symptoms in schizophrenia," *Am J Psychiatry*, Vol 161(9), 2004, pp. 1705–8

72. J. Levine et al., "Elevated homocysteine levels in young male patients with schizophre-

nia," *Am J Psychiatry*, Vol 159(10), 2002, pp. 1790–2

73. J. Applebaum et al., "Homocysteine levels in newly admitted schizophrenic patients," *J Psychiatr Res*, Vol 38(4), 2004, pp. 413–16

74. P. Godfrey et al., "Enhancement of recovery from psychiatric illness by methylfolate," *Lancet*, Vol 336(8712), 1990, pp. 392–5

75. B. Regland et al., "Homocysteinemia and schizophrenia as a case of methylation deficiency," *J Neural Transm Gen Sect*, Vol 98(2), 1994, pp. 143–52

76. O. Shumaico et al., "Homocysteine-reducing strategies improve symptoms in chronic schizophrenic patients with hyperhomocysteinemia," *Biol Psychiatry*, Vol 60 (3), 2006, pp. 265–9

77. J. Levine et al., "Homocysteine-reducing strategies improve symptoms in chronic schizophrenic patients with hyperhomocysteinemia," *Biol Psychiatry*, Vol 60(3), 2006, pp. 265–9.

78. A. Hoffer, "Megavitamin B3 therapy for schizophrenia," *Canad Psychiatric Ass J*, Vol 16, 1971, pp. 499–504

79. J.R. Wittenborn, "Niacin in the long term treatment of schizophrenia," *Arch Gen Psychiatry*, Vol 28, 1973, pp. 308–15

80. J.R. Wittenborn, "A search for responders to niacin supplementation," *Arch Gen Psychiatry*, Vol 31, 1974, pp. 547–52

81. P.O. O'Reilly et al., "The mauve factor: an evaluation," *Dis Nerv Syst*, Vol 26(9), 1965, pp. 562–8

82. W. McGinnis et al., "Discerning the mauve factor" (awaiting publication)

83. W. McGinnis et al., "Discerning the mauve factor"

84. L. Bender, "Childhood schizophrenia," *Psychiatric Quarterly*, Vol 27, 1953, pp. 3–81

85. H. Graff and A. Handford, "Celiac syndrome in the case history of five schizophrenics," *Psychiatric Quarterly*, Vol 35, 1961, pp. 306–13

86. F.C. Dohan et al., "Relapsed schizophrenics: more rapid improvement on a milk and cereal-free diet," *Brit J Psychiat*, Vol 115, 1969, pp. 595–6

87. D.S. King, "Can allergic exposure provoke psychological symptoms? A double-blind test," *Biol Psychiatry*, Vol 16(1), 1981, pp. 3–19

88. W. Philpott and D. Kalita, *Brain Allergies*, Keats Publishing (1980)

89. C.S. Hourigan, "The molecular basis of celiac disease," *Clin Exp Med*, Vol 6(2), 2006, pp. 53–9

90. T. Gerarduzzi et al., "Celiac disease in U.S.A. among risk groups and general population in U.S.A.," *J Pediatr Gastroeneterol Nutr*, Vol 31 (suppl), 2000, S29, Abstr 104

91. W. Eaton et al., "Celiac disease and schizophrenia: Population based case control study with linkage of Danish national registers," *BMJ*, Vol 328(7446), 2004, pp. 438–9

92. A. Hoffer, "Megavitamin B3 therapy for schizophrenia"

93. R. Cade. See http://paleodiet.com/autism/cadelet.txt

94. H. Karlsson, R.H. Yolken et al., "Retroviral RNA identified in the cerebrospinal fluids and brains of individuals with schizophrenia," *Proc Natl Acad Sci*, Vol 98(8), 2001, pp. 4634–9

95. T. Soutzos, unpublished 2002 study of 40 patients at Guy's and St. Thomas's Hospitals, London, in which 90 percent had high sulphite levels in their urine, compared with none of the healthy individuals used as controls, the majority of whom had none. See http://news.bbc.co.uk/hi/english/health/newsid_117000/117990.stm

96. B.F. El-Khodor and P. Boksa, "Birth insult increases amphetamine-induced behavioral responses in the adult rat," *Neuroscience*, Vol 87(4), 1998, pp. 893–904

Part 6: Mental Health in the Young (Chapters 27–34)

1. National Institutes of Health, Bethesda, NIH Consensus Statement 1998, "Diagnosis and Treatment of ADHD"
2. A. Richardson, "Fatty acids in dyslexia, dyspraxia, ADHD and the autistic spectrum," *The Nutrition Practitioner*, Vol 3(3), 2001, pp. 18–24
3. A. Lucas, R. Morley and T. Cole, "Randomized trial of early diet in preterm babies and later intelligence quotient," *BMJ*, Vol 317, 28 November 1998, pp. 1481–7
4. A.L. Kubala and M.M. Katz, "Nutritional factors in psychological test behavior," *J Genet Psychol*, Vol 96, 1960, p. 343–52
5. A. Schauss, "Nutrition and behavior," *J App Nutr*, Vol 35, 1983, p. 30–5
6. S.J. Schoenthaler et al., "The effect of randomized vitamin-mineral supplementation on violent and non-violent antisocial behavior among incarcerated juveniles," *J Nut Env Med*, Vol 7, 1997, pp. 343–52
7. S.J. Schoenthaler et al., "The effect of vitamin-mineral supplementation on the intelligence of American schoolchildren: a randomized, double-blind placebo-controlled trial," *J Altern Complement Med*, Vol 6(1), 2000, pp. 19–29
8. R.M. Carlton et al., "Rational dosages of nutrients have a prolonged effect on learning disabilities," *Altern Ther Health Med*, Vol 6(3), 2000, pp. 85–91
9. M. Colgan and L. Colgan, "Do nutrient supplements and dietary changes affect learning and emotional reactions of children with learning difficulties? A controlled series of 16 cases," *Nutr Health*, Vol 3, 1984, pp. 69–77
10. L. Rogers and R. Pelton, "Effects of glutamine on IQ scores of mentally deficient children," *Tex Rep Biol Med*, Vol 15, 1957, pp. 84–90
11. A.J. Richardson and J. Wilmer, "Association between fatty acid symptoms and dyslexic and ADHD characteristics in normal college students," paper given at British Dyslexia Association International Conference, University of York, April 2001
12. A. Richardson and B. Puri, "A randomized double-blind, placebo-controlled study of the effects of supplementation with highly unsaturated fatty acids on ADHD-related symptoms in children with specific learning difficulties," *Prog Neuropsychopharmacol Biol Psychiatry*, Vol 26(2), 2002, pp. 233–9
13. A.J. Richardson et al., "Fatty acid deficiency signs predict the severity of reading and related problems in dyslexic children," paper given at British Dyslexia Association International Conference, University of York, April 2001
14. A.J. Richardson and P. Montgomery, "The Oxford-Durham study: A randomized, controlled trial of dietary supplementation with fatty acids in children with developmental coordination disorder," *Pediatrics*, Vol 115(5), 2005, pp. 1360–6
15. C.M. Absolon et al., "Psychological disturbance in atopic eczema: the extent of the problem in school-aged children," *Br J Dermatol*, Vol 137(2), 1997, pp. 241–5
16. A.J. Richardson et al., "Abnormal cerebral phospholipid metabolism in dyslexia indicated by phosphorus-31 magnetic resonance spectroscopy," *NMR Biomed*, Vol 10,

1997, pp. 309–14

17. B.J. Stordy, "Dyslexia, attention deficit hyperactivity disorder, dyspraxia—do fatty acids help?," *Dyslexia Review*, Vol 9(2), 1997, pp. 1–3

18. B.J. Stordy, "Benefit of decosahexanoic acid supplements to dark adaptation in dyslexia," *Lancet*, Vol 346, 1995, p. 385

19. M. Portwood, "The role of dietary fatty acids in children's behavior and learning," *Nutr Health*, Vol.18(3), 2006, pp. 233–47

20. M. Portwood, "The role of dietary fatty acids in children's behavior and learning," *Nutr Health*, Vol.18(3), 2006, pp. 233–47

21. M. Colgan and L. Colgan, "Do nutrient supplements and dietary changes affect learning and emotional reactions of children with learning difficulties?," 1984

22. H.L. Needleman and C.A. Gatsonis, "Low level lead exposure and the IQ of children," *JAMA*, Vol 263(5), 1990, pp. 673–8

23. I.D. Capel et al., "Comparison of concentrations of some trace, bulk, and toxic metals in the hair of normal and dyslexic children," *Clin Chem*, Vol 27(6), 1981, pp. 879–81

24. J. Biederman and S.V. Faraone, "Attention-deficit hyperactivity disorder," *Lancet*, vol 366(9481), 2005 pp. 237–48

25. N.D. Volkow et al., "Therapeutic doses of oral methylphenidate significantly increase extracellular dopamine in the human brain," *J Neuroscience*, Vol 21(RC121), 2001, pp. 1–5

26. E. Costello et al., "10-year research update review: The epidemiology of child and adolescent psychiatric disorders: 11. Developmental Epidemiology," *J Am Acad Child Adolesc Psychiatr*, Vol 45 (1), 2005, pp. 8–25

27. Dr. Joan Baizer of the State University of New York at Buffalo at the Annual Meeting of the Society for Neuroscience, 11 November 2001

28. See www.blockcenter.com/articles2/ritalin_dea.htm and R.D. Ciaranello, "Attention deficit-hyperactivity disorder and resistance to thyroid hormone—a new idea?," *N Engl J Med*, Vol 328(14), 1993, pp. 1038–9

29. *NIH Consensus Statement: Diagnosis and Treatment of Attention Deficit Hyperactivity Disorder (ADHD)*, National Institutes of Health, Bethesda (1998)

30. Oregon Health & Science University, "Drug Class Review on Pharmacologic Treatments for ADHD Final Report." See www.ohsu.edu/drugeffectiveness (click on Documents, then Final Reports), Healthy Skepticism, www.healthyskepticism. org/home.php? and Medco Health Solutions Associated Press 15 September 2005

31. N. Lambert and C. Hartsough, "Prospective study of tobacco smoking and substance dependencies among samples of ADHD and non-ADHD participants," *Journal of Learning Disabilities*, Vol 31, 1998, pp. 533–44

32. A. Hoffer, "Vitamin B3 dependent child," *Schizophrenia*, Vol 3, 1971, pp. 107–13.

33. See the Optimal Wellness Centre website www.mercola.com/2001/jan/7/ lendon_smith.htm, and www.smithsez.com/ADHDandADD.html

34. N.I. Ward, "Assessment of clinical factors in relation to child hyperactivity," *J Nutr Environ Med*, Vol 7, 1997, pp. 333–42

35. N.I. Ward, "Hyperactivity and a previous history of antibiotic usage," *Nutrition Practitioner*, Vol 3(3), 2001, p. 12

36. B. Starobrat-Hermelin and T. Kozielec, "The effects of magnesium physiological supplementation on hyperactivity in children with attention deficit hyperactivity disorder

(ADHD): Positive response to magnesium oral loading test," *Magnes Res*, Vol 10(2), 1997, pp. 149–56

37. S.J. Schoenthaler et al., "The effect of randomized vitamin-mineral supplementation on violent and non-violent antisocial behavior among incarcerated juveniles," *J Nut Env Med*, Vol 7, 1997, pp. 343–52

38. I. Colquhon and S. Bunday, "A lack of essential fatty acids as a possible cause of hyperactivity in children," *Medical Hypotheses*, Vol 7, 1981, pp. 673–9

39. L.J. Stevens et al., "Essential fatty acid metabolism in boys with attention-deficit hyperactivity disorder," *Am J Clin Nutr*, Vol 65, 1995, pp. 761–8

40. J.R. Burgess, "ADHD; observational and interventional studies," NIH workshop on omega-3 EFAs in psychiatric disorder, National Institutes of Health, Bethesda, 1998

41. A.J. Richardson et al., "Treatment with highly unsaturated fatty acids can reduce ADHD symptoms in children with specific learning difficulties: a randomized controlled trial," paper given at British Dyslexia Association International Conference, University of York, April 2001

42. A. Richardson and B. Puri, "A randomized double-blind, placebo-controlled study of the effects of supplementation with highly unsaturated fatty acids on ADHD-related symptoms in children with specific learning difficulties," *Prog Neuropsychopharmacol Biol Psychiatry*, Vol 26(2), 2002, pp. 233–9

43. A. Richardson and B. Puri, "A randomized double-blind, placebo-controlled study of the effects of supplementation with highly unsaturated fatty acids on ADHD," 2002

44. B. O'Reilly, paper given at Hyperactive Childrens Support Group Conference, June 2001, U.K.

45. N.I. Ward et al., "The influence of the chemical additive tartrazine on the zinc status of hyperactive children—a double-blind placebo controlled study," *J Nutr Med*, Vol 1, 1990, pp. 51–7

46. M.D. Boris and F.S. Mandel, *Annals of Allergy*, Vol 72, 1994, pp. 462–8

47. R.J. Theil, "Nutrition based interventions for ADD and ADHD," *Townsend Letter for Doctors and Patients*, April 2000, pp. 93–5

48. C.M. Carter et al., "Effects of a few food diet in attention deficit disorder," *Arch Dis Child*, Vol 69, 1993, pp. 564–8

49. Swain et al., "Salicylates, oligoantigenic diet and behavior," *Lancet*, Vol 2(8445), 1985, p. 41–2

50. R.J. Prinz et al., "Dietary correlates of hyperactive behavior in children," *J Consulting Clin Psychol*, Vol 48, 1980, pp. 760–9

51. S.J. Schoenthaler et al., "The effect of randomized vitamin-mineral supplementation on violent and non-violent antisocial behavior among incarcerated juveniles," 1997

52. L. Langseth and J. Dowd, "Glucose tolerance and hyperkinesis," *Fd Cosmet Toxicol*, Vol 16, 1978, p. 129

53. D. Papalos and J. Papalos, *The Bipolar Child*, Broadway Books (2000)

54. K. Blum and J. Holder, 2002, "The Reward Deficiency Syndrome," American College of Addictionology and Compulsive Disorders, pub. Amereon Ltd, Mattituck, NY

55. N.D. Volkow et al., "Therapeutic doses of oral methylphenidate significantly increase extracellular dopamine in the human brain," 2001

56. R. Huff, *U.S. State Department of Developmental Services Report on Autism*, 1999

57. G. Baird et al., "Prevalence of disorders of the autism spectrum in a population cohort

of children in South Thames: The Special Needs and Autism Project (SNAP)," *Lancet*, Vol 368, 2006, pp. 210–15

58. B. Rimland et al., "The effect of high doses of vitamin B6 on autistic children: a double-blind crossover study," *Am J Psychiatry*, Vol 135(4), 1978, pp. 472–5

59. S.I. Pfeiffer et al., "Efficacy of vitamin B6 and magnesium in the treatment of autism: a methodology review and summary of outcomes," *J Autism Dev Disord*, Vol 25(5), 1995, pp. 481–93

60. J. Martineau et al., "Vitamin B6, magnesium, and combined B6-Mg: therapeutic effects in childhood autism," *Biol Psychiatry*, Vol 20(5), 1985, pp. 467–78

61. S. Vancassel et al., "Plasma fatty acid levels in autistic children," *Prostaglandins Leukot Essent Fatty Acids*, Vol 65, 2001, pp. 1–7

62. J.G. Bell et al., "Red blood cell fatty acid compositions in a patient with autism spectrum disorder: a characteristic abnormality in neurodevelopmental disorders?," *Prostaglandins Leukot Essent Fatty Acids*, Vol 63(1–2), 2000, p. 21–5.

63. J.G. Bell, "Fatty acid deficiency and phospholipase A2 in autistic spectrum disorders," report given at research workshop on fatty acids in neurodevelopmental disorders, St. Anne's College, Oxford, September 2001

64. M. Megson, "Is autism a G-Alpha protein defect reversible with natural vitamin A?," *Medical Hypotheses*, Vol 54(6), 2000, pp. 979–83

65. M. Megson, "The biological basis for perceptual deficits in autism: vitamin A and G-proteins," lecture given at Ninth International Symposium on Functional Medicine, May 2002

66. P. Whiteley, the Sunderland University Autism Unit, talk given at the Autism Unravelled Conference, London, May 2001

67. P. Whitely et al., "A gluten free diet as an intervention for autism and associated disorders: preliminary findings," *Autism: International J of Research and Practice*, Vol 3, 1999, pp. 45–65

68. J. Robert Cade, University of Florida Department of Medicine and Physiology, at www.panix.com/~paleodiet/autism/cadelet.txt

69. Letter to the Editor, "Anti-fungal drugs more helpful than Ritalin in autistic children," *Townsend Letter for Doctors and Patients*, April 2001, p. 99

70. A. Wakefield et al., "Enterocolitis in children with developmental disorders," *Am J Gastroenterol*, Vol 95(9), 2000, pp. 2285–95

71. P. Ashwood and A. Wakefield, "Immune activation of peripheral blood and mucosal CD3 lymphocyte Cytokine profiles in children with autism and gastrointestinal symptoms," *J Neuroimmunol*, Vol 173(1–2), 2006, pp. 126–34

72. V.K. Singh et al., "Abnormal measles-mumps-rubella antibodies and CNS autoimmunity in children with autism," *J Biomed Sci*, Vol 9, 2002, pp. 359–64

73. J.J. Bradstreet et al, "Detection of measles virus genomic RNA in cerebrospinal fluid of children with regressive autism: A report of three cases," *JAPS*, Vol 9(2), pp. 38–45

74. H.S. Singer, "Antibrain antibodies in children with autism and their unaffected siblings," *J Neuroimmunol*, Vol 178(1–2), 2006, pp. 149–55

75. M.A. Brudnak, "Application of genomeceuticals to the molecular and immunological aspects of autism," *Med Hypotheses*, Vol 57(2), 2001, pp. 186–91

76. P. Varmanen et al., "S54X-prolyl dipeptidyl aminopeptidase gene (pepX) is part of the

glnRA operon in *Lactobaccilus rhamnosus*," *J Bacteriol*, Vol 182(1), 2000, pp. 146–54

77. Whitely et al., "A gluten free diet as an intervention for autism and associated disorders: preliminary findings," *Autism: International J of Research and Practice*, Vol 3, 1999, pp. 45–65.

78. J. Robert Cade, University of Florida Department of Medicine and Physiology, at www.panix.com/~paleodiet/autism/cadelet.txt

79. M. Ash and E. Gilmore, "Modifying autism through functional nutrition" paper given at Allergy Research Group conference, January 2001

80. Dr. Rosemary Waring, University of Birmingham School of Biosciences, speaking at the Autism Unravelled Conference, London, May 2001

81. W. Walsh et al., *Metallothionein and Autism*, Pfeiffer Treatment Center, Naperville, Illinois (2001). See www.hriptc.org

82. J.K. Kern and A.M. Jones, "Evidence of toxicity, oxidative stress, and neuronal insult in autism," *J Toxicol Environ Health, Part B*, Vol 9, 2006, pp. 485–99. Also see W. McGinnis, "Oxidative stress in autism," *Altern Ther Health Med*, Vol 10, 2004, pp. 22–36

83. S.J. James et al., "Metabolic endophenotype and related genotypes are associated with oxidative stress in children with autism," *Am J Med Genet B Neuropsychiatr Genet*, Vol 141(8), 2006, pp. 947–56

84. S.J. James et al., Metabolic biomarkers of increased oxidative stress and impaired methylation capacity in children with autism. *Am J Clin Nutr*, Vol 80(6), 2004, pp. 1611–17

85. S.P. Pasca et al, "High levels of homocysteine and low serum paraoxonase 1 arylesterase activity in children with autism," *Life Sci*, Vol 78(19), 2006, pp. 2244–8

86. A.J. Wakefield et al., "Ileal-lymphoid hyperplasia, non-specific colitis, and pervasive developmental disorder in children," *Lancet*, Vol 351, 1998, pp. 637–41

87. Andrew Wakefield, speaking at the Allergy Research Foundation conference, November 1999

88. D. Thrower, "Autism and MMR—Summary of Published Research," available from www.foodforthebrain.org under "reports'

89. P. Shattock, presentation, *Food for The Brain Conference*, 1 October 2006

90. F.E. Yazbak, "Autism—is there a vaccine connection?" See www.autisme.net/Yazbak1.htm

91. B. Rimland, *J Nut Env Med*, Vol 10, 2000, pp. 267–9

92. See ref 72 (B. Rimland). See also Ashcraft & Gerel (law firm), "Autism caused by childhood vaccinations containing Thimerosal or mercury," which considers the litigation of individual claims www.ashcraftandgerel.com/thimerosal.html

93. B. Rimland, "Parents' ratings of the effectiveness of drugs and nutrients," *Autism Research Review International*, October 1994

94. H. Turkel, et al., "Intellectual improvement of a retarded patient treated with the 'U' series," *J Orthomol Psychiatry*, Vol 13(4), 1984, pp. 272–6

95. R.F. Harrell et al., "Can nutritional supplements help mentally retarded children? an exploratory study," *Proc Natl Acad Sci*, Vol 78(1), 1981, pp. 574–8

96. T. Tuormaa, *An Alternative to Psychiatry*, The Book Guild Ltd (1991). Also see B. Rimland, "Parents' ratings of the effectiveness of drugs and nutrients," 1994

97. M. Pogribna et al., "Homocysteine metabolism in children with Down syndrome: in

vitro modulation," *Am J Hum Genet*, Vol 69(1), 2001, pp. 88–95

98. Study reported on www.tri21.org/leichtman/

99. R. Bidder et al., "Multivitamins and minerals for children with Downs syndrome," *Dev Med Child Neurol*, Vol 31, 1989, pp. 532–7

100. N.J. Lobaugh et al., "Piracetam therapy does not enhance cognitive functioning in children with Down syndrome," *Arch Paedatr Adolesc Med*, Vol 155(4), 2001, pp. 442–8

101. S.L. Black, "Piracetam therapy for Down syndrome: a rush to judgment?," Letter, *Archives of Paediatric and Adolescent Medicine*, 155(10), 2001

102. B. Gesch, "The SCASO project," *Int J Biosocial Med Res*, Vol 12(1), pp. 41–68

103. M. Virkunnen, "Reactive hypoglycemic tendency among habitually violent offenders," *Nutrition Reviews*, Vol 44(suppl), 1986, pp. 94–103

104. S.J. Schoenthaler, "The Northern California diet-behavior program: An empirical evaluation of 3,000 incarcerated juveniles in Stanislaus County Juvenile Hall," *Int J Biosocial Res*, Vol 5(2), 1983, pp. 99–106

105. S.J. Schoenthaler, "The Los Angeles probation department diet-behavior program: An empirical analysis of six institutional settings," *Int J Biosocial Res*, Vol 5(2), 1983, pp. 107–17

106. R. Freeman et al., *Lead Burden of Sydney Schoolchildren*, University of New South Wales (1979)

107. H. Needleman et al., 1979, "Deficits in psychological and classroom performance of children with elevated dentine lead levels," *New England J of Med*, Vol 300, pp. 689–95

108. G. Thomson et al., "Blood lead levels and children's behavior: results from the Edinburgh lead study," *J Child Psychol Psychiatry*, Vol 30(4), 1989, pp. 515–28

109. R. Pihl and O. Ervin, "Lead and cadmium levels in violent criminals," *Psychol Rep*, Vol 66(3:1), 1990, pp. 839–44

110. G. Schauss, "Comparative hair-mineral analysis results of 21 elements, in a randomly selected behaviorally 'normal' 19–59 year old population and violent adult offenders," *Int J Biosocial Res*, Vol 1(2), 1981, pp. 21–41

111. S.J. Schoenthaler, "The northern-California diet-behavior program: An empirical evaluation of 3,000 incarcerated juveniles in Stanislaus County Juvenile Hall," *Int J Biosocial Res*, Vol 5(2), 1983, pp. 107–17

112. S.J. Schoenthaler et al., "The effect of randomized vitamin-mineral supplementation on violent and non-violent antisocial behavior among incarcerated juveniles," *J Nut Env Med*, Vol 7, 1997, pp. 343–52

113. T. Hamazaki et al., "The effect of docosahexaenoic acid on aggression in young adults: a placebo-controlled double-blind study," *J Clin Invest*, Vol 97, 1996, pp. 1129–33

114. I. Menzies, "Disturbed children: The role of food and chemical sensitivites," *Nutr Health*, Vol 3, 1984, pp. 39–45

115. J. Egger et al., "Controlled trial of oligoantigenic treatment in the hyperkinetic syndrome," *Lancet*, Vol 1(8428), 1985, pp. 540–5

116. A.G. Schauss and C.E. Simonsen, "A critical analysis of the diets of chronic juvenile offenders," Part 1, *J Orthomol Psychiatry*, Vol. 8(3), 1979, pp. 149–57

117. B. Gesch, SCASO pilot study data, unpublished

118. See ref. 104 (S.J. Schoenthaler, 1983) and features on www.mentalhealthproject.com

119. B. Gesch, "Influence of supplementary vitamins, minerals and essential fatty acids on the antisocial behavior of young adult prisoners," *Brit J Psychiatry*, Vol 181, 2002,

pp. 22–8

120. E. Noble, "The gene that rewards alcoholism," *Scientific American*, Science and Medicine, March/April 1996, pp. 52–61

121. U.D. Register et al., "Influence of nutrients in intake of alcohol," *J Am Diet Assoc*, Vol 61(2), 1972, pp. 159–62

122. A.F. Libby et al., "The junk food connection—alcohol and drug lifestyle adversely affect metabolism and behavior," *Orthomolecular Psychiatry*, Vol 11(2), 1982, pp. 116–27

123. Personal communication with Dr. Abram Hoffer. See also W.E. Beebe and O.W. Wendel, *Preliminary Observations of Altered Carbohydrate Metabolism in Psychiatric Patients*, D. Hawkins and L. Pauling (eds), W.H. Freeman and Co. (1973), pp. 435–51

124. U.D. Register et al., "Influence of nutrients in intake of alcohol," 1972

125. W. Philpott and D. Kalita, *Brain Allergies*, Keats Publishing (1980)

126. Society for the Study of Addiction. See www.addiction-ssa.org/

127. M.R. Werbach, *Nutritional Influences on Mental Illness*, Third Line Press (1991)

128. B. Spittle and J. Parker, "Wernicke's encephalopathy complicating schizophrenia," *Aust and NZ J Psych*, Vol 27, 1993, pp. 638–52

129. K. Eriksson et al., "Effects of thiamine deprivation and antagonism on voluntary ethanol intake in rats," *J Nutr*, Vol 110, 1980, p. 937

130. L.L. Rogers et al., "Voluntary alcohol consumption by rats following administration of glutamine," *J Biol Chem*, Vol 220(1), 1956, pp. 321–3

131. H. Ikeda, "Effects of taurine on alcohol withdrawal," *Lancet*, Sept. 1977, Vol. 2(8036), p. 509

132. R.M. Guenther, "Role of nutritional therapy in alcoholism treatment," *Int J Biosocial Res*, Vol 4(1), 1983, pp. 5–18

133. R.F. Smith, "A five year field trial of massive nicotinic acid therapy of alcoholics in Michigan," *J Orthomolec Psych*, Vol 3, 1974, pp. 327–31

134. A. Hoffer and H. Osmond et al., "Treatment of schizophrenia with nicotinic acid and nicotinamide," *J Clin Exper Psychopathol*, Vol 18, 1957, pp. 131–58

135. A.F. Libby and I. Stone, "The Hypoascorbemia-Kwashiorkor approach to drug addiction therapy: pilot study," *Orthomolecular Psychiatry*, Vol 6(4), 1977, pp. 300–8

136. K.M. Hambidge and A. Silverman, "Pica with rapid improvement after dietary zinc supplementation," *Arch Dis Child*, Vol 48, 1973, pp. 567–8

137. R. Bakan, "The role of zinc in anorexia nervosa: etiology and treatment," *Med Hypotheses*, Vol 5(7), 1979, pp. 731–6

138. D. Horrobin et al., *Med Hyp*, Vol 6, 1980, pp. 277–96

139. Casper and Prasad, 1980, later confirmed by L. Humphries et al., "Zinc deficiency and eating disorders," *J Clin Psychiatry*, Vol 50(12), 1989, pp. 456–9

140. P.R. Flanagan, "A model to produce pure zinc deficiency in rats and its use to demonstrate that dietary phytate increases the excretion of endogenous zinc," *J Nutr*, Vol 114, 1984, pp. 493–502 and A. Grider et al., "Age-dependent influence of dietary zinc restriction on short-term memory in male rats," *Physiology and Behaviour*, Vol 72(3), 2001, pp. 339–48

141. A. Arcasoy, N. Akar et al., "Ultrastructural changes in the mucosa of the small intestine in patients with geophagia (Prasad's syndrome)," *J Pediatr Gastroenterol Nutr*, Vol 11(2), 1990, pp. 279–82

142. D. Bryce-Smith and R.I. Simpson, "Case of anorexia nervosa responding to zinc sul-

phate," *Lancet*, Vol 2(8398), 1984, p. 350

143. Katz et al., *J Adol Health Care*, Vol 8, 1987, pp. 400–6

144. L. Humphries et al., "Zinc deficiency and eating disorders," *J Clin Psychiatry*, Vol 50(12), 1989, pp. 456–9

145. C. Birmingham et al., "Controlled trial of zinc supplementation in anorexia nervosa," *Int J Eat Disord*, Vol 15(3), 1994, pp. 251–5

146. N.F. Shay and H.F. Mangian, "Neurobiology of zinc-influenced eating behavior," *J Nutr*, Vol 130(5S Suppl), 2000, pp. 1493S–9S

147. R. Bakan et al., "Dietary zinc intake of vegetarian and non-vegetarian patients with anorexia nervosa," *Int J Eat Disord*, Vol 13(2), 1993, pp. 229–33

148. F. Askenazy et al., "Whole blood serotonin content, tryptophan concentrations, and impulsivity in anorexia nervosa," *Biological Psychiatry*, Vol 43(3), 1998, pp. 188–95

149. A. Favaro, "Tryptophan levels, excessive exercise, and nutritional status in anorexia nervosa," *Psychosomatic Medicine*, Vol 62(4), 2000, pp. 535–8

150. P.J. Cowen and K.A. Smith, "Serotonin, dieting, and bulimia nervosa," *Advances in Experimental Medicine and Biology*, Vol 467, 1999, pp. 101–4

151. W.H. Kaye et al., "Effects of acute tryptophan depletion on mood in bulimia nervosa," *Biol Psychiatry*, Vol 47(2), 2000, pp. 151–7

152. D.B. Smith and E. Obbens, "Antifolate-antiepileptic relationships," in M. I. Botez and E.H. Reynolds, eds, *Folic Acid in Neurology, Psychiatry and Internal Medicine*, Raven Press (1979)

153. F.B. Gibberd et al., "The influence of folic acid on the frequency of epileptic attacks," *Europ J Clin Pharmacology*, Vol 19(1), 1981, pp. 57–60

154. See ref 152

155. M. Nakazawa, "High dose vitamin B6 therapy in infantile spasms—the effect of adverse reactions," *Brain and Development*, Vol 5(2), 1983, p. 193

156. J. Pietz et al., "Treatment of infantile spasms with high-dosage vitamin B6," *Epilepsia*, Vol 34(4), 1993, pp. 757–63

157. A. Sohler and C. Pfeiffer, "A direct method for the determination of managanese in whole blood: patients with seizure activity have low blood levels," *J Orthomol Psychiat*, Vol 12, 1983, pp. 215–34

158. C.L. Dupont and Y. Tanka, "Blood manganese levels in children with convulsive disorder," *Biochem Med*, Vol 33(2), 1985, pp. 246–55

159. P.S. Papavasiliou et al., "Seizure disorders and trace metals: Manganese tissue levels in treated epileptics," *Neurology*, Vol 29, 1979, p. 1466

160. Y. Tanaka, "Low manganese level may trigger epilepsy," *JAMA*, Vol 238, 1977, p. 1805

161. C. Pfeiffer et al., "Zinc and manganese in the schizophrenias," *J Orthomol Psychiat*, Vol 12, 1983, pp. 215–34

162. Y. Shoji, "Serum magnesium and zinc in epileptic children," *Brain and Development*, Vol 5(2), 1983, p. 200

163. S.K. Gupta et al., "Serum Magnesium levels in idiopathic epilepsy," *J Assoc Physicians India*, Vol 42(6), 1994, pp. 456–7

164. L.F. Gorges et al., "Effect of magnesium on epileptic foci," *Epilepsia*, Vol 19(1), 1978, pp. 81–91

165. *Pediatria Romania*, Vol 31(4), 1982, pp. 343–7

166. C.L. Zhang et al., "Paroxysmal epileptiform discharges in temporal lobe slices after pro-

longed exposure to low magnesium are resistant to clinically used anticonvulsants," *Epilepsy Res*, Vol 20(2), 1995, pp. 105–11

167. Y. Shoji, "Serum magnesium and zinc in epileptic children," 1983

168. A. Barbeau et al., "Zinc, taurine and epilepsy," *Arch Neurol*, Vol 30, 1974, pp. 52–8

169. M.I. Botez et al., "Thiamine and folate treatment of chronic epileptic patients: a controlled study with the Wechsler IQ scale," *Epilepsy-Res*, Vol 16(2), 1993, pp. 157–63, and A. Keyser, "Epileptic manifestations and vitamin B1 deficiency," *Eur-Neurol*, Vol 31(3), 1991, pp. 121–5

170. V.T. Ramaeckers, "Selenium deficiency triggering intractable seizures," *Neuropediatrics*, Vol 25(4), 1994, pp. 217–23

171. I.R. Tupeev, "The antioxidant system in the dynamic combined treatment of epilepsy patients with traditional anticonvulsant preparations and an antioxidant—alpha-tocopherol," *Biull Eksp Biol Med*, Vol 116(10), 1993, pp. 362–4

172. S. Yehuda, "Essential fatty acid preparation (SR-3) raises the seizure threshold in rats," *Eur J Pharmacol*, Vol 254(1–2), 1994, pp. 193–8

173. S. Schlanger, M. Shinitzky and D. Yam, "Diet enriched with omega-3 fatty acids alleviates convulsion symptoms in epilepsy patients," *Epilepsia*, Vol 43(1), 2002, pp. 103–4

174. E.S. Roach et al., "N,N-dimethylglycine for epilepsy," Letter to the Editor, *N Engl J Med*, Vol 307, 1982, pp. 1081–2

175. R. Huxtable et al., "The prolonged anticonvulsant action of taurine on genetically determined seizure-susceptibility," *Canadian J Neurol Sci*, Vol 5, 1978, p. 220

176. D.A. Richards et al., "Extracellular GABA in the ventrolateral thalamus of rats exhibiting spontaneous absence epilepsy: a microdialysis study," *J Neurochem*, Vol 65(4), 1995, pp. 1674–80

177. J. Schmidt, "Comparative studies on the anti-convulsant effectiveness of nootropic drugs in kindled rats," *Biomed Biochim Acta*, Vol 49(5), 1990, pp. 413–9

178. J.W. Crayton et al., "Epilepsy precipitated by food sensitivity: Report of a case with double-blind placebo-controlled assessment," *Clinical Electroencephalo*, Vol 12(4), 1981, pp. 192–8

179. W.J. Rea and C.W. Suits, "Cardiovascular disease triggered by foods and chemicals," in J.W. Gerrard, *Food Allergy: New Perspectives*, Charles C. Thomas (1980)

Part 7: Mental Health in Old Age (Chapters 35–38)

1. V.L. Davidson and D.B. Sittman, *Biochemistry: The National Medical Series for Independent Study*, Harawl Publishing (1994), pp. 477–8

2. L. Fleming et al., "Parkinson's disease and brain levels of organochlorine pesticides," *Ann Neurol*, Vol 36(1), 1994, pp. 100–3

3. M. Thiruchelvam et al., "The Nigrostriatal Dopaminergic System as a preferential target of repeated exposures to combined paraquat and maneb: implications for Parkinson's Disease," *Journal of Neuroscience*, Vol 20(24), 2000, pp. 9207–14 and J. Corell et al., "The risk of Parkinson's disease with exposure to pesticides, farming, well water and rural living," *Neurology*, Vol 67, 1998, pp. 1210–18

4. L. Leader, *Parkinson's Disease—The Way Forward*, Denor Press (2000), p. 77

5. W. Duan et al., "Dietary folate deficiency and elevated homocysteine levels endanger

dopaminergic neurons in models of Parkinson's Disease," *J Neurochemistry*, Vol 80, 2002, pp. 101–10

6. S. Hassin-Baer et al., "Plasma homocysteine levels and Parkinson's disease: Disease progression, carotid intima-media thickness and neuropsychiatric complications," *Clin Neuropharmacol*, Vol 29(6), 2006, pp. 305–11

7. R.B. Postuma et al., "Vitamins and entacapone in levodopa-induced hyperhomocysteinemia: A randomized controlled study," *Neurology*, Vol 66(12), 2006, pp. 1941–3

8. L.M. de Lau et al., "Dietary folate, vitamin B12, and vitamin B6 and the risk of Parkinson's disease," *Neurology*, Vol 67(2), 2006, pp. 315–18

9. L. Leader, *Parkinson's Disease—The Way Forward* (2001), p. 87, "Optimizing Function by Nutritional Manipulation," p. 145, "Liver Detoxification and Optimal Liver Function," Helen Kimber

10. G.B. Steventon et al., "Plasma cysteine and sulphate levels in patients with motor neurone, Parkinson's and Alzheimer's Disease," *Neurosci Letts*, Vol 110, 1990, pp. 216–20

11. S. Fahn, "A pilot trial of high dose alpha-tocopherol and ascorbate in early Parkinson's Disease," *Ann Neurol*, Vol 32(S), 1992, pp. 128–32

12. J.S. Bland and J.A. Bralley, "Nutritional upregulation of hepatic detoxification enzymes," *J Applied Nutrition*, Vol 4, 1992, pp. 3–15

13. R.B. D'Agostino et al., "Plasma homocysteine as a risk factor for dementia and Alzheimer's disease," *N Engl J Med*, Vol 346(7), 2002, pp. 476–83

14. W. Duan, M.P. Mattson et al., "Dietary folate deficiency and elevated homocysteine levels endanger dopaminergic neurons in models of Parkinson's disease," *J Neurochem*, Vol 80(1), 2002, pp. 101–10

15. G. Leader and L. Leader, *Parkinson's Disease—The New Nutritional Handbook* , Denor Press (1996/7), p. 96

16. *ABPI Compendium of Data Sheets and Summaries of Product Characteristics (1999–2000)*, pp. 371, 1333, Datapharm Publications Limited

17. *ABPI Compendium*, pp. 1105–6

18. G. Leader and L. Leader, *Parkinson's Disease—The New Nutritional Handbook*, p. 96

19. I.R. Bell et al., "Brief communication. Vitamin B1, B2, and B6 augmentation of tricyclic antidepressant treatment in geriatric depression with cognitive dysfunction," *J Am College of Nutrition*, Vol 11(2), 1992, pp. 159–63

20. H. Refsum et al., "The Hordaland Homocysteine Study: A Community-Based Study of Homocysteine, Its Determinants, and Associations with Disease," *J Nutr*, Vol 136, 2006, pp. 1731S–40S

21. K. Tucker et al., "High homocysteine and low B vitamins predict cognitive decline in aging men: The Veterans Affairs Normative Aging Study," *Am J Clin Nutr*, Vol 82, 2005, pp. 627–35

22. J. Durga et al., "Folate and the methylenetetrahydrofolate reductase mutation correlate with cognitive performance," *Neurobiol Aging*, Vol 27(2), 2006, pp. 334–43

23. W.J. Perrig et al., "The relation between antioxidants and memory performance in the old and very old," *J Am Geriatr Soc*, Vol 45(6), 1997, pp. 718–24

24. A.J. Perkins et al., "Association of antioxidants with memory in a multiethnic elderly sample using the Third National Health and Nutrition Examination Survey," *Am J Epidemiol*, Vol 150(1), 1999, pp. 37–44

25. J.W. Miller, "Vitamin E and memory: is it vascular protection?," *Nutr Rev*, Vol 58(4),

2000, pp. 109–11

26. D. Edwin et al., "Cognitive impairment in alcoholic and nonalcoholic cirrhotic patients," *Hepatology*, Vol 30(6), 1999, pp. 1363–7

27. F. Calon et al., "Docosahexaenoic acid protects from dendritic pathology in an Alzheimer's disease mouse model," *Neuron*, Vol 43, 2004, pp. 633–45

28. C.H. Wilkins et al., "Vitamin D deficiency is associated with low mood and worse cognitive performance in older adults," *Am J Geriatr Psychiatry*, Vol 14, 2006, pp. 1032–40

29. R. Wurtman et al., "Effect of oral CDP-choline on plasma choline and uridine levels in humans," *Biochem Pharm*, Vol 60, 2000, pp. 989–92

30. S. Suzuki et al., "Oral administration of soybean lecithin transphosphatidylated phosphatidylserine improves memory impairment in aged rats," *J Nutr*, Vol 131(11), 2001, pp. 2951–6

31. J. Kleijnin and P. Knipschild, "Ginkgo biloba," *Lancet*, Vol 340(8828), 1992, pp. 1136–9

32. P.L. Le Bars, "A placebo-controlled, double-blind, randomized trial on an extract of Ginkgo Biloba for dementia," *JAMA*, Vol 278(16), 1997, pp. 1327–32

33. F. Huguet et al., "Decreased cerebral 5-HT1A receptors during aging: reversal by Ginkgo biloba extract," *J Pharm Pharmacol*, Vol 46, 1994, pp. 316–18

34. J. Birks, "Ginkgo biloba for cognitive impairment and dementia," *Cochrane Database Syst Rev*, Vol 4, 2002, CD003120

35. M. Van Dongen et al., "Ginkgo for elderly people with dementia and age-associated memory impairment: A randomized clinical trial," *J Clin Epidemiol*, Vol 56, 2003, 367–76

36. P.R. Solomon et al., "Ginkgo for memory enhancement: A randomized controlled trial," *JAMA*, Vol 288, 2002, pp. 835–40

37. J.A. Mix and W.D. Crews, "A double-blind, placebo-controlled, randomized trial of Ginkgo biloba extract EGb 761 in a sample of cognitively intact older adults: Neuropsychological findings," *Hum Psychopharmacol*, Vol 17(6), 2002, pp. 267–77

38. R.M. Sapolsky, "Why stress is bad for your brain," *Science*, Vol 273(5276), 1995, pp. 749–50

39. T. Satoh et al., "Walking exercise and improved neuropsychological functioning in elderly patients with cardiac disease," *J Intern Med*, Vol 238(5), 1995, pp. 423–8

40. R. Clarke et al., "Folate, vitamin B12, and serum total homocysteine levels in confirmed Alzheimer's disease," *Arch Neurol*, Vol 55, 1998, pp. 1449–55

41. E. Hogervorst et al., "Plasma homocysteine levels, cerebrovascular risk factors, and cerebral white matter changes (leukoaraiosis) in patients with Alzheimer disease," *Arch Neurol*, Vol 59, 2002, pp. 787–93

42. J.H. Williams et al., "Minimal hippocampal width relates to plasma homocysteine in community-dwelling older people," *Age Ageing*, Vol 31, 2002, pp. 440–4

43. A. McCaddon et al., "Alzheimer's disease and total plasma aminothiols," *Biol Psychiatry*, Vol 53, 2003, pp. 254–60

44. J.W. Green et al., "Homocysteine, vitamin B6, and vascular disease in AD patients," *Neurology*, Vol 58, 2002, pp. 1471–5

45. M. Esiri et al., "Cerebrovascular disease and threshold for dementia in the early stages of Alzheimer's disease," *Lancet*, Vol 354, 1999, pp. 919–20

46. S. Seshadri et al., "Plasma homocysteine as a risk factor for dementia and Alzheimer's

disease," *New Engl J Med*, Vol. 346(7), 2002, pp. 466–8

47. P.S. Sachdev et al., "Relationship between plasma homocysteine levels and brain atrophy in healthy elderly individuals," *Neurology*, Vol. 58, 2002, pp. 1539–41

48. T. den Heijer, "Homocysteine and brain atrophy on MRI of non-demented elderly," *Brain*, Vol 126, 2003, pp. 170–5

49. H.X. Wang et al., "Vitamin B(12) and folate in relation to the development of Alzheimer's disease," *Neurology*, Vol 56(9), 2001, pp. 1188–94

50. S.J. Duthie et al., "Homocysteine, B vitamin status, and cognitive function in the elderly," *Am J Clin Nutr*, Vol. 75(5), 2002, pp. 908–13

51. D. Kado et al., "Homocysteine levels and decline in physical function," *Am J Med*, Vol 113(7), 2002, pp. 537–42

52. A. McCaddon and C. Kelly, "Alzheimer's disease: A 'cobalaminergic' hypothesis," *Med Hypotheses*, Vol 37(3), 1992, pp. 161–5

53. A. McCaddon et al., "Total serum homocysteine in senile dementia of Alzheimer's type," *Int J Geriatr Psychiatr*, Vol 13, 1998, pp. 235–9

54. A. McCaddon et al., "Homocysteine and cognitive decline in healthy elderly," *Dement Geriatr Cognit Disord*, Vol 12, 2000, pp. 309–13

55. A. McCaddon et al., "Analogues, aging and aberrant assimilation of vitamin B12 in Alzheimer's disease," *Dement Geriatr Cognit Disord*, Vol 12, 2001, pp. 133–7

56. V. Herbert and B. Herzlich, "A proposed model of sequential stages in the development of vitamin B12 deficiency," *Blood*, Vol 66(suppl1), 1985, p. 45a

57. A. McCaddon et al., "Total serum homocysteine in senile dementia of Alzheimer's type," *Int J Geriatr Psychiatry*, Vol 13, 1998, pp. 235–9

58. A. McCaddon et al., "Functional vitamin B12 deficiency and Alzheimer disease," *Neurology*, Vol 58, 2002, pp. 1395–9

59. M. Toshifumi et al., "Elevated plasma homocysteine levels and risk of silent brain infarction in elderly people," *Stroke*, Vol 32, 2001, p. 1116

60. S.A. Lipton et al., "Neurotoxicity associated with dual actions of homocysteine at the N-methyl-D-aspartate receptor," *Proc Natl Acad Sci U.S.A.*, Vol 94, 1997, pp. 5923–8

61. M.F. Beal et al., "Neurochemical characterization of excitotoxin lesions in the cerebral cortex," *J Neurosci*, Vol 11, 1991, pp. 147–58

62. R. Clarke et al., "Folate, vitamin B12 and total serum homocysteine levels in confirmed Alzheimer's disease," *Arch Neurol*, Vol 55, 1998, pp. 1449–55

63. T. Bottiglieri et al., "Plasma total homocysteine levels and the C677T mutation in the methylenetetrahydrofolate reductase (MTHFR) gene: A study in an Italian population with dementia," *Mech Ageing Dev*, Vol. 122(16), 2001, pp. 2013–23

64. D.A. Snowdon et al., "Serum folate and the severity of atrophy of the neocortex in Alzheimer disease: Findings from the Nun Study," *Am J Clin Nutr*, Vol 71(4), 2000, pp. 993–8

65. K. Eto et al, "Brain hydrogen silphide is severely decreased in Alzheimer's disease," *Biochem Biophys Res Commun*, Vol 293, 2002, pp. 1485–8

66. R. Clarke et al., "Folate, vitamin B12, and serum total homocysteine levels in confirmed Alzheimer disease," *Arch Neurol*, Vol 55(11), 1998, pp. 1449–55

67. H. Refsum, "Low vitamin B-12 status in confirmed Alzheimer's disease as revealed by serum holotranscobalamin," *J Neurol Neurosurg Psychiatr*, Vol 74, 2003, pp. 959–61

68. G. Ravaglia et al., "Folate, but not homocysteine, predicts the risk of fracture in elderly

persons," *J Gerontol A Biol Sci Med Sci*, Vol 60(11), 2005, pp. 1458–62

69. R. Clarke et al., "Folate, vitamin B12, and serum total homocysteine levels in confirmed Alzheimer disease," *Arch Neurol*, Vol 55, 1998, pp. 1449–55

70. K. Koyama et al., "Efficacy of methylcobalamin on lowering total homocysteine plasma concentrations in haemodialysis patients receiving high-dose folate supplementation," *Nephrol Dial Transplant*, Vol 17, 2002, pp. 916–22

71. D. McGregor et al., "Betaine supplementation decreases post-methionine hyperhomocysteinemia in chronic renal failure," *Kidney Int*, Vol 61(3), 2002, pp. 1040–6

72. M.M. Corrada et al., "Reduced risk of Alzheimer's disease with high folate intake: The Baltimore longitudinal study of aging." *Alzh Dement*, Vol 1, 2005, pp. 11–18

73. N. Scarmeas, "Mediterranean diet, Alzheimer disease and vascular mediation," *Arch Neurol*, Vol 63(12), 2006, pp. 1709–17

74. Y. Freund-Levi et al., "Omega 3 fatty acid treatment in 174 patients with mild to moderate Alzheimer disease: OmegAD study: a randomized double blind trial," *Arch Neurol*, Vol 63(10), 2006, pp. 1402–8

75. J.G. Crawford, "Alzheimer's disease risk factors as related to cerebral blood flow," *Med Hypotheses*, Vol 46, 1996, pp. 367–77

76. A. Osawa et al., "Relationship between cognitive function and regional cerebral blood flow in different types of dementia," *Disabil Rehabil*, Vol 26, 2004, pp. 739–45

77. D. Laurin et al., "Physical activity and risk of cognitive impairment and dementia in elderly persons," *Arch Neurol*, Vol 58, 2001, pp. 498–504

78. T. Satoh et al., "Walking exercise and improved neuropsychological functioning in elderly patients with cardiac disease," *J Intern Med*, vol 238, 1995, pp. 423–8

79. E. Larson et al., "Exercise is associated with reduced risk for incident dementia among persons 65 years and older," *Ann Intern Med*, Vol 144, 2006, pp. 73–81

80. S.J. Colcombe et al., "Aerobic fitness reduces brain tissue loss in aging humans," *J Gerontol A Biol Sci Med Sci*, Vol 58, 2003, pp. 176–80

81. L. Teri et al., "Exercise plus behavioral management in patients with Alzheimer disease: A randomized controlled trial," *JAMA*, Vol 290, 2003, pp. 2015–22

82. J.D. Elsworth et al., "Deprenyl administration in man: A selective MAO-B inhibitor without the 'cheese effect'," *Psychopharmacology (Berl)*, Vol 57(1), 1978, pp. 33–8

83. Knoll research reported in W. Dean et al., *Smart Drugs II—The Next Generation*, Health Freedom Publications (1993)

84. D.S. Khalsa, *Altern Ther Health Med*, Vol 4(6), 1998, pp. 38–43 and R.M. Wu et al., *Ann NY Acad Sci*, Vol 786, 1996, pp. 379–90

85. D. Ward and J. Morgenthaler, *Smart Drugs and Nutrients*, B and J Publications (1990), pp. 42–3

86. P. Mindus et al., "Piracetam-induced improvement of mental performance. A controlled study on normally aging individuals," *Acta Psychiat Scand*, Vol 54, 1976, pp. 150–60

87. L. Israel et al., "Drug therapy and memory training programs: a double-blind randomized trial of general practice patients with age-associated memory impairment," *Int Psychogeriatr*, Vol 6(2), 1994, pp. 155–70

88. L.S. Schneider and J.T. Olin, "Overview of clinical trials of hydergine in dementia," *Arch Neurol*, Vol 51(8), 1994, pp. 787–98

89. L.S. Schneider and J.T. Olin, "Overview of clinical trials of hydergine in dementia,"

1994

90. D. Ward and J. Morgenthaler, *Smart Drugs and Nutrients*
91. I. Zhdanova et al., "Sleep-inducing effects of low doses of melatonin ingested in the evening," *Clinical Pharmacology and Therapeutics*, Vol 57(5), 1995, pp. 552–8
92. R. Nave et al., "Melatonin improves evening napping," *Eur J Pharmacol*, Vol 275(2), 1995, pp. 213–16

General

Recommended reading

Child, S., *An A–Z of Child Health: A Nutritional Approach*, Argyll, 2002

Hoffer, A., *Adventures in Psychiatry: The Scientific Memoirs of Dr. Abram Hoffer*, KOS Publishing Inc., 2005

Holford, P., *The New Optimum Nutrition Bible*, Piatkus, 2005

Holford, P., *The Holford Low-GL Diet*, Piatkus, 2004

Holford, P. and Braly, J., *Hidden Food Allergies*, Piatkus, 2005

Holford, P. and Burne, J., *Food is Better Medicine than Drugs*, Piatkus, 2006.

Holford, P. and Cass, H., *Natural Highs*, Piatkus, 2001

Holford, P. and Colson, D., *Optimum Nutrition for Your Child's Mind*, Piatkus, 2006

Holford, P. with Heaton, S. and Colson, D., *The Alzheimer's Prevention Plan*, Piatkus, 2005

Holford, P. and Lawson, S., *Optimum Nutrition Before, During and After Pregnancy*, Piatkus, 2004

Holford, P. and McDonald Joyce, F., *The Holford Low-GL Diet Cookbook*, Piatkus, 2005

Holford, P. and McDonald Joyce, F., *The Holford Low-GL Diet Made Easy*, Piatkus, 2006

Holford, P. and Ridgeway, J., *The Optimum Nutrition Cookbook*, Piatkus, 2000

Papolos, D. and Papolos, J., *The Bipolar Child*, Broadway Books, 1999

Pfeiffer, C.C., *Mental and Elemental Nutrients*, Keats Publishing, 1975

Richardson, A., *They Are What You Feed Them: How Food Can Improve Your Child's Behaviour, Mood and Learning*, Harper Thorsons, 2006

Werbach, M., *Nutritional Influences on Mental Illness*, Third Line Press, 1991

Wigmore, A., *The Sprouting Book*, Avery, 1986

Chapters 4 and 5—Smart fats and phospholipids

Schmidt, M.A., *Smart Fats*, Frog Ltd, 1997

Stoll, A.L. *The Omega 3 Connection*, Simon and Schuster, 2002

Chapter 6—Amino acids

Braverman, E.R. et al., *The Healing Nutrients Within*, Keats Publishing, 1997

Chapter 13—Boosting intelligence

Benton, D., *Food for Thought*, Penguin, 1996

Chapters 14, 36 and 37—Memory enhancement, preventing memory decline, and Alzheimer's

Hoffer, A., *Smart Nutrients—A Guide to Nutrients That Can Prevent and Reverse Senility*, Avery Publishing, 1994
Khalsa, D.S. and Stauth, C., *Brain Longevity*, Warner Books, 1997
Lombard, J. and Germano, C., *The Brain Wellness Plan*, Kensington Books, 1997
Warren, T., *Beating Alzheimer's*, Avery, 1991

Chapters 15 and 23—Beating the blues and depression

Brown, M. and Robinson, J., *When Your Body Gets the Blues*, Rodale Press, 2002
Cass, H., *St. John's Wort—Nature's Blues Buster*, Avery Publishing, 1998
Ross, J., *The Mood Cure*, Thorsons, 2003

Chapter 16—Hormonal mood swings

Carruthers, M., *The Testosterone Revolution*, Thorsons, 2001
Colgan, M., *Hormonal Health*, Apple Publishing Canada, 1996
Lee, J., *What Your Doctor Didn't Tell You About Menopause*, Warner Books, 1996

Chapter 17—Unwinding anxiety

Cass, H. and McNally, T., *Kava—Nature's Answer to Stress, Anxiety, Insomnia*, Prima Health, 1998

Chapters 24–26—Manic depression and schizophrenia

Dryden, W. and Gordon, J., *Think Your Way to Happiness—How to Help Yourself with Cognitive Therapy*, Sheldon Press, 1990
Hoffer, A., *Vitamin B-3, Schizophrenia, Discovery, Recovery and Controversy*, Quarry Health Books, 2000
Horrobin, D., *The Madness of Adam and Eve—How Schizophrenia Shaped Humanity*, Bantam Press, 2001

Lawson, V., *Inside Out*, 2001. This is a good, practical self-help guide for people with manic depression, available from the Manic Depression Fellowship (in the U.K., call 020 7793 2600).

Chapter 28—Attention deficit disorders

ADHD—Hyperactive Children: A Parents' Guide, Hyperactive Children's Support Group, 2002. To order, see www.hacsg.org.uk
Block, M., *No More ADHD*, Block Books, 2001
Papolos, D. and M., *The Bipolar Child*, Broadway Books, 2000
Weintrub, S., *Natural Treatments for ADD and Hyperactivity*, Woodland Publishing, 1997

Chapter 29—Autism

Gillberg, C. and Coleman, M., *Biology of the Autistic Syndrome*, Mac Keith Press, 2000
McCandless, J., *Children with Starving Brains*, Bramble Books, 2002

Chapter 32—Beating addictions

Holford, P., *Beat Stress and Fatigue*, Piatkus Books, 1999
Mathews Larson, J., *Seven Weeks to Sobriety*, Random House, 1997
Miller, M. and Miller, D., *Staying Clean and Sober*, Woodland Publishing, 2006

Chapter 33—Eating disorders

Woodman, M., *The Owl Was a Baker's Daughter—Obesity, Anorexia Nervosa, and the Repressed Feminine*, Inner City Books, 1980

Chapter 35—Parkinson's disease

Leader, G. and L., *Parkinson's Disease: Reducing Symptoms with Nutrition and Drugs*, Denor Press, 2006
Leader, G. and L., *Parkinson's Disease—The Way Forward*, Denor Press, 1999. See www.parkinsonsdisease-the-way-forward.com for more details.

Chapter 38—Smart drugs and hormones

Dean, W. and Morgenthaler, J., *Smart Drugs and Nutrients*, B&J Publications, 1990
Dean, W., Morgenthaler, J. and Fowkes, S.W., *Smart Drugs II—The Next Generation*, Health Freedom Publications, 1993

Useful addresses

Addictions

Alcoholics Anonymous (AA) is a fellowship of men and women who share their experience, strength, and hope with each other so that they may solve their common problem and help others to recover from alcoholism using a 12-step program. The only requirement for membership is a desire to stop drinking. Alcoholics Anonymous is worldwide with A.A. meetings in almost every community. You can find times and places of local A.A. meetings or events by contacting a nearby central office, intergroup or answering service of U.S. and Canada.

Contact www.aa.org for a comprehensive list of locations throughout the United States. The General Service Office does not maintain local meeting information.

Narcotics Anonymous (NA) is a nonprofit society of recovering addicts who meet regularly to help each other stay clean. Recovery in NA focuses on the problem of addiction, rather than on any particular drug, using the same 12-step program as Alcoholics Anonymous. Membership is not limited to addicts who use one drug or another. Those who feel they may have a problem with any drugs—legal or illegal, including alcohol—are welcome in Narcotics Anonymous.

Contact Narcotics Anonymous, PO Box 9999, Van Nuys, CA 91409 / Tel: (818) 773-9999 / Fax: (818) 700-0700 / Website: www.na.org

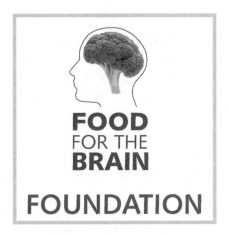

ADHD/Hyperactivity

Children and Adults with Attention-Deficit/Hyperactivity Disorder (CHADD) is a national non-profit organization providing education, advocacy, and support for individuals with AD/HD. In addition to its informative website, CHADD also publishes a variety of printed materials to keep members and professionals current on research advances, medications and treatments affecting individuals with AD/HD.

Contact CHADD, 8181 Professional Place, Suite 150, Landover, MD 20785 / Tel: (800) 233-4050 / Fax: (301) 306-7090 / Website: www.chadd.org

Feingold Association of the United States is an organization of families and professionals, dedicated to helping children and adults apply proven dietary techniques for better behavior, learning, and health.

Contact Feingold Association of the United States, 554 East Main Street, Suite 301, Riverhead, NY 11901 / Tel: (800) 321-3287 / Fax: (631) 369-2988 / Website: www.feingold.org / Email: Help@feingold.org

Allergies

Food allergy testing is available through your nutritional therapist or doctor.

Immuno Laboratories offers food allergy testing (IgG ELISA) through your doctor or health practitioner.

Contact Immuno Laboratories, 6801 Powerline Road, Fort Lauderdale, FL 33309 / Tel: (954) 691-2500 or (800) 231-9197 / Fax: (954) 691-2505 / Website: www.immunolab.com

YorkTest Laboratories also offer IgG testing. Using a home-test kit, you can take your own pinprick blood sample and return it to the lab for analysis. These test kits are available worldwide.

Contact www.yorktest.com

Alzheimer's

Alzheimer's Research and Prevention Foundation (ARPF) is dedicated to reducing the incidence of Alzheimer's disease by conducting clinical research and providing educational outreach.

Contact ARPF, 6300 E. El Dorado Plaza, Suite 400, Tucson, AZ 85715 / Tel: (520) 749-8374 / Fax: (520) 296-6640 / Website: www.alzheimersprevention. org / Email: Info@alzheimersprevention.org

The Alzheimer's Research Trust is the U.K.'s leading non-profit group for dementia research. It is dedicated to funding scientific studies to find ways to treat, cure, or prevent Alzheimer's disease, vascular dementia, Lewy Body disease, and fronto-temporal dementias.

Contact www.alzheimers-research.org for more details

See also CERI (page 481).

Autism

The Autism Collaboration provides information about autism to parents and professionals, and conducts research on the efficacy of various therapeutic interventions, in collaboration with the Autism Research Institute (see following).

Contact www.autism.org

Autism Research Institute (ARI), founded by Bernard Rimland, Ph.D., is the hub of a worldwide network of parents and professionals concerned with autism. The only organization of its kind, ARI was founded in 1967 to conduct and foster scientific research designed to improve the methods of diagnosing, treating, and preventing autism. ARI also disseminates research findings to parents and others all over the world that are seeking help. The ARI data bank, the world's largest, contains nearly 40,000 detailed case histories of autistic children from more than sixty countries. ARI publishes Autism Research International.

Contact ARI, 4182 Adams Avenue, San Diego, CA 92116 / Tel: (866) 366-3361 / Website: www.autism.com

Autism Society of America (ASA) was founded in 1965 by a small group of parents working on a volunteer basis out of their homes. Over the last 35 years, the Society has developed into the leading source of information and referral on autism. Today, over 20,000 members are connected through a working network of over 200 chapters in nearly every state. Membership in ASA continues to grow as more and more parents and professionals unite to form a collective voice representing the autism community.

Contact ASA, 7910 Woodmont Avenue, Suite 300, Bethesda, MD 20814-3067 / Tel: (800) 328-8476 / Website: www.autism-society.org

Depression and Manic Depression

The Depression and Bipolar Support Alliance (DBSA) is the nation's leading patient-directed organization focusing on the most prevalent mental illnesses—depression and bipolar disorder. The organization fosters an understanding about the impact and management of these life-threatening illnesses by providing up-to-date, scientifically based tools and information written in language the general public can understand. DBSA supports research to promote more timely diagnosis, develop more effective and tolerable treatments, and discover a cure. The organization works to ensure that people living with mood disorders are treated equitably.

Contact DBSA, 730 North Franklin Street, Suite 501, Chicago, IL 60654-7225 / Tel: (800) 826-3632 / Fax: (312) 642-7243 / Website: www.dbsalliance.org

Down's Syndrome

Friends of Trisomy 21 Research is a voluntary support group set up by parents of children with Down's syndrome to back the Trisomy 21 Research Foundation. Friends aim to raise the necessary funding for research into Down's syndrome and nutrition intervention, and to improve the availability of information for parents and caregivers so they are able to make informed choices about treatment and care. They publish a newsletter for members packed with invaluable information and advice.

Contact Friends of Trisomy 21 Research, 11718 Barrington Court, #511, Los Angeles, CA 90049 / Tel: (310) 472-8778

Also contact Trisomy 21 Research Foundation, 933 First Colonial Road, Suite 109, Virginia Beach, VA 23454 / Tel: (310) 425-1969 / Website: www.tri21.org. Also see some good articles on The Down's Syndrome Page at www.ceri.com/downhome.htm

Dyslexia

The International Dyslexia Association (IDA) was established to continue the pioneering work of Dr. Samuel T. Orton, a neurologist who was one of the first to identify dyslexia as a neurological difference and, along with Anna Gillingham, develop effective teaching approaches. For over 50 years it has fought for the rights of people with dyslexia while fending off critics who said that there was no such thing as dyslexia—that children who exhibited signs of dyslexia and other learning disabilities were lazy, stupid or worse, developmentally disabled, and therefore incapable of learning. During this time the organization has tested and tutored hundreds of thousands of children so that they would grow up to lead productive and fulfilling lives. Nowhere else can a person discover such a full range of useful information, practices, and research about dyslexia than through The International Dyslexia Association.

Contact IDA, 40 York Road, 4th Floor, Towson, MD 21204/ Tel: (410) 296-0232 / Fax: (410) 321-5069 / Voice Message Requests for Information: (800) ABCD123 / Website: www.interdys.org

Eating Disorders

National Eating Disorders Association (NEDA) is the largest not-for-profit organization in the United States working to prevent eating disorders and provide treatment referrals to those suffering from anorexia, bulimia and binge eating disorder and those concerned with body image and weight issues.

Contact NEDA, 603 Stewart Street, Suite 803, Seattle, WA 98101 / Tel: (206) 382-3587 / Information Helpline: (800) 931-2237 / Website: www.National EatingDisorders.org / Email: info@NationalEatingDisorders.org

Laboratory Testing

Laboratory tests are becoming increasingly available for measuring a person's status for vitamins, essential fats, hormones, and even neurotransmitters. The following is an up-to-date list of the best laboratories in the U.S.

The Bio-Center Lab carries out blood tests for essential fats, urine tests for pyroluria, chemical sensitivity panels, toxic element screens, and more. Only available through qualified practitioners.

Contact Bio-Center Lab, 3100 North Hillside Avenue, Wichita, KS 67219-3904 / Tel: (316) 684-7784 / (800) 494-7785 / Fax: (316) 682-2062 / Website: www.bio-centerlab.org / Email: biocenterlab@brightspot.org

Diagnos-Techs, Inc., a clinical and research laboratory, offers a range of tests, including salivary tests for DHEA, melatonin, estrogen, progesterone, and testosterone, among others. A nutritionist can arrange for you to have these tests.

Contact Diagnos-Techs, Inc., 6620 South 192nd Place, Building J, Kent, WA 98032 / Tel: (800) 878-3787 / Fax: (425) 251-0637 / Website: www.diagnos-techs.com / Email: diagnos@diagnostechs.com

Doctor's Data, Inc., is an independent reference laboratory providing data on levels of toxic and essential elements in hair, and elements, amino acids, and metabolites in blood and urine. DDI uses ICP-MS, HPLC, and photometric analyses to measure elements, amino acids and metabolites. DDI's specialized instrumentation can detect ultratrace levels of analytes.

Contact Doctor's Data, Inc., 3755 Illinois Avenue, St. Charles, IL 60174-2420 / Tel: (800) 323-2784 / Fax: (630) 587-7860 / Website: www.doctorsdata.com / Email: inquiries@doctorsdata.com

Genova Diagnostics (formerly Great Smokies Diagnostic Laboratory) is a full-service testing company dealing with digestion, nutrition, detoxification, oxidative stress, immunology, allergy, hormones and endocrine regulation, and cardiovascular function. Client services are available 8 AM to 8 PM EST.

Contact Genova Diagnostics, 63 Zillicoa Street, Asheville, NC 28801 / Tel: (800) 522-4762 / Fax: (828) 252-9303 / Website: www.genovadiagnostics.com

Optimum Health Resource Laboratories, Inc., (formerly York Nutritional Laboratories) specialize in testing for allergies and intolerances, and offer a FoodScan test that tests you for IgG sensitivity to a wide range of foods. It involves a home kit that enables you to send a pinprick of blood that is then used to test your food intolerances, giving you a clear indication of your food intolerances. They also test for IgE sensitivity and homocysteine.

Contact Optimum Health Resource Laboratories, Inc., 419 South Federal Highway, Dania Beach, FL 33004 / Tel: (954) 926-8020 / Website: www.optimumhealthresource.com

Trace Elements, Inc., a leading laboratory for hair mineral analysis for healthcare professionals worldwide.

Contact Trace Elements, Inc., 4501 Sunbelt Drive, Addison, TX 75001-5130 / Tel: (972) 250-6410 / (800) 824-2314 / Fax: (972) 248-4896 / Website: www.traceelements.com / Email: teilab@traceelements.com

Vitamin Diagnostics, Inc., performs an up-to-19-item assay of vitamins and micronutrients in their metabolically available forms. Includes vitamins A, B1, B2, B3, B5, B6, B12, C, E, beta-carotene, biotin, lipoate, biopterin, carnitine, acyl-carnitine, folic acid, free and total choline, and inositol.

Contact Vitamin Diagnostics, Inc., Route 35 & Industrial Drive, Cliffwood Beach, NJ 07735 / Tel: (732) 583-7773 / Fax: (732) 583-7774 / Email: lab@vitdiag.com

Memory

The Cognitive Enhancement Research Institute (CERI) is the best way to keep up to date on mind and memory boosters. This website has many interesting features, and international listings for suppliers of smart drugs and nutrients, and will keep you updated on topical issues.

Contact CERI, PO Box 4029, Menlo Park, CA 94026 / Tel: (650) 321-CERI (2374) / Fax: (650) 323-3864 / Website: www.ceri.com / For books and products: www.smart-publications.com

Mental Health General

Food for the Brain is an educational non-profit group that promotes the link between optimum nutrition and mental health (see page 000). The Food for the Brain Schools Campaign also gives schools and parents advice on how to make kids smarter by improving the quality of food they eat in and outside of school. It has a free mental health e-news service, an online library of new research and special reports, a listing of frequent seminars and conferences, and a free online mental health questionnaire and the Food for the Brain Child Questionnaire, which helps you identify imbalances correctable by optimum nutrition.

Contact www.foodforthebrain.org

The International Society for Orthomolecular Medicine exists to further the advancement of orthomolecular medicine throughout the world, and to unite the many and various groups already operating in eighteen countries. Orthomolecular Medicine describes the practice of using the most appropriate nutrients, including vitamins, minerals, and other essential compounds, in the most therapeutic amounts, according to an individual's particular biochemical requirements to establish optimum health. The Society serves to educate health professionals and the public in the benefits and practice of orthomolecular medicine through publications, including the Journal of Orthomolecular Medicine (formerly the Journal of Orthomolecular Psychiatry).

Contact www.orthomed.org

The National Alliance on Mental Illness (NAMI), founded in 1979, is a non-profit, grass-roots, self-help, support and advocacy organization of consumers, families, and friends of people with severe mental illnesses, such as schizophrenia, schizoaffective disorder, bipolar disorder, major depressive disorder, obsessive-compulsive disorder, panic and other severe anxiety disorders, autism and pervasive developmental disorders, attention deficit/hyperactivity disorder, and other severe and persistent mental illnesses that affect the brain.

Contact NAMI, Colonial Place Three, 2107 Wilson Boulevard, Suite 300, Arlington, VA 22201-3042 / Tel: (703) 524-7600 / Fax: (703) 524-9094 / TDD: (703) 516-7227 / Information Helpline: (800) 950-NAMI (6264) / Website: www.nami.org

The National Institute of Mental Health's (NIMH) mission is to reduce the burden of mental illness and behavioral disorders through research on mind, brain, and behavior. This public health mandate demands that we harness powerful scientific tools to achieve better understanding, treatment, and eventually, prevention of these disabling conditions that affect millions of Americans.

Contact NIMH Office of Communications, 6001 Executive Boulevard, Room 8184, MSC 9663, Bethesda, MD 20892-9663 / Tel: (301) 443-4513 or (866) 615-NIMH (6464) / Toll-free TTY: (301) 443-8431 / Fax: (301) 443-4279 / Fax: (301) 443-5158 / Website: www.nimh.nih.gov / Email: nimhinfo@nih.gov

Mental Health America (MHA) (formerly the National Mental Health Association) is the country's oldest and largest nonprofit organization addressing all aspects of mental health and mental illness. With more than 340 affiliates nationwide, MHA works to improve the mental health of all Americans, especially the 54 million people with mental disorders, through advocacy, education, research and service.

Contact MHA, 2000 N. Beauregard Street, 6th Floor, Alexandria, Virginia 22311 / Tel: (703) 684-7722 / or (800) 969-6642 / Fax: (703) 684-5968 / Website: nmha.org

Safe Harbor Project collects and distributes information on non-pharmaceutical approaches to mental disorders via their website, which is full of useful information and articles. You can also subscribe to their free e-newsletter.

Contact Safe Harbor, 787 W. Woodbury Road, Suite 2, Altadena, CA 91001 / Tel: (626) 204-0161 / Fax: (626) 791-7867 / Website: www.AlternativeMental Health.com / Email: mail@alternativementalhealth.com

Nutritional Treatment and Nutrition Practitioners

The Brain Bio Centre is a UK-based treatment center, putting the optimum nutrition approach into practice for those with mental health problems, including depression, learning difficulties, dyslexia, ADHD, autism, schizophrenia, dementia and Alzheimer's, and addiction recovery.

Contact www.brainbiocentre.com

The Pfeiffer Treatment Center (PTC) is a private, non-profit clinic providing extensive biochemical analysis and individualized nutrient-based treatment to both children and adults for over 20 years. PTC specializes in treating learning and behavior problems, such as ADD and ADHD, and developmental disorders, such as autism, as well as depression, bipolar disorder and schizophrenia. PTC is staffed by a team of physicians, chemists, and other professionals who specialize in the effects of biochemistry on behavior, thought, or mood. The individualized biochemical treatment that PTC provides, based on the fact that each person has unique biochemistry, is a result of extensive research and has been shown to be effective through many outcome studies.

Contact PTC, 4575 Weaver Parkway, Warrenville, IL 60555-4039 / Tel: (630) 505-0300 or (866) 504-6076 / Website: www.hriptc.org / Email: info@hriptc.org

One-on-one nutrition consultations are available in the U.S. through naturopathic physicians, nutritionists, and physicians trained in the optimum nutrition approach. The following organizations can help you find a practitioner in your area.

American Association for Health Freedom, 1350 Connecticut Avenue, NW, 5th Floor, Washington, DC 20036 / Tel: (880) 230-2762 / Fax: (202) 315-5837 / Website: www.healthfreedom.net / Email: office@healthfreedom.net

American Association of Naturopathic Physicians (AANP), 4435 Wisconsin Avenue, NW, Suite 403, Washington, DC 20016 / Tel: (202) 237-8150 or (866) 538-2267 / Fax: (202) 237-8152/ Website: www.naturopathic.org / Email: member.services@naturopathic.org

American College for Advancement in Medicine (ACAM), 8001 Irvine Center Drive, Suite 825, Irvine CA 92618 / Tel: (800) 532-3688 / Fax: (949) 309-3538 / Website: www.acam.org

American Holistic Medical Association (AHMA), 23366 Commerce Park, Suite 101B, Beachwood, OH 44122 / Tel: (216) 292-6644 / Fax: (216) 292-6688 / Website: www.holisticmedicine.org / Email: info@holisticmedicine.org

Bastyr University, 14500 Juanita Drive, NE, Kenmore, WA 98028 / Tel: (425) 823-1300 / Fax: (425) 823-6222 / Website: www.bastyr.edu

Institute for Functional Medicine (IFM), 4411 Pt. Fosdick Drive, NW, Suite 305, Gig Harbor, WA 98335 / Tel: (253) 858-4724 or (800) 228-0622 / Fax: (253) 853-6766 / Website: www.functionalmedicine.org

Parkinson's Disease

Dr. Geoffrey Leader and **Lucille Leader** have specialized in the nutritional support of Parkinson's disease and have written *Parkinson's Disease: The Way Forward.*

Contact www.parkinsonsdisease-the-way-forward.com

Psychotherapy

Your health insurance provider can put you in touch with a well-qualified professional in your area. I have been impressed by people trained in psychosynthesis and also in a highly effective technique called Eye Movement Desensitization and Reprocessing, an information processing therapy. When you are looking for a psychotherapist you can ask them if they are trained in these approaches.

American Psychology Association (APA) offers a list of clinical psychologists by area.

Contact APA, 750 First Street, NE, Washington, DC 20002 / Tel: (202) 336-5500 or (800) 374-2721 / Website: www.apa.org

Association for the Advancement of Psychosynthesis (AAP) is a resource for psychotherapists trained in psychosynthesis, a wholistic approach to psychological health that involves self-development and personal growth.

Contact AAP, PO Box 414, Somerset, KY 42502 / Tel: (646) 320-3914 / Website: www.aap-psychosynthesis.org

Eye Movement Desensitization and Reprocessing Institute (EMDR) offers a list of licensed clinicians specifically trained in EMDR, a therapy that helps to process and let go off charged events that make us anxious, angry, and depressed.

Contact EMDR, PO Box 750, Watsonville, CA 95077 / Tel: (831) 761-1040 / Fax: (831) 761-1204 / Website: www.emdr.com / Email: inst@emdr.com

Schizophrenia

International Schizophrenia Foundation (ISF) works for improved diagnosis, treatment, preventive work and research into schizophrenia and related disorders. Research in Orthomolecular Medicine has led to the positive treatment of degenerative illnesses such as diabetes, cancer, allergies, and learning problems as well. The Foundation publishes the *Journal of Orthomolecular Medicine,* free archive online: http://orthomolecular.org/library/jom/index.shtml, and sponsors the annual Orthomolecular Medicine Today Conference.

Contact International Schizophrenia Foundation, 16 Florence Avenue, Toronto, Ontario, Canada M2N 1E9 / Tel: (416) 733-2117 / Fax: (416) 733-2352 / Website: www.orthomed.org/isf/isf.html / Email: centre@orthomed.org

Sleep

Silence of peace is a music CD, composed by John Levine, which induces alpha brain waves, the prerequisite for a good night's sleep. This highly effective CD is available from www.patrickholford.com under "books and CDs."

Stress Reduction—T'ai Chi, Yoga, Meditation

The T'ai Chi Foundation is a nonprofit international educational organization that supports the teaching and study of t'ai chi.

Contact T'ai Chi Foundation, PO Box 575, Midtown Station, New York, NY 10018 / Tel: (212) 645-7010 / Website: www.TaiChiFoundation.org

Anusara Yoga is a dynamic form of hatha yoga that is taught throughout the U.S. by certified teachers.

Contact Anusara Yoga, 9400 Grogans Mill Road, Suite 200, The Woodlands, TX 77380 / Tel: (281) 367-9763 or (888) 398-9642 / Fax: (281) 367-2744 / Website: www.anusara.com

Siddha Yoga Meditation offers one-day courses in meditation and free weekly meditation programs in different centers throughout the U.S.

Contact SYDA, 371 Brickman Road, PO Box 600, South Fallsburg, NY 12779 / Tel: (845) 434-2000 / Website: www.siddhayoga.org

Product and supplement directory

Good-quality supplements are produced by the following companies and are widely available in the U.S. To find the nearest retail store or for online ordering, contact:

Enzymatic Therapy at (800) 783-2286 or www.enzy.com

Nature's Plus at (800) 645-9500 or www.naturesplus.com

Solgar at (877)-765-4274 or www.solgar.com

Source Naturals at (800) 815-2333 at www.sourcenaturals.com

Twinlab Corporation at (800) 645-5626 or www.twinlab.com

NuTriVene, the formula designed for children with Down's syndrome, is available by mail order. Contact NuTriVene at (800) 899-3413 or www.nutrivene.com

Smart drugs and nutrients can be bought by mail order. For details of suppliers, see www.ceri.com.

Verilux lighting is a good source for full-spectrum bulbs and lamps. Verilux products are carried at some retail stores, including Sharper Image, Brookstone, Ace Hardware, and True Value. Contact Verilux at (888) 544-4865 or www.verilux.net

Index

(page numbers in italics refer to illustrations)